INSTRUCTOR'S MANUAL AND TEST BANK TO ACCOMPANY
UNDERSTANDING NORMAL & CLINICAL NUTRITION

FOURTH EDITION

Eleanor Noss Whitney

Corinne Balog Cataldo

Sharon Rady Rolfes

PREPARED BY

Lori Waite Turner, M.S., R.D.
Tallahassee Community College

Roberta Anding, M.S., R.D./L.D., C.D.E.
The University of Texas Health Science Center School of Nursing

Frances D. Moncure, Ph.D., R.N.
Georgia State University

Harry S. Sitren, Ph.D.
Center for Nutritional Sciences-University of Florida

Margaret Hedley, M. Sc., R.P. Dt.
University of Guelph

West Publishing Company
Minneapolis/St. Paul   New York   Los Angeles   San Francisco

WEST'S COMMITMENT TO THE ENVIRONMENT

In 1906, West Publishing Company began recycling materials left over from the production of books. This began a tradition of efficient and responsible use of resources. Today, up to 95% of our legal books and 70% of our college texts and school texts are printed on recycled, acid-free stock. West also recycles nearly 22 million pounds of scrap paper annually—the equivalent of 181,717 trees. Since the 1960s, West has devised ways to capture and recycle waste inks, solvents, oils, and vapors created in the printing process. We also recycle plastics of all kinds, wood, glass, corrugated cardboard, and batteries, and have eliminated the use of Styrofoam book packaging. We at West are proud of the longevity and the scope of our commitment to the environment.

Production, Prepress, Printing and Binding by West Publishing Company.

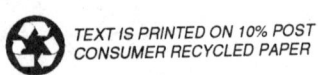 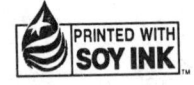

COPYRIGHT © 1994 by WEST PUBLISHING CO.
　　　　　　　　　　　 610 Opperman Drive
　　　　　　　　　　　 P.O. Box 64526
　　　　　　　　　　　 St. Paul, MN 55164–0526

All rights reserved
Printed in the United States of America
01 00 99 98 97 96 95 94　　8 7 6 5 4 3 2 1 0

ISBN 0–314–04931–2

IMPORTANT NOTICE...IMPORTANT NOTICE...IMPORTANT NOTICE

This manual provides additional information and material which may be of help to you in teaching your nutrition course. We do hope you will find the manual useful, and we do ask that you let us know how we can offer even better materials in the future.

While this manual is intended for use by adopters of **UNDERSTANDING NORMAL AND CLINICAL NUTRITON**, Fourth Edition, you may also find parts of it helpful for courses where you have adopted other West nutrition texts written or edited by Ellie Whitney. There is no permission charge for using and/or reproducing any material in this manual, but we do ask that you fill in the information below and return this page to us. It's pre-addressed for your convenience; simply remove this sheet from the manual, fold it where indicated on the reverse side and tape or staple closed. We also welcome your suggestions for improvement or evaluation of this manual. Please feel free to send your comments to us.

Thank you

West Publishing Company

I have adopted:

___ **UNDERSTANDING NORMAL AND CLINICAL NUTRITION**, 4/e by Whitney, Cataldo, and Rolfes

___ **NUTRITION AND DIET THERAPY**, 4/e by Cataldo, DeBruyne and Whitney

___ **UNDERSTANDING NUTRITION**, 6/e by Whitney and Rolfes

___ **PERSONAL NUTRITION**, 2/e by Boyle and Zyla

___ **LIFE SPAN NUTRITION**, by Rolfes and DeBruyne (edited by E. Whitney)

for classroom use beginning_____, 19_____

Course Name_____Your Enrollment_____

Your Name_____

Department_____

Street Address/Building_____

Place
Stamp
Here

WEST PUBLISHING COMPANY
College Marketing, D4-13
610 Opperman Drive
P.O. Box 64526
St. Paul, MN 55164-0526

ATTN: Nutrition Editor

CONTENTS OF INSTRUCTOR'S MANUAL

Chapter 1	An Overview Of Nutrition
Chapter 2	Food Choices And Diet-Planning Guides
Chapter 3	Digestion, Absorption, And Transport
Chapter 4	The Carbohydrates: Sugars, Starch, And Fibers
Chapter 5	The Lipids: Triglycerides, Phospholipids, And Sterols
Chapter 6	Protein: Amino Acids
Chapter 7	Metabolism: Transformations And Interactions
Chapter 8	Energy Balance And Weight Control
Chapter 9	The Water-Soluble Vitamins: B Vitamins And Vitamin C
Chapter 10	The Fat-Soluble Vitamins: A, D, E, And K
Chapter 11	The Body Fluids And The Major Minerals
Chapter 12	The Trace Minerals
Chapter 13	Fitness: Physical Activity, Nutrients, And Body Adaptations
Chapter 14	Consumer Concerns About Foods
Chapter 15	Nutrition Assessment
Chapter 16	Nutrition Care Strategies
Chapter 17	Life Cycle Nutrition: Pregnancy, Lactation, And Infancy
Chapter 18	Life Cycle Nutrition: Childhood, Adolescence, And The Later Years
Chapter 19	Nutrition And Illness
Chapter 20	Nutrition And Severe Stress
Chapter 21	Enteral Nutrition
Chapter 22	Parenteral Nutrition
Chapter 23	Nutrition And Disorders Of The Upper GI Tract
Chapter 24	Nutrition And Disorders Of The Lower GI Tract
Chapter 25	Nutrition And Disorders Of The Liver
Chapter 26	Nutrition, Diabetes, And Hypoglycemia
Chapter 27	Nutrition And Disorders Of The Blood Vessels, Heart, And Lungs
Chapter 28	Nutrition And Disorders Of The Kidneys
Chapter 29	Nutrition And Wasting Disorders: Cancer And Aids

HANDOUTS

Handout 2-1	Compare Your Food Intake to the Daily Food Guide
Handout 3-1	Digestive Secretions and Their Actions
Handout 3-2	Transport of Nutrients into Blood
Handout 4-1	Sweetness of Sugars
Handout 4-2	Foods to Include on a High Fiber Diet
Handout 5-1	Exposing Hidden Fat
Handout 5-2	How to Modify a Recipe
Handout 6-1	Protein Sources
Handout 7-1	Glycolysis
Handout 7-2	Self-Assessment for Alcoholism
Handout 8-1	Medical Problems Associated With Obesity
Handout 11-1	Osmotic Pressure
Handout 11-2	Choosing a Milk Substitute
Handout 13-1	Ways to Include Exercise in a Day
Handout 13-2	How to Evaluate a Fitness Program
Handout 14-1	Safe Internal Temperatures for Meat and Poultry
Handout 17-1	Effects of Nutrient Deficiencies During Pregnancy
Handout 17-2	Supervised Food Activities for Preschoolers
Handout 18-1	Changes with Age: Preventable versus Unavoidable

TRANSPARENCY ACETATE (TA) LIST

TRANSPARENCY ACETATE NUMBER   **TITLE**

1	Elements in the Six Classes of Nutrients
2	Setting the RDA for a Nutrient
3	Naive vs Accurate View of Nutrient Needs
4	The Nutrient RDA and the Energy RDA
5	Stages in the Development of a Nutrient Deficiency
6	The Ten Leading Causes of Illness & Death in the United States
7	The USDA Food Pyramid
8	Canada's Food Guide to Healthy Eating
9	The Gastrointestinal Tract
10	Peristalsis
11	The Small Intestinal Villi
12	The Vascular System
13	A Nephron
14	The Liver
15	Atoms and Their Bonds
16	Condensation
17	Hydrolysis
18	The Major Sugars
19	Chemical Structures of Glucose, Galactose, and Fructose
20	Glycogen and Starch Molecules Compared
21	Digestion and Absorption of Starch and Disaccharides
22	Regulation of Blood Glucose Concentration
23	Condensation of Glycerol and Fatty Acids
24	A Mixed Triglyceride
25	Comparison of Dietary Fats
26	Hydrogenation
27	Structural Formulas for Omega-3 and Omega-6 Fatty Acids
28	A Lecithin
29	Cholesterol
30	Emulsification of Fat by Bile
31	Absorption and Transport of Lipids
32	Amino Acid Structure
33	Formation of A Dipeptide

34	Enzyme Action
35	Transport Proteins
36	Protein Synthesis
37	Anabolic and Catabolic Reactions: Glycogen
38	Anabolic and Catabolic Reactions: Triglycerides
39	Anabolic and Catabolic Reactions: Protein
40	Glycolysis
41	Pyruvate-to-Acetyl CoA
42	Glucose Retrieval via the Cori Cycle
43	The Paths of Pyruvate and Acetyl CoA
44	The Breakdown of Acetyl CoA
45	The Glucose to Energy Pathway
46	The Fats to Energy Pathway
47	Fatty Acid Oxidation
48	Amino Acid-to-Energy Pathway
49	Transamination to Make a Nonessential Amino Acid
50	Urea Synthesis
51	Urea Excretion
52	Electron Transport Chain
53	The Central Pathways of Energy Metabolism
54	How Carbohydrate, Eaten in Excess, Contributes to Body Fat
55	How Fat, Eaten in Excess, Contributes to Body Fat
56	How Protein, Eaten in Excess, Contributes to Body Fat
57	Feasting
58	Fasting
59	Continued Fasting
60	Ketone Body Formation
61	One Pathway for the Degradation of Ethanol
62	BMI Silhouettes
63	Weight Cycling Effect of Repeating Dieting
64	Coenzyme Action
65	Riboflavin Coenzyme
66	Niacin Coenzyme in Action
67	Dose Levels and Effects
68	Metabolic Pathways Involving B Vitamins
69	Vitamin C's Role in Hydroxyproline
70	Vitamin C Intake
71	Three Forms of Vitamin A
72	Vision
73	Mucous Membrane Integrity
74	Vitamin A Deficiency and Toxicity
75	Vitamin A Compounds
76	Vitamin D Synthesis and Activation
77	Blood Clotting Process

78	The Amounts of Minerals in a 60-Kilogram Human Body
79	How the Body Regulates Water Excretion
80	Water Follows Salt
81	Osmotic Pressure
82	pH's of Common Substances and Body Fluids
83	Calcium Balance in Bones
84	Iron Routes in the Body
85	Zinc Routes in the Body
86	Cobalt With Vitamin B12
87	Delivery of Oxygen by the Heart and Lungs
88	The Effect of Diet on Physical Endurance
89	Incomplete Breakdown of Glucose
90	Information Gathered During Nutrition Assessment Helps Determine a Person's Nutrition Status
91	How to Measure Triceps Fat Fold
92	How to Measure Midarm Circumference
93	Communication Channels
94	The Placenta
95	Stages of Embryonic and Fetal Development
96	The Concept of Critical Periods
97	Comparison of Nutrient RDA of Nonpregnant, Pregnant and Lactating Women
98	Weight Gain of Human Infants
99	Examples of Growth Charts
100	Nutrient RDA of a Five-Month-Old Infant and an Adult Male
101	The Aging of the U.S. Population
102	Diet/Lifestyle Risk Factors and Degenerative Disease
103	Interrelationships Between Illness and Malnutrition
104	Nutrition and Immunity
105	Two Antivitamins Used As Drugs
106	Phases of a Stress Response
107	Different Degrees of Burn Wounds
108	Immune Cells and Intestinal Villi
109	Selection of the Feeding Method
110	Feeding Tube Placement Sites
111	Selection of Formulas
112	The Central Veins Used for TPN
113	Effect of Gastric Pressure on Reflux
114	Relationship of the Upper GI Tract to the Diaphragm
115	Typical Gastric Surgery Restrictions
116	Dumping Syndrome
117	Steatorrhea
118	Surgical Procedures to Control Obesity
119	The Effects of Fat Malabsorption

120	Nutrient Absorption in the GI Tract
121	Ileostomy and Colostomy
122	The Liver's Circulatory System
123	The Consequences of Cirrhosis
124	Ammonia Production in the Body
125	Examples of Aromatic and Branched-Chain Amino Acids
126	Obesity Diagram
127	Metabolic Consequences of Untreated IDDM and NIDDM
128	The Formation of Plaques in Arteries
129	How Normal Blood Pressure Supports Fluid Exchange
130	HDL and LDL Compared
131	Events Leading to Osteodystrophy
132	Consequences of the Nephrotic Syndrome
133	Causes of the Cancer Cachexia Syndrome

CANADIAN NUTRITION INFORMATION

CONTENTS

INTRODUCTION	1
CANADIAN GOVERNMENT DEPARTMENTS AND LEGISLATION	3
SI METRIC UNITS	5
TEACHING CANADIAN INFORMATION: *CHAPTER 1: AN OVERVIEW OF NUTRITION	7
Adjusting for SI Metric Units	7
Nutrition Recommendations in Canada	7
Surveys of Populations	8
HIGHLIGHT 1: WHO SPEAKS ON NUTRITION? THE QUALIFIED VERSUS THE QUACKS	10
Dietitians' Credentials in Canada	10
CHAPTER 2: FOOD CHOICES AND DIET-PLANNING GUIDES	11
Canada's Food Guide to Healthy Eating	11
Good Health Eating Guide	12
Nutrient Enrichment in Canada	12
The Guidelines Applied to Ethnic Diets	16
Self-Study - Calculate Your Nutrient Intakes	16

* All subsequent chapters refer to **Teaching Canadian Information**

x

HIGHLIGHT 2: FOOD LABELS	19
Food Labelling in Canada	19
Nutrition Labelling in Canada	21
CHAPTER 4: THE CARBOHYDRATES: SUGAR, STARCH AND FIBERS	23
Carbohydrate and Dietary Fibre Recommendations	23
Estimating Carbohydrate using Food Groups of Good Health Eating Guide	23
HIGHLIGHT 4: ALTERNATIVES TO SUGAR	26
CHAPTER 5: THE LIPIDS: TRIGLYCERIDES, PHOSPHOLIPIDS, AND STEROLS	27
Recommendations about Fats	27
Estimating Fat using Food Groups of Good Health Eating Guide	28
HIGHLIGHT 5: ALTERNATIVES TO FATS	29
CHAPTER 6: PROTEIN: AMINO ACIDS	31
Protein and Health	31
Estimating Protein using Food Groups of Good Health Eating Guide	31
Amino Acid Supplements	33
HIGHLIGHT 6: HEALTH ASPECTS OF A MEATLESS DIET	34
HIGHLIGHT 7: ALCOHOL AND NUTRITION	35
CHAPTER 8: ENERGY BALANCE AND WEIGHT CONTROL	37
SI Energy Units	37
Healthy Weights	37
Eating Plans with the Good Health Eating Guide	38
HIGHLIGHT 8: EATING DISORDERS - ANOREXIA AND BULIMIA	40
CHAPTER 9: THE WATER-SOLUBLE VITAMINS: B VITAMINS AND VITAMIN C	41
Vitamins in Canadian Foods	41
Vitamin Recommendations	41
CHAPTER 10: THE FAT-SOLUBLE VITAMINS: A, D, E, AND K	43
Fat Soluble Vitamins in Canadian Foods	43
HIGHLIGHT 10: VITAMIN AND MINERAL SUPPLEMENTS	44

CHAPTER 11: THE BODY FLUIDS AND THE MAJOR MINERALS   45
  Sodium and Potassium Recommendations   45
  Sodium Content of Packaged Food   45
  Calcium   45
  Phosphorus   46

CHAPTER 12: THE TRACE MINERALS   47
  Trace Mineral Recommendations   47
  Iron Enrichment   47

HIGHLIGHT 12: OUR CHILDREN'S DAILY LEAD   49

CHAPTER 13: FITNESS: PHYSICAL ACTIVITY, NUTRIENTS AND BODY ADAPTATIONS   51
  Canadian Programs and Studies   51

HIGHLIGHT 13: SUPPLEMENTS AND ERGOGENIC AIDS ATHLETES USE   53

CHAPTER 14: CONSUMER CONCERNS ABOUT FOODS   55
  Food-Borne Illnesses   55
  Environmental Contaminants, Natural Toxicants and Pesticides   56
  Food Additives and Allergens   56
  Food Irradiation   57
  Consumer Concerns about Food Safety and Nutrition   58

HIGHLIGHT 14: ENVIRONMENTALLY CONSCIOUS FOODWAYS   58
  Agricultural Methods in Canada   58

CHAPTER 15: NUTRITION ASSESSMENT   59
  SI Units in Nutrition Assessment   59

HIGHLIGHT 15: U.S. AND WORLD HUNGER   60
  Hunger in Canada   60

CHAPTER 16: NUTRITION CARE STRATEGIES   61
  Diet Manuals in Canada   61

CHAPTER 17: LIFE CYCLE NUTRITION: PREGNANCY, LACTATION AND INFANCY   63
  Canadian Guidelines and Programs   63

HIGHLIGHT 17: FETAL ALCOHOL SYNDROME   65

CHAPTER 18: LIFE CYCLE NUTRITION: CHILDHOOD, ADOLESCENCE,
AND THE LATER YEARS ... 67
Dietary Fat and Children ... 67
School Food Policy ... 67
Child Hunger ... 67
Programs for the Elderly ... 68

HIGHLIGHT 18: CAFFEINE: THE BREWING CONTROVERSY ... 69

HIGHLIGHT 19: DIET AND HEALTH ... 71
Nutrition Recommendations ... 71
Canadian Consensus Conference on Cholesterol ... 71
Health Promotion ... 71

CHAPTER 26: NUTRITION, DIABETES, AND HYPOGLYCEMIA ... 73
Canadian Food Choice System ... 73

CHAPTER 29: NUTRITION AND WASTING DISORDERS: CANCER
AND AIDS ... 75

HIGHLIGHT 29: HEALTH CARE REFORM, COST CONTAINMENT,
AND NUTRITION SERVICES ... 76

RESOURCE GROUPS ... 77

REFERENCES ... 82

CONTENTS OF TEST BANK

Chapter 1	An Overview Of Nutrition
Chapter 2	Food Choices And Diet-Planning Guides
Chapter 3	Digestion, Absorption, And Transport
Chapter 4	The Carbohydrates: Sugars, Starch, And Fibers
Chapter 5	The Lipids: Triglycerides, Phospholipids, And Sterols
Chapter 6	Protein: Amino Acids
Chapter 7	Metabolism: Transformations And Interactions
Chapter 8	Energy Balance And Weight Control
Chapter 9	The Water-Soluble Vitamins: B Vitamins And Vitamin C
Chapter 10	The Fat-Soluble Vitamins: A, D, E, And K
Chapter 11	The Body Fluids And The Major Minerals
Chapter 12	The Trace Minerals
Chapter 13	Fitness: Physical Activity, Nutrients, And Body Adaptations
Chapter 14	Consumer Concerns About Foods
Chapter 15	Nutrition Assessment
Chapter 16	Nutrition Care Strategies
Chapter 17	Life Cycle Nutrition: Pregnancy, Lactation, And Infancy
Chapter 18	Life Cycle Nutrition: Childhood, Adolescence, And The Later Years
Chapter 19	Nutrition And Illness
Chapter 20	Nutrition And Severe Stress
Chapter 21	Enteral Nutrition
Chapter 22	Parenteral Nutrition
Chapter 23	Nutrition And Disorders Of The Upper GI Tract
Chapter 24	Nutrition And Disorders Of The Lower GI Tract
Chapter 25	Nutrition And Disorders Of The Liver
Chapter 26	Nutrition, Diabetes, And Hypoglycemia
Chapter 27	Nutrition And Disorders Of The Blood Vessels, Heart, And Lungs
Chapter 28	Nutrition And Disorders Of The Kidneys
Chapter 29	Nutrition And Wasting Disorders: Cancer And Aids

INTRODUCTION TO INSTRUCTOR'S MANUAL

This manual is designed to guide the development and organization of lecture content for the chapters in the text, <u>Understanding Normal and Clinical Nutrition</u>.

Scope

The scope provides an overview of the major concepts or main ideas presented in the chapters.

Objectives

The objectives provide a list of competencies expected of the students after completion of readings and other supplementary aids provided in each chapter. Additionally, these objectives can be used to develop a syllabus and can serve as unit objectives.

Outline

The outline is designed to aid the instructor in lecture preparation and structure. Transparency acetates relevant to the material being discussed are listed to the right of the outline.

Teaching Strategies/Other Resources

The teaching strategies provide an opportunity to enhance the traditional lecture material with discussion questions, films, and slides; most of the resources selected are free, available on loan or for sale at a nominal price.

Key to Clinical Application Questions and Case Studies
(In chapters 15, 16 and 19 through 29)

These provide one possible answer to these text features. A discussion of them will also be found in the student's Study Guide, although the latter are more geared to helping the student arrive at answers for her or himself.

Other Features

For the normal nutrition chapters, there are handout masters, which may be copied as needed.

There is a list of the transparency acetates with their titles. These are available through

Margaret Hedley has prepared a section of the manual giving the Canadian information corresponding to the US standards and explaining where the information is different.

We wish to acknowledge the contribution of Mary Rhiner Ashbacher, who did the chapter outlines upon which are based the outlines for chapters 1 through 14 and 17 and 18.

Note About Page Numbering

Since the efforts of 6 different people in far-flung locations were combined for this Instructor's Manual and Test Bank, the numbering for the pages was done within chapters, rather than consecutively from start to end. Since there are running heads with the chapter titles throughout the volume, we think this will cause few, if any, problems.

>Lori Turner
>Roberta Anding
>Mary Ann Neeley
>Frances Moncure
>Harry Sitren
>Margaret Hedley

INTRODUCTION TO TEST BANK

A Note on Test Bank Style and Use
For the Normal Nutrition Chapters
(1-14, 17 and 18)

The test bank consists of the two major types of test questions, own thoughts (creativity) and organize a response to reveal their level of recall knowledge, comprehension, evaluation, application, and/or reasoning. In this test bank, two types of essay questions are offered: restricted response (e.g., Compare and contrast...) and extended response (e.g., Describe...; Discuss...).

Among the various types of objective tests, measurement professionals overwhelmingly prefer multiple-choice over completion, true-false, and matching items. Multiple-choice items are the most flexible and adaptable. When properly written, they are capable of assessing not only recall knowledge but also application of knowledge. In turn, the application of knowledge may require certain levels of comprehension and analytical reasoning.

The inclusion of other types of objective questions in a test composed primarily of multiple choice items may be viewed as adding variety to the test. However, combining different types of questions in the same test will more likely result in distractions that affect efficient use of available test time. Since assessment of student learning from objective tests is more reliable as the number of questions increases, the elimination of as many distractions as possible will promote better use of time, thus allowing more items to be included in the same time period.

While reading through these questions, you will notice the consistency of style and format. With few exceptions, each question is composed of a stem followed by four options - one and only one correct option and three distractors. The stem is presented in either question form or as an incomplete statement. In keeping with recommendations of measurement professionals, there are no options with "All of the above" or "None of the above" as responses. Where appropriate, two or more correct answers are combined into a compound response within the same option.

Finally, the symbol (K) refers to questions that require simple recall of knowledge whereas the symbol (A) refers to questions that require application of knowledge. Underneath each question, will be found the correct response and the page number where it can be found in the text.

Harry Sitren

INTRODUCTION TO TEST BANK

For The Clinical Nutrition Chapters
(15, 16 and 19 through 29

The Test Bank has different levels of test questions depending on the level of the student in your program. Each question is labeled as knowledge, comprehension, application analysis, synthesis or evaluation. As a general rule, knowledge questions are the easiest and evaluation questions the most difficult. Therefore, dietetic programs should choose questions from all levels, whereas licensed vocational nursing programs and dietetic technician programs should choose the knowledge or comprehension questions. Definitions of the question types are provided below:

LEVELS OF QUESTIONS

Knowledge (K)

Identify something on the test <u>already stated</u> in the book whether it is a fact, a reason, an example, a comparison, an intervention or an evaluation.

Comprehension (C)

Identify a new example, not already stated in the book but which illustrates a concept in the book. Also given new examples, identify the concept which they illustrate.

Application (AP)

Identify an example of something from a short case study in the test. This could be a defined nutrition status or a recommended intervention. This goes above the comprehension level because the student has to determine which information in the case study is relevant to the question and its impact on the decision as to the correct answer.

Analysis (AN)

Identify the parts of some person's nutritional status or disease state from information in the case study. Materials with charts, grids, and percentile graphs are included with the test. Reasons for some things in the case data can be induced from other things in the data. Calculations may be needed to arrive at conclusions about nutrition status (on a multiple choice test it is really selection of the best of four analyses).

Synthesis (S)

Identify from information in a case study some predictions about the person's nutrition status or disease state in the future. The student uses information from social and natural science pre-requisite courses, supplementary readings, and current course content. Synthesis level questions could also require the student to select new interventions that could be predicted to work based on the above information combined. These could also ask the student to derive hypotheses from findings of several studies presented with the test. (For a multiple choice test these would still be only selection of the best one of four ready made syntheses). Achievement of synthesis level objectives should be evaluated by additional methods such as case studies and term projects.

Evaluation (E)

From information in a case follow-up, in a nutrition plan, and given criteria, students identify areas where client nutritional status is improved and why. This level also includes making statements of desired outcomes and setting criteria. The students have to know how to determine how realistic a certain level of accomplishment is, given information in the assessment and their knowledge from past courses and chapters (Evaluation questions require the processing of information. Recall of an evaluation already stated in the book is at the knowledge level).

Roberta Anding
Mary Ann Neeley
Frances Moncure

Chapter 1
AN OVERVIEW OF NUTRITION

CHAPTER SUMMARY

    Nutrition plays a significant role in health and disease. The science of nutrition studies the nutrients in food and the body's handling of those nutrients. Nutrients include carbohydrate, fat, protein, vitamins, minerals and water.

    Protein, fat and carbohydrate are classified as energy-yielding nutrients. Alcohol, though not a nutrient, also contributes food energy. Vitamins and minerals play a different role from the energy-yielding nutrients. They are consumed in much smaller quantities and serve as helpers of chemical processes or function structurally. Water is needed in the most abundant quantity and is indispensable to body activities.

    The Recommended Dietary Allowances (RDA) set amounts of energy and selected nutrients considered to be adequate to meet the nutrient needs of practically all healthy people. Other recommendations for nutrients include The Estimated Minimum Requirements and The Estimated Safe and Adequate Daily Dietary Intakes. Recommendations are based on scientific research.

    Nutritional assessment evaluates the many factors that influence or reflect nutritional health. Nutrition plays a direct role in four of the ten leading causes of illness and death in the United States. Government and other agencies have developed diet recommendations to prevent or forestall disease.

    Highlight 1 describes the characteristics of nutrition misinformation and scientific research.

CHAPTER 1, AN OVERVIEW OF NUTRITION

Learning Objectives

1. What is a nutrient? Name the six classes of nutrients found in foods.
2. Which nutrients are inorganic and which are organic? Discuss the significance of that distinction.
3. Which nutrients yield energy? How is energy measured?
4. What factors must be included in the full definition of a healthy diet? Which are covered by the RDA? To whom do they apply? How are they used? In your description, address the issues of whether the RDA represent the minimum requirements, whether the RDA need to be met daily, and whether the RDA apply to individuals.
6. What judgement factors are involved in setting the energy and nutrient intake recommendations?
7. What balance of energy-yielding nutrients is recommended to meet energy need?
8. What happens when people don't get enough or get too much energy or nutrients? Describe the methods used to detect energy and nutrient deficiencies and excesses.
9. What methods are used in nutrition surveys? What kinds of information can these surveys provide?
10. Describe the differences between the population approach and the individual approach to making dietary recommendations. Which approach do today's dietary guidelines take?
11. What recommendations are made in the *Diet and Health Report*? What recommendations appear in the *Dietary Guidelines for Americans*? How are they similar? How are they different?

Chapter Outline   Acetates/Handouts

I. Introduction

II. The Nutrients

    A. Essential nutrients must be supplied by food

    B. The chemical composition of foods and the human body are similar

    C. Chemical composition of nutrients   TA1 Elements in the Six Classes of Nutrients

D. Energy-yielding nutrients

1. Energy is measured as kCalories
   a. carbohydrate - 4 kCal/gram
   b. fat - 9 kCal/gram
   c. protein - 4 kCal/gram
   d. alcohol - 7 kCal/gram

2. Energy in almost all foods is provided by a mixture of energy yielding nutrients

3. The body uses the energy-yielding nutrients to:
   a. help build new compounds
   b. help move the body
   c. escape as heat
   d. excrete as waste

E. Fiber

1. Yields little or no energy
2. Largely undigested
3. Beneficial to health

F. Vitamins

1. Organic compounds
2. Consumed in smaller quantities
3. Assist in body processes
4. Vulnerable to destruction

G. Minerals

1. Inorganic elements
2. Consumed in varying quantities
3. Structural component
4. Indestructible yet can be bound by substances

H. Water

1. Indispensable and abundant
2. Often taken for granted
3. Enormous consumption compared to other nutrients
4. Participates in many chemical reactions
5. Provides environment for many body activities

CHAPTER 1, AN OVERVIEW OF NUTRITION

III. Recommended Nutrient Intakes

    A. Recommended Dietary Allowances

        1. Energy intake is set at the population average
        2. Protein is based on body weight
        3. Fiber has no specific quantitative recommendations
        4. Eleven vitamins and seven minerals
            a. specific recommendations
            b. based on valid scientific studies
            c. vary among individuals

TA2 Setting the RDA for a Nutrient
TA3 Naive vs Accurate View of Nutrient Needs

TA4 The Nutrient RDA and the Energy RDA

    B. Estimated Minimum Requirements for three minerals

    C. Estimated Safe and Adequate Daily Dietary Intakes for two vitamins and five minerals

    D. Other recommendations

        1. Carbohydrate to provide one-half of kCalories
        2. Fat to provide less than one-third of kCalories
        3. Water needs are related to energy expenditure

    E. Using the RDA

        1. Healthy people only
        2. Safe and adequate recommendations, not requirements
        3. Intended to be met by consuming a variety of foods
        4. Average daily intakes
        5. Used to plan and evaluate diets for populations
        6. Guidelines for nutritional labeling of foods
        7. Safety margins

    F. FAO/WHO recommended energy and nutrient intakes for use worldwide

    G. Malnutrition

IV. Nutrition Assessment

    A. Methods

        1. Historical information
- a. medical
- b. socioeconomic
- c. drug
- d. diet

        2. Anthropometric measures
- a. height
- b. weight
- c. limb circumferences

        3. Physical examinations

        4. Laboratory tests
- a. blood
- b. urine

    B. Nutritional deficiency stages   *TA5 Stages in the Development of a Nutrient Deficiency*

    C. Population surveys

        1. Food consumption surveys to determine what people eat
        2. Nutrition status surveys to examine the people themselves

V. Nutrition and Disease Prevention

    A. Relationship of nutrition to the ten leading causes of illness and death in the United States   *TA6 The Ten Leading Causes of Illness and Death in the United States*

    B. Role of nutrition in degenerative disease

        1. Poor nutrition can accelerate disease development
        2. Healthful nutrition can help prevent or forestall disease
        3. Nutrition therapy can ease impact of disease

C. Dietary recommendations against disease

    1. Vary food choices
    2. Maintain an appropriate body weight
    3. Include starch and fiber in the diet
    4. Limit sugar intake
    5. Limit fat and cholesterol intake
    6. Limit salt intake
    7. Limit alcohol intake

D. Diet and Health Recommendations

E. Dietary Guidelines

VI. Highlight: Who Speaks on Nutrition?

Chapter 2
FOOD CHOICES AND DIET-PLANNING GUIDES

CHAPTER SUMMARY

People have many reasons for choosing the foods they eat. These include personal preferences, habit, ethnic heritage or tradition, social interactions, availability, convenience, economy, positive and negative associations, values, physical appearance and nutrition.

Basic diet planning principles include choosing an adequate diet that provides enough energy and nutrients to meet the needs of healthy people. Secondly, the diet must be balanced - using enough but not too much of each type of food. Overeating must be avoided. Foods should deliver the most nutrients for the least amount of food energy thus being nutrient dense. Variety and moderation contribute to all of these factors.

A tool for successful diet planning includes the four food group plan. This familiar plan sorts foods into groups based on nutrient content and origin. The daily food guide divides food into five groups and suggested servings are more generous. The USDA's food pyramid illustrates these concepts.

The exchange lists categorize foods by their nutrient and energy content.

Ethnic diets provide variety thus helping to ensure nutritional adequacy, but moderation to control energy and fat intake is still important.

Highlight 2 describes revised food labeling regulations.

2 CHAPTER 2, FOOD CHOICES AND DIET-PLANNING GUIDES

Learning Objectives

1. Give several reasons (and examples) why people make the food choices that they do. Can you think of other reasons why you, or others, might choose certain foods?
2. Name the diet-planning prinicples and briefly describe each prinicple. Explain how each principle might help to achieve another principle.
3. Name the five food groups in the Daily Food Guide and identify several foods typical of each group. Explain how such plans group foods and what diet-planning principles the plans best accommodate. How are food group plans used, and what are some of their strengths and weaknesses?
4. Name the exchange lists and a food typical of each list. Explain how the exchange system groups foods and what diet-planning principles the system best accommodates. How are exchange systems used, and what are some of their strengths and weaknesses?
5. Review the *Dietary Gudelines* from Chapter 1. What types of grocery selections would you make to achieve those recommendations?
6. How many servings from each food group are represented in Tuesday's meals (from Figure 2-4)? How does this compare with the recommendations?

Chapter Outline   Acetates/Handouts

I. Food Selection: Practices and Principles

   A. Food choices are based on many aspects

      1. Personal preference
      2. Habit
      3. Ethnic heritage or tradition
      4. Social interactions
      5. Availability, convenience, and economy
      6. Positive and negative associations
      7. Emotional comfort
      8. Religious, political, or environmental values
      9. Physical appearance
      10. Nutritional value

   B. Diet-planning principles

      1. Adequacy of diet to provide nutrients to meet the needs of healthy people
      2. Balance the diet using sufficient yet moderate quantities of each type of food
      3. KCalorie control to avoid kcalorie control overeating

CHAPTER 2, FOOD CHOICES AND DIET-PLANNING GUIDES

4. Nutrient density is selecting nutrient dense foods that deliver the most nutrients for the least food energy
5. Moderation - providing enough but not too much of a dietary constituent
6. Variety - using different foods on different occasions

II. Diet-Planning Guides

    A. Food group plans sort foods according to nutrient content

        1. Four food group plan
            a. advantages
            b. disadvantages
        2. Daily food guide
            a. lists range for suggested number of servings based on activity levels
            b. fruits and vegetables are divided
            c. categorizes foods by nutrient density
        3. USDA Food Pyramid   TA7 The USDA Food Pyramid
        4. Vegetarian food group plan suggests meat and milk alternates   TA8 Canada's Food Guide to Healthy Eating

    B. Exchange lists sort foods by their proportions of carbohydrate, fat, and protein

        1. The six exchange lists
            a. starch/bread
            b. meat
            c. vegetables
            d. fruit
            e. milk
            f. fat
        2. The added sugar list indicates concentrated sweets equivalent to 1 teaspoon of white sugar
        3. The foods on the exchange lists may be found in unexpected places
        4. Controlling energy and fat
            a. fruit portion sizes vary
            b. bread list specifies foods with added fat
            c. foods on the meat and milk lists are categorized based on their fat content

    C. Combining food group plans and exchange lists

CHAPTER 2, FOOD CHOICES AND DIET-PLANNING GUIDES

    D. A comparison of two days' meals   H2-1 Compare Your Food Intake to the Daily Food Guide

III. The Guidelines Applied

    A. From guidelines to groceries- choose nutrient dense foods

        1. Breads, cereals, and other grain products
            a. choose whole grains
            b. choose enriched products
            c. some cereals are fortified
        2. Vegetables
            a. choose green and yellow/orange vegetables for vitamin content
            b. choose fresh vegetables when possible
        3. Fruit
            a. choose citrus and yellow/orange fruits for vitamin content
            b. choose fresh fruits when possible
            c. fruit juices without added sugar are acceptable choices
        4. Meat, fish, and poultry
            a. choose lean cuts
            b. use low fat cooking methods
        5. Milk
            a. choose low fat or non-fat substitute milk and milk products
            b. fortified with vitamins A and D

    B. The guidelines applied to ethnic diets

        1. Northern Europe
        2. Southern Europe
        3. West Africa
        4. Mexico
        5. China
        6. Religious dietary traditions

IV. Highlight: Food Labels

Chapter 3
DIGESTION, ABSORPTION, AND TRANSPORT

CHAPTER SUMMARY

The gastrointestinal tract is a flexible muscular tube that prepares nutrients for absorption. Food enters the mouth, where it is reduced to a coarse mash. Peristalsis passes this bolus through the esophagus to the stomach. The stomach retains the bolus, adds water, and grinds it to a suspension of small particles. The semiliquid mass (chyme) passes to the small intestine where it is further broken down. Undigested and unabsorbed nutrients as well as water, pass through the large intestine to be eliminated. Various glands and organs work together secreting digestive juices containing hormones and enzymes that assist in breaking down foods to absorbable units.

Nutrients absorbed through the microvilli of the small intestine travel to one of two systems - the bloodstream directly or the lymphatic system then the bloodstream. Once inside the vascular system, nutrients travel freely and can be used by any cells in the body.

Details of the gastrointestinal system are regulated by the endocrine (hormone) and nervous system. PH levels, sphincters, digestive and enzymatic secretions all assist in making the digestive tract responsive to conditions in its environment. A healthy digestive tract will help to promote proper functioning of the system. Balance, variety, moderation and adequacy of the diet promote optimal utilization of foods consumed.

Highlight 3 reviews common digestive problems.

CHAPTER 3, DIGESTION, ABSORPTION, AND TRANSPORT

Learning Objectives

1. Describe the problems involved with digesting food and the solutions offered by the human body.
2. Describe the path food follows as it travels through the digestive system. Summarize the muscular actions that take place along the way.
3. Name five organs that secrete digestive juices. How do the juices and enzymes facilitate digestion?
4. Describe the problems involved with absorbing nutrients and the solutions offered by the small intestine.
5. How is blood routed through the digestive system? Which nutrients enter the bloodstream directly? Which are first absorbed into the lymph?
6. Describe how the body regulates the processes of digestion and absorption.
7. What steps can you take to help your GI tract function at its best?

Chapter Outline   Acetates/Handouts

I. Digestion

    A. Anatomy of the digestive tract

        1. Mouth
        2. Esophagus to stomach
        3. Small intestine   TA9 The
        4. Large intestine (colon)   Gastrointestinal
        5. Rectum   Tract

    B. The muscular action of digestion

        1. Peristalsis
        2. Stomach action   TA10 Peristalsis
        3. Segmentation
        4. Sphincter contractions

    C. The secretions of digestion

        1. Saliva
        2. Gastric juice
        3. Pancreatic juice and intestinal enzymes   H3-1 Digestive
        4. Bile   Secretions and Their
        5. Protective factors   Actions

CHAPTER 3, DIGESTION, ABSORPTION, AND TRANSPORT

    D.   The final stage of digestion

        1.   Nutrients disassembled to their basic building blocks are ready for absorption
        2.   Undigested residues continue through the digestive tract and enter the large intestine
        3.   Intestinal bacteria

II.   Absorption

    A.   Anatomy of the absorptive system

    B.   Intestinal cells - A closer look

    C.   Villi and microvilli are responsible for trapping nutrient particles to be absorbed   TA11 The Small Intestinal Villi

    D.   Cells are able to handle all kinds and combinations of foods and nutrients   H3-2 Transport of Nutrients into Blood

III.   The Circulatory System   TA12 The Vascular System

    A.   The blood circulatory system

        1.   General route to body tissues is heart to arteries to capillaries to veins to heart
        2.   Digestive system route is heart to arteries to capillaries (in intestine) to vein to capillaries (in liver) to vein to heart
        3.   Functions of the liver   TA13 A Nephron
                                                                                                                              TA14 The Liver

    B.   The lymphatic system

        1.   One way route for fluid from the tissue spaces to enter subclavian vein the blood
        2.   Similar to blood but lacking red blood cells and platelets
        3.   Sponge like system

IV.   Regulation of Digestion and Absorption

    A.   Gastrointestinal hormones and pathways

CHAPTER 3, DIGESTION, ABSORPTION, AND TRANSPORT

        1. Hormonal (endocrine) system and nervous system work together
        2. Stimulus/response mechanism

    B. The system is affected by lifestyle factors

        1. Rest
        2. Physical activity
        3. Mental state
        4. Diet of balance, moderation, variety and adequacy

V. Highlight: Common Digestive Problems

Chapter 4
THE CARBOHYDRATES: SUGARS, STARCH, AND FIBER

CHAPTER SUMMARY

The carbohydrate family includes simple carbohydrates (the sugars) and complex carbohydrates (starch and fiber). The sugars include the monosaccharides (glucose, fructose and galactose) and the disaccharides (sucrose, lactose and maltose). The starches include the polysaccharides (glycogen, starch, and fiber).

Carbohydrate digestion involves hydrolyzing bonds to absorbable forms. This process begins in the mouth and continues through the stomach and small intestine. After absorption, nutrients circulate to the liver whose cells convert fructose and galactose to glucose.

The main function of glucose in the body is to provide energy. Glycogen is the storage form of glucose - found only in the liver and muscle cells. Extra glucose can be converted to fat.

It is recommended that the diet contain 55-60% of total calories from carbohydrate. Refined sugars should contribute 10% or less of total calories. Exchange lists provide guidelines to estimate carbohydrate intake.

Water-soluble and water-insoluble fibers produce diverse health effects. Weight control, large intestine functioning, decreased risk of colon cancer, lowered blood cholesterol and better control of diabetes are positive benefits of fiber. Excessive fiber may result in abdominal discomfort, low nutrient availability, and bulk production.

Highlight 4 classifies the list of FDA approved artificial sweeteners, their properties, and allowable intakes and uses.

CHAPTER 4, THE CARBOHYDRATES: SUGARS, STARCH, AND FIBER

Learning Objectives

1. Which carbohydrates are described as simple and which are complex?
2. Describe the structure of a monosaccharide and name the three disaccharides important in nutrition and their component monosaccharides. In what foods are these sugars found?
3. What happens in a condensation reaction? In a hydrolysis reaction?
4. Describe the structure of polysaccharides and name the ones important in nutrition. How are starch and glycogen similar and how do they differ?
5. Describe starch and sugar digestion and absorption.
6. What are the possible fates of glucose?
7. How does the body maintain blood glucose concentrations? What happens when it rises too high or falls too low?
8. What are the health effects of sugars?
9. What are the dietary recommendations regarding complex carbohydrate and concentrated sugar intakes.
10. Demonstrate how the exchange system can help you estimate the carbohydrate content of a meal.
11. How do the fibers differ from the other polysaccharides?
12. Describe fiber digestion.
13. What are the health effects of fibers?
14. What are the dietary recommendations regarding fibers?
15. What foods provide fiber?

Chapter Outline   Acetates/Handouts

I. The Chemist's View of Carbohydrates   TA15 Atoms and Their
                                                     Bonds

    A. Carbon

    B. Nitrogen

    C. Oxygen

    D. Hydrogen

II. The Simple Carbohydrates

    A. Monosaccharides

        1. Glucose
        2. Fructose
        3. Galactose

CHAPTER 4, THE CARBOHYDRATES: SUGARS, STARCH, AND FIBER

    B.   Disaccharides

        1.   Chemical reactions
            a.   Condensation   TA16 Condensation
            b.   Hydrolysis   TA17 Hydrolysis
        2.   Sucrose (fructose and glucose)   TA18 The Major Sugars
        3.   Lactose (galactose and glucose)   TA19 Chemical Structures of Glucose, Galactose, and Fructose
        4.   Maltose (glucose and glucose)

III.   The Complex Carbohydrates

    A.   Glycogen - storage form of glucose in animals   TA20 Glycogen and Starch Molecules Compared

    B.   Starch - long branched or unbranched chains of glucose

IV.   Digestion and Absorption of Starch and Sugars   TA21 Digestion and Absorption of Starch and Disaccharides

    A.   Mouth - salivary enzymes

    B.   Small intestine - enzymes

    C.   Large intestine - indigestible carbohydrates remain

    D.   Absorption into the bloodstream

        1.   Through the small intestine
        2.   To the liver
        3.   Converted to glucose

    E.   Sugar by any other name   H4-1 Sweetness of Sugars

        1.   Honey versus sugar
        2.   Fruit sugars

    F.   Lactose intolerance

4   CHAPTER 4, THE CARBOHYDRATES: SUGARS, STARCH, AND FIBER

        1. lack of lactase
        2. hereditary
        3. other reasons
        4. individualized diets
        5. use of milk products
        6. use of special foods or enzyme tablets

V. Glucose in the Body

    A. Carbohydrate metabolism

        1. Storing glucose as glycogen
        2. Using glucose for energy
        3. Converting glucose to fat if large quantities are consumed

    B. The constancy of blood glucose

        1. High glucose concentration may cause confusion and difficulty with breathing
        2. Low glucose concentration may cause dizziness and weakness
        3. Homeostasis is best   TA22 Regulation of
        4. Insulin responds to high blood   Blood Glucose
           glucose   Concentration
        5. Glucagon responds to low blood glucose
        6. The glycemic index of foods

VI. Health Effects and Recommended Intakes of Sugars and Starches

    A. Health effects of sugars

        1. Accusations about sugar:
           a. Unnatural
           b. Additive
        2. Accusation: Sugar causes malnutrition
           a. Sugar can displace needed nutrients
           b. Caloric allowance is important in determining amount of empty-calorie foods to consume
        3. Accusation: Sugar causes obesity
           a. Sugar can contribute
           b. High fat intake and lack of exercise are greater contributing factors

4. Accusation: Sugar causes diabetes
    a. Dietary sugar does not cause diabetes
    b. Controlling sugar in diabetes is important
5. Accusation: Sugar raises blood lipids levels and increases the risk of heart disease
    a. For most people sugar has little influence on blood sugar
    b. For carbohydrate-sensitive people, sugar can change blood lipid levels in favor of heart disease
6. Accusation: Sugar causes ulcers
    a. A strong relationship has been found in one study
    b. A low refined sugar intake may protect against ulcers
7. Accusation: Sugar causes dental caries
    a. Strong positive relationship
    b. Sticky foods especially susceptible
    c. Time of exposure to foods is also important
8. Accusation: Sugar causes misbehavior in children and criminal behavior in adults
    a. These beliefs are based on speculations
    b. These statements have not been confirmed by scientific research

B. Health effects of starch

1. Diets high in complex carbohydrate also tend to be low in fat, low in energy and high in fiber, vitamins and minerals
2. Effects of starch are difficult to separate

C. Recommended intakes of sugars and starch

1. No RDA
2. 55-60% of total kcalories
3. 10% of total kcalories from refined sugars
4. Increase starch and fiber intake through vegetables, grains, legumes and fruits

D. Using the exchange system to estimate carbohydrate content of foods

1. Starch/bread group provides 15 grams per serving
2. Vegetable group provides 5 grams per serving
3. Fruit group provides 15 grams per serving

CHAPTER 4, THE CARBOHYDRATES: SUGARS, STARCH, AND FIBER

        4. Milk group provides 12 grams per serving

VII. Fibers: benefit of high fiber diets might include the prevention of diseases and obesity

VIII. The Chemist's View of Fibers

    A. The Major fibers

        1. Cellulose occurs in fruits, vegetables, and legumes
        2. Hemicelluloses are found in cereal fiber
        3. Pectins are found in vegetables and fruits
        4. Gums and mucilages are added to foods as stabilizers
        5. Lignin is the woody part of carrots and fruits with small seeds

    B. Other classifications of fibers

        1. Water soluble fiber
            a. Gums, pectin, some hemi-cellulose, and mucilages
            b. Found in fruits, barley, oats, and legumes
            c. Lowers blood cholesterol
            d. Delays stomach emptying
            e. Delays transit time of chyme in small intestine
        2. Water-insoluble fiber
            a. Cellulose, some hemi-cellulose, and lignin
            b. Found in vegetables, wheat, and cereals
            c. Increases fecal weight
            d. Speeds transit time of chyme in the small intestine
        3. Water-soluble and water-insoluble fibers
            a. Slow starch breakdown
            b. Delay glucose absorption into the blood
            c. Fermented by microorganisms in the digestive tract
        4. Physical properties of fiber
            a. Water-holding capacity
            b. Viscosity
            c. Cation-exchange capacity
            d. Bile-binding capacity
            e. Fermentability

CHAPTER 4, THE CARBOHYDRATES: SUGARS, STARCH, AND FIBER   7

IX. Digestion and Absorption of Fibers

   A. Stimulates saliva

   B. Delays gastric emptying

   C. Delays absorption of fats and carbohydrates in the small intestine

   D. Large intestine action

      1. Attracts water to soften stools
      2. Fibers are fermented by bacteria
      3. Short-chained fatty acids that are generated are absorbed and used for energy

X. Health Effects and Recommended Intakes of Fibers

   A. Positive health effects of fiber

      1. Weight control
      2. Improving large intestine function and health
      3. Preventing colon cancer
      4. Lowering blood cholesterol
      5. Glycemic response and diabetes control

   B. Negative health effects of fibers

      1. Bulk effect may prevent sufficient intake of kcalories
      2. Abdominal discomfort
      3. Low nutrient availability

   C. Recommended intakes of fiber

      1. 35 grams per day
      2. Select from a variety of sources
      3. Daily food guide plan
         a. 2-4 servings fruit
         b. 3-5 servings vegetables
         c. 6-11 servings of breads
      4. Increase fiber slowly in diet to avoid discomfort

H4-2 Foods to Include on a High Fiber Diet

XI. Highlight: Alternatives to Sugar

Chapter 5
THE LIPIDS: TRIGLYCERIDES, PHOSPHOLIPIDS, AND STEROLS

CHAPTER SUMMARY

The lipids include triglycerides (fats and oils), phospholipids, and sterols all important to nutrition. In foods fats provide palatability, tenderness, and flavor. Fats provide satiety in meals.

Triglycerides are composed of fatty acids and glycerol. Triglycerides and fatty acids provide energy, insulation, and protection from shock. Triglycerides in the diet provide fat-soluble vitamins, add satiety, and deliver flavor, texture and tenderness to foods.

Phospholipids are used as emulsifiers in foods. Sterols are found in both plant and animals foods, but cholesterol is found only in animal foods. Sterols include vital body compounds such as bile acids, sex and adrenal hormones, and Vitamin D.

Fat is emulsified by bile acids in the small intestine. Enzymes digest the fat. After absorption, fats are transported in the bloodstream by lipoproteins. These include chylomicrons, very-low-density lipoproteins, low-density lipoproteins, and high-density lipoproteins. The distinction between the lipoproteins has important implications for health.

Lipid profiles are important to evaluate risk of heart disease. Fat contributes to obesity, cancer, hypertension, and diabetes. Current recommendations include reducing fat intake to an average of 30% of energy or less and average saturated fat intake to less than 10% of energy among people aged two years and older.

Highlight 5 describes the use of the fat substitutes Simplesse and Olestra.

2 CHAPTER 5, THE LIPIDS: TRIGLYCERIDES, PHOSPHOLIPIDS, AND STEROLS

LEARNING OBJECTIVES

1. Describe the the structure of a triglyceride. What are the differences between saturated, unsaturated, monounsaturated, and polyunsaturated fats?
2. What does hydrogenation do to fats?
3. What does the term "omega" mean with respect to fatty acids? How is this relevant to health?
4. Which of the fatty acids are essential?
5. How do phospholipids differ from triglycerides in structure? How does cholesterol differ?
6. Explain fat digestion, absorption, and transport.
7. What do lipoproteins do? What are the differences among the chylomicrons, VLDL, LDL, and HDL?
8. What roles does cholesterol play in the body?
9. Describe the routes cholesterol takes in the body.
10. What roles do the triglycerides and phospholipids perform in the body?
11. How does excessive fat intake influence health?
12. What features do fats bring to food?
13. What are the dietary recommendations regarding fat and cholesterol intake?
14. What food lists of the exchange system supply fat in abundance? In moderation? Not at all?

Chapter Outline   Acetates/Handouts

I. Introduction

II. The Triglycerides

   A. The chemist's view of fatty acids   TA23 Condensation of
                                                   Glycerol and Fatty
                                                   Acids
       1. The carbon chain   TA24 A Mixed
       2. Triglyceride formation   Triglyceride
       3. Degree of saturation
          a. saturated fatty acid
          b. unsaturated fatty acid
          c. monounsaturated fatty acid
          d. polyunsaturated fatty acid
       4. Oils and fats   TA25 Comparison of
          a. vegetable and fish oils are high in   Dietary Fats
             monounsaturated fat

CHAPTER 5, THE LIPIDS: TRIGLYCERIDES, PHOSPHOLIPIDS, AND STEROLS

        b. olive and canola oils are high in polyunsaturated fat
        c. animal fats are high in saturated fat
        d. coconut and palm oil are plant oils high in saturated fat - an exception to the general rule

   B. Processed fat in foods

      1. Hydrogenation of fats affects texture of foods   TA26 Hydrogenation
      2. Trans-fatty acids are stable but safety is questioned

   C. Role of triglycerides and fatty acids

      1. In the body
        a. provide energy
        b. provide insulation against temperature extremes
        c. provide protection against shock
      2. In the diet
        a. bring fat-soluble vitamins
        b. deliver flavor, aroma, and tenderness
        c. slow digestion, adding satiety and a sense of fullness

   D. The essential polyunsaturated fatty acids   TA27 Structural Formulas for Omega-3 and Omega-6 Fatty Acids

      1. Debate over essentiality   TA28 Lecithin
      2. Polyunsaturated fatty acid deficiencies
      3. Role of polyunsaturated fatty acids

III. The phospholipids and sterols

   A. The chemist's view of phospholipids

   B. Phospholipids in foods are used as emulsifiers

   C. Role of phospholipids in cell membranes

   D. The chemist's view of sterols

CHAPTER 5, THE LIPIDS: TRIGLYCERIDES, PHOSPHOLIPIDS, AND STEROLS

- E. Sterols in food
    1. Cholesterol found only in animal foods — TA29 Cholesterol
    2. Eggs and organ meats are particularly high in cholesterol

- F. Role of sterols
    1. bile acids
    2. sex hormones
    3. adrenal hormones
    4. vitamin D

IV. Digestion, Absorption, Transport, and Metabolism

- A. Emulsification — TA30 Emulsification of Fat by Bile
- B. Digestion occurs in small intestine
- C. Absorbed in the form of glycerol and fatty acids — TA31 Absorption and Transport of Lipids
- D. Transport
    1. Chylomicrons
    2. Very low density lipoproteins
    3. Low density lipoproteins
    4. High density lipoproteins
    5. Other routes for cholesterol
- E. A Preview of Lipid Metabolism
    1. Storing fat as fat
    2. Using fat for energy

V. Health Effects and Recommended Intakes of Lipids

- A. Health effects of lipids
    1. Omega-3 fatty acids reduce blood clotting tendencies and reduce blood pressure
    2. High lipid levels in blood relate to heart problems

B. Recommended fat intakes

1. 30% of total caloric intake
2. 10% of total caloric intake for saturated fat
3. 300 mg or less of cholesterol
4. Reduce fat in diet by:
   a. no fat in cooking   H5-1 Exposing Hidden
   b. lean meats   Fat
   c. decrease meat portions and frequency
   d. substitute lower fat products
   e. increase fruits and vegetables

C. Using the exchange system to estimate fats

1. The milk list
2. The meat list
3. The fat list
4. Vegetables, fruit and grains
5. Miscellaneous foods
6. Low fat meals

D. Availability of low fat foods   H5-2 How to Modify a
                                          Recipe

VI. Highlight 5 - Alternatives To Fat

Chapter 6
PROTEIN: AMINO ACIDS

CHAPTER SUMMARY

Protein is vital to the structural and working materials of all cells. Protein contains nitrogen atoms as well as oxygen, hydrogen and carbon atoms. Amino acids are the basic building blocks of protein. Essential amino acids are those the body cannot synthesize in amounts sufficient to meet needs.

Protein functions in the growth and maintenance of tissues. Enzymes, hormones and antibodies are proteins. Proteins assist with fluid and acid-base balance. Protein assists in the transport of nutrients, clotting of blood and sight.

Egg protein is used as the standard to measure protein quality. Proteins of high quality are easily digested and offer the body all the essential amino acids. Chemical scoring, biological value, net protein utilization, and protein efficiency ratio are measures used to evaluate protein quality.

Nitrogen balance studies help to determine the amount of protein needed in the body. Recommendations include allowing 15% of total calories as protein.

Highlight 6 covers the advantages and disadvantages of the meatless diet.

CHAPTER 6, PROTEIN: AMINO ACIDS

Learning Objectives

1. Describe the structure of amino acids, and explain how their sequence in proteins affects the proteins' shapes.
2. How does the chemical structure of protein differ from the structures of carbohydrates and fats?
3. Describe protein digestion and absorption.
4. Descibe some of the roles proteins play in the human body.
5. What are enzymes? What roles do they play in chemical reactions?
6. How does the body use amino acids? What is deamination?
7. Describe protein synthesis.
8. What factors affect the quality of dietary protein?
9. What are the health consequences of ingesting inadequate protein and energy? Describe marasmus and kwashiorkor. How can you distinguish between the two conditions, and in what ways do they overlap?
10. How might protein excess, or the type of protein eaten, influence health?
11. What factors are considered in establishing recommended protein intakes? Define nitrogen balance.
12. Which food lists of the exchange system supply protein in abundance? In moderation? Not at all?
13. What are the benefits and risks of taking protein and amino acid supplements?
14. How can vegetarians meet their protein needs without eating meat?

Chapter Outline   Acetates/Handouts

I. Introduction

II. The Chemist's View of Proteins

    A. Amino acid structure   TA32 Amino Acid Structure
                                                                   TA33 Formation of a Dipeptide

    B. Essential amino acids

    C. Amino acid sequence

    D. Folding of the chain

    E. The completed protein

III. Digestion and Absorption

IV. Roles of Proteins and Amino Acids in the Body

    A. Protein in growth and maintenance

        1. Growth
        2. Repair
        3. Replacement
        4. Protein turnover

    B. Enzymes   TA34 Enzyme Action

    C. Fluid balance

    D. Acid-base balance

    E. Antibodies

    F. Hormones

    G. Transport proteins   TA35 Transport Proteins

    H. Blood clotting

    I. Visual pigments

    J. Amino acids in the body

        1. Using amino acids for protein or non-essential amino acids
        2. Using amino acids for other gluconeogenesis compounds
        3. Using amino acids for energy
        4. Deaminating amino acids
        5. Using excess amino acids for fat

V. Protein in the Body

    A. Protein synthesis   TA36 Protein Synthesis

    B. Protein quality

        1. Complete protein
        2. Complementary protein
        3. Digestibility
        4. Reference protein - egg

CHAPTER 6, PROTEIN: AMINO ACIDS

    C. Measurement of protein quality

        1. Chemical scoring
        2. Biological value
        3. Net protein utilization
        4. Protein efficiency ratio

VI. Health Effects of Protein

    A. Protein-energy malnutrition

        1. Kwashiorkor
        2. Marasmus
        3. Malnutrition and infection

    B. Protein excess

        1. Contributes to obesity
        2. Promotes calcium losses
        3. Stresses kidney and liver

    C. Animal versus vegetable protein

VII. Recommended Protein Intakes

    A. Nitrogen balance studies

    B. Protein recommendations

        1. 15% of total kcalories
        2. 0.8 grams per kilogram body weight

VIII. Protein in Food   H6-1 Protein Sources

    A. Meat eaters' protein sources

    B. Vegetarian protein sources

    C. Protein and amino acid supplements

IX. Highlight: Health Aspects of Meatless Diets

Chapter 7
METABOLISM: TRANSFORMATIONS AND INTERACTIONS

CHAPTER SUMMARY

After a balanced meal, the energy yielding nutrients are digested and absorbed. Carbohydrate yields glucose which is used by the brain cells and other cells, and is broken down to pyruvate and acetyl CoA to provide energy. Some is stored as glycogen. Fat yields glycerol and fatty acids. These are also broken down to acetyl CoA, enter the TCA cycle and provide energy. Some are reassembled and stored as fat. Protein yields amino acids which primarily function to build body protein. Although, if needed for energy, amino acids will be broken down through the same pathways as carbohydrate and fat.

Surplus carbohydrate is stored as glycogen. When glycogen stores are filled, excess is routed to fat. Surplus fat is stored as fat with seemingly unlimited capacity. Surplus protein is deaminated. It is used for energy, if needed. If not needed for energy, it is stored as fat.

Stored energy is drawn upon as the body shifts from a fed state to a fasting state. Fat stores last longer than carbohydrate. It is important that the nervous system and brain cells have glucose available to them. Protein may be called upon to meet this need. Ketosis, a condition of high blood ketone bodies and ketone bodies in the urine, is a danger sign. Ketosis helps to prolong life in life threatening situations.

Highlight 7 describes the relationship of nutrition and alcohol.

CHAPTER 7, METABOLISM: TRANFORMATIONS AND INTERACTIONS

Learning Objectives

1. Define metabolism, anabolism, and catabolism; give an example of each.
2. Name one of the body's quick-energy molecules, and describe how it is used.
3. What are coenzymes, and what service do they provide in metabolism?
4. Name the four basic units, derived from foods, used by the body in metabolic transformations. How many carbons are in the "backbones" of each?
5. Summarize the main steps in the metabolism of glucose, glycerol, fatty acids, and amino acids.
6. How does the body dispose of excess nitrogen?
7. Describe how a surplus of the three energy nutrients contributes to body fat stores.
8. What adaptations does the body make during a fast? What are ketone bodies? Define ketosis.
9. Distinguish between a loss of *fat* and a loss of *weight*, and describe how both might happen.

Chapter Outline   Acetates/Handouts

I. Chemical Reactions in the Body

    A. Introduction

        1. carbohydrates to glucose
        2. fats to glycerol and fatty acids
        3. protein to amino acids

    B. Anabolism - building up reactions

        1. Requires energy
        2. Glucose to glycogen   TA37 Anabolic and Catabolic Reactions Glycogen
        3. Glycerol and fatty acids to triglycerides   TA38 Anabolic and Catabolic Reactions Triglycerides
        4. Amino acids to protein   TA39 Anabolic and Catabolic Reactions Protein

    C. Catabolism - breaking down reactions

        1. Release energy
        2. Glycogen to glucose
        3. Triglycerides to glycerol and fatty acids
        4. Protein to amino acids

CHAPTER 7, METABOLISM: TRANSFORMATIONS AND INTERACTIONS

   D. The transfer of energy in reactions

   E. Enzymes and coenzymes are helpers in reactions

II. Breaking Down Nutrients for Energy

   A. Glucose

   1. Glucose-to-pyruvate pathway — H7-1 Glycolysis
   2. Glucose-to-pyruvate, an anaerobic pathway — TA40 Glycolysis
   3. Pyruvate-to-acetyl CoA — TA41 Pyruvate-to-Acetyl CoA
   4. Glucose retrieval via the Cori Cycle — TA42 Glucose Retrieval via the Cori Cycle
   5. Muscle's needs for oxygen for energy metabolism
   6. Pyruvate-to-acetyl CoA, an irreversible step — TA43 The Paths of Pyruvate and Acetyl CoA
   7. Acetyl CoA-to-carbon dioxide: The TCA cycle makes more energy available — TA44 The Breakdown of Acetyl CoA
   8. Acetyl CoA-to-fat

   TA45 The Glucose-to-Energy Pathway

   B. Glycerol and fatty acids — TA46 The Fats-to-Energy Pathway

   1. Glycerol-to-pyruvate
   2. Fatty acids-to-acetyl CoA — TA47 Fatty Acid Oxidation
   3. Glucose not retrievable from fatty acids

   C. Amino acids

   1. Amino acid catabolism — TA48 Amino Acid-to-Energy Pathway
      a. Deamination occurs first
      b. Different metabolic pathways
   2. Glucose retrievable from animo acids
   3. Amino acids-to-fat

4 CHAPTER 7, METABOLISM: TRANFORMATIONS AND INTERACTIONS

        4. Deamination
        5. Transamination   TA49 Transamination to Make a Nonessential Amino Acid

        6. Ammonia-to-urea in the liver   TA50 Urea Synthesis
        7. Urea excreted via the kidneys   TA51 Urea Excretion
        8. Water needed to excrete urea

    D. The final steps of catabolism

        1. The TCA cycle
        2. The electron transport chain   TA52 Electron Transport Chain

        3. Summary   TA53 The Central Pathways of Energy Metabolism

III. The Body's Energy Budget

    A. The economics of feasting

        1. Surplus carbohydrate   TA54 How Carbohydrate, Eaten in Excess, Contributes to Body Fat

        2. Surplus fat   TA55 How Fat, Eaten in Excess, Contributes to Body Fat

        3. Surplus protein   TA56 How Protein, Eaten in Excess, Contributes to Body Fat

        4. The body's use of stored energy

    B. The economics of fasting

        1. Drawing on energy stores   TA57 Feasting
        2. Fat stores last longer   TA58 Fasting
        3. Glucose needed for the brain
        4. Protein called on to meet brain's glucose need
        5. Fat's small glucose contribution from glycerol
        6. The shift to ketosis   TA60 Ketone Body Formation

        7. Suppression of appetite

CHAPTER 7, METABOLISM: TRANSFORMATIONS AND INTERACTIONS

8. Slowing of metabolism
9. Symptoms of starvation
10. The low-carbohydrate diet
11. The protein-sparing fast

IV. Highlight: Alcohol and Nutrition

H7-2 Self-Assessment for Alcoholism
TA61 One Pathway for the Degradation of Ethanol

Chapter 8
ENERGY BALANCE AND WEIGHT CONTROL

CHAPTER SUMMARY

Energy balance is a simple yet complex formula. Energy in (food and beverages) is measured by use of the bomb calorimeter computed from the amounts of carbohydrate, fat and protein, or estimated by use of the food exchange system. The energy expended includes basal metabolism, physical activity, thermal effect of food and adaptive thermogenesis.

A variety of techniques are used to measure body weight and body composition. Height/weight charts and body mass index are used as guidelines for weight. Fatfold measures and waist/hip ratios are the common methods used to measure body composition.

Choices for treatment of obesity are many. Poor choices include pills, over-the-counter products, surgery, and other gimmicks. Recommended treatments for obesity involve planning a well balanced reduced calorie diet, with exercise. Behavior and attitude are important aspects.

Problems of underweight pose health problems also. Strategies for weight gain include consuming energy-dense foods, three meals a day, large portions, snacks, and exercise to build muscles.

Highlight 8 discusses anorexia nervosa and bulimia, eating disorders characterized by sociological, neurochemical and psychological problems.

CHAPTER 8, ENERGY BALANCE AND WEIGHT CONTROL

Learning Objectives

1. What are the consequences of an unbalanced energy budget?
2. What types of activites does the body spend energy on? How can energy expenditure be estimated?
3. Distinguish between body weight and body composition. What assessment techniques are used to measure each?
4. What problems are involved in defining "ideal" body weight?
5. What risks are associated with excess body weight and excess body fat? What is central obesity and what is its relationship to disease?
6. What factors are thought to cause obesity?
7. List several ill-advised ways to lose weight and explain why such methods are not recommended.
8. Discuss dietary strategies suitable for achieving and maintaining a healthy body weight.
9. What are the benefits of increased physical activity in a weight-loss program?
10. Describe the behavior-modification techniques recommended for changing an individual's dietary habits. What role does personal attitude play?
11. What are the problems of underweight?
12. Describe strategies for successful weight gain.

Chapter Outline   Acetates/Handouts

I. Energy Balance

   A. Change in energy stores = energy in minus energy out

   B. 1 lb body fat = 3500 kcal

   C. Recommended weight loss is 1/2 lb to 1 lb per week

   D. Energy intake for weight loss is 10 kcal per body weight

   E. Quick weight loss does not always reflect change in body fat

II. Energy in: The kcalories in food

   A. Estimating food energy

   B. Determinants of food intake

III. Energy out: The kcalories the body spends

   A. The generation of heat

      1. Basal thermogenesis (metabolism)
      2. Exercise-induced thermogenesis (physical activity)
      3. Diet-induces thermogenesis (thermal effect of food)
      4. Adaptive thermogenesis (energy of adaptation)

   B. Components of energy expenditure

      1. Basal metabolism
      2. Physical activity
      3. Thermic effect of food
      4. Adaptive thermogenesis

   C. Estimating energy requirements

IV. Body Weight and Body Composition

   A. Body weight

      1. Definitions
      2. Weight for height
      3. Body mass index

   B. Body composition

      1. Fatfold measures
      2. Waist-to-hip ratio
      3. Other measures of body composition

   C. Ideal body composition

V. Causes of Obesity

   H8-1 Medical Problems Associated with Obesity

   A. Fat cell development

   B. Genetics

   C. Fat cell metabolism

   D. Set-point theory

CHAPTER 8, ENERGY BALANCE AND WEIGHT CONTROL

    E. The "fattening power" of fat

    F. Inactivity

VI. Controversies in Obesity Treatment

    A. Dangers of weight loss

        1. Fad diets
        2. Weight cycling   TA63 Weight Cycle Effects of Repeated Dieting
        3. Psychological problems

    B. Benefits of weight loss and maintenance

        1. Gradual permanent weight will improve health
        2. Prevention is the key

VII. Treatments of Obesity: Poor Choices

    A. Pills, procedures, and other possibilities

    B. Very-low-kcalorie diets

VIII. Treatments of obesity: Good Choices

    A. Eating plans

        1. Energy intakes
            a. approximately 10 kcal per lb of current weight
            b. nutrient dense foods
            c. no less than 1200 kcal per day
            d. complex carbohydrates
            e. eat slowly
            f. select low fat foods
            g. limit concentrated sweets
            h. limit alcoholic beverages
            i. drink plenty of water
        2. Physical activity
            a. increases energy output
            b. speeds up basal metabolism
            c. controls appetite

d. reduces stress
e. psychological well being
f. self-esteem

B. Behavior and attitude

1. Behavior modification
   a. antecedents
      (1) eliminate inappropriate eating cues
      (2) suppress cues
      (3) strengthen cues
   b. behavior
      (1) desired eating behavior
      (2) desired exercise behavior
   c. consequences
      (1) positive
      (2) negative
2. Personal attitude
   a. learn to deal with feelings
   b. positive self-talk
   c. positive thinking
   d. use support groups

IX. Underweight

A. Problems

1. Health consequences
2. Infertility
3. Diverse causes
4. Body not prepared to deal with stressful conditions

B. Weight-gain strategies

1. Energy dense foods
2. Three meals daily
3. Large portions
4. Snacks between meals
5. Plenty of juice and milk
6. Exercise to build muscle

X. Highlight: Anorexia Nervosa and Bulimia   H8-2 Eating Attitudes Test

Chapter 9
THE WATER-SOLUBLE VITAMINS: B VITAMINS AND VITAMIN C

CHAPTER SUMMARY

The structure and function of vitamins differ from the energy-yielding nutrients. The amounts needed by the body are considerably less as compared to the energy-yielding nutrients. Vitamins are essential nutrients with unique characteristics.

The water soluble vitamins are needed in frequent, small amounts. They are absorbed directly into blood, and travel freely. They are excreted in the urine, so are unlikely to reach toxic levels.

Thiamin, riboflavin, niacin, pantothenic acid, biotin, Vitamin B_6, folate, Vitamin B_{12} and Vitamin C are reviewed. Functions, intake recommendations, deficiency symptoms and diseases, problems with toxicity and significant food sources are outlined in detail. The unique characteristics of each vitamin is given. Interrelationships are discussed.

Highlight 9 reviews characteristics of properly designed experimental research studies. Readers are cautioned to examine claims made about Vitamin C from the media. Research indicates that the effect of Vitamin C on the common cold is small. New evidence is helping to understand the role of Vitamin C in more detail.

CHAPTER 9, THE WATER SOLUBLE VITAMINS: B VITAMINS AND VITAMIN C

Learning Objectives

1. For thiamin, riboflavin, niacin, biotin, pantothenic acid, vitamin B_6, folate, vitamin B_{12}, and vitamin C, state:
    - Its chief function in the body.
    - Its characteristic deficiency symptoms.
    - Its significant food sources.
2. What is the relationship of tryptophan to niacin?
3. Which B vitamins are involved in energy metabolism? Protein metabolism? Cell division?
4. What risks are associated with high vitamin C doses?

Chapter Outline   Acetates/Handouts

I. The Vitamins

    A. Functions

        1. Vitamins act singly
        2. Vitamins assist enzymes with energy production and help cells multiply
        3. Amounts consumed are measured in micrograms or milligrams   TA64 Coenzyme Action

    B. Classification

        1. Water-soluble
            a. absorbed directly into the blood
            b. travel freely in the blood
            c. freely circulate into the water-filled compartments of the body
            d. excreted in the urine
            e. needed in frequent small doses
            f. unlikely to reach toxic levels
        2. Fat-soluble
            a. absorbed into the lymph system then the blood
            b. require protein carriers for transport
            c. become trapped in cells associated with fat
            d. remain in fat storage sites in the body
            e. needed in periodic doses

CHAPTER 9, THE WATER SOLUBLE VITAMINS: B VITAMINS AND VITAMIN C

II. The Water-Soluble Vitamins

III. The B Vitamins - As Individuals

    A. Thiamin

        1. Function
- a. Part of TPP (thiamin pyrophosphate)
- b. coenzyme in energy metabolism
- c. supports appetite and nerve function

        2. Thiamin recommendations
- a. RDA 0.5 mg/1000 kcal/day
  1 mg/day minimum
- b. men (19-50 yr) 1.5 mg/day
- c. women (19-50 yr) 1.0 mg/day

        3. Thiamin deficiency
- a. beriberi
- b. heart problems
- c. muscle and nerve problems

        4. Thiamin food sources
- a. pork, ham, bacon, liver
- b. whole-grain and enriched breads
- c. legumes and nuts

    B. Riboflavin

        1. Function   TA65 Riboflavin Coenzyme
- a. facilitates release of energy
- b. part of FAD and FMN

        2. Riboflavin recommendations
- a. RDA 0.6 mg/1000 kcal/day
  1.2 mg/day minimum
- b. men (19-50 yr) 1.7 mg/day
- c. women (19-50 yr) 1.3 mg/day

        3. Riboflavin deficiency
- a. ariboflavinosis
- b. mouth, gums and tongue
- c. nervous system and eyes
- d. skin rash

        4. Riboflavin food sources
- a. milk, yogurt, cottage cheese
- b. meat
- c. leafy green vegetables
- d. whole grain and enriched breads and cereals

CHAPTER 9, THE WATER SOLUBLE VITAMINS: B VITAMINS AND VITAMIN C

5. Unique characteristic: destroyed by light and irradiation

C. Niacin

1. Functions
   a. part of NAD and NADH
   b. coenzyme in energy metabolism   TA66 Niacin Coenzyme in Action
   c. supports skin, nervous and digestive system
2. Niacin recommendations
   a. RDA 6.6 NE/1000 kcal/day 13 NE/day minimum
   b. made from tryptophan
   c. men (19-50 yr) 19 mg NE/day
   d. women (19-50 yr) 15 mg NE/day
3. Niacin deficiency
   a. pellagra
   b. digestive problems
   c. affects nervous system
   d. skin problems
4. Niacin toxicity
   a. affects nervous system
   b. lowers LDL and increases HDL
   c. increases blood glucose
5. Niacin food sources
   a. milk and eggs
   b. meat, poultry, fish
   c. whole grain and enriched breads and cereals
   d. nuts and all protein containing foods

D. Biotin

1. Function
   a. coenzyme in energy metabolism
   b. coenzyme in fat metabolism
   c. coenzyme in amino acid metabolism
   d. coenzyme in glycogen synthesis
2. Biotin recommendations
   a. no RDA
   b. estimated safe and adequate intake 30-100 micrograms/day
3. Biotin deficiency
   a. abnormal heart function
   b. loss of appetite

CHAPTER 9, THE WATER SOLUBLE VITAMINS: B VITAMINS AND VITAMIN C

                c.   muscle pain and weakness
                d.   dry, scaly intake
        4.   Biotin food sources are widespread
        5.   Unique characteristics
                a.   egg white protein avidin binds biotin
                b.   synthesized by GI tract

E.   Pantothenic acid

        1.   Function
                a.   part of CoA
                b.   used in energy metabolism
        2.   Pantothenic acid recommendations
                a.   no RDA
                b.   estimated safe and adequate intake 4-7 mg/day
        3.   Pantothenic acid deficiency
                a.   intestinal distress
                b.   vomiting
                c.   fatigue
                d.   insomnia
        4.   Pantothenic acid food sources are widespread
        5.   Unique characteristic: easily destroyed by heat

F.   Vitamin B_6

        1.   Function
                a.   part of PLP (pyridoxal phosphate)
                b.   coenzyme
                c.   converts tryptophan to serotonin
                d.   red blood cells antagonist
        2.   Vitamin B_6 recommendations
                a.   RDA 0.016 mg/g protein/day
                b.   men (19-50 yr) 2.0 mg/day
                c.   women (19-50 yr) 1.6 mg/day
        3.   Vitamin B_6 deficiency
                a.   weakness, irritability, insomnia
                b.   growth failure, impaired motor function, and convulsions
        4.   Vitamin B_6 toxicity   TA67 Dose Levels and
                a.   nerve damage   Effects
                b.   numbness of mouth
        5.   Vitamin B_6 food sources
                a.   green leafy vegetables
                b.   meats, fish, poultry, shellfish, legumes
                c.   fruits, whole grains

CHAPTER 9, THE WATER SOLUBLE VITAMINS: B VITAMINS AND VITAMIN C

      6. Other information
         a. Does not cure PMS
         b. bioavailability

G. Folate

    1. Function
       a. Part of THF (tetrahydrofolate), and DHF (dihydrofolate)
       b. coenzyme in DNA synthesis
    2. Folate recommendations
       a. RDA 3 micrograms/kg body weight
       b. higher for pregnancy
    3. Folate deficiency
       a. impairs cell division
       b. impairs protein synthesis
       c. interactions with drugs
    4. Folate food sources
       a. leafy green vegetables and fruits
       b. legumes and seeds
       c. liver

H. Vitamin B_{12}

    1. Function
       a. coenzyme in cell synthesis
       b. maintains nerve cells
       c. re-forms folate coenzyme
    2. Vitamin B_{12} Recommendations: RDA 2 micrograms/day
    3. Vitamin B_{12} Deficiency
       a. lack of intrinsic factor
       b. paralysis of nerve and muscles
       c. large cell type anemia
    4. Vitamin B_{12} food sources
       a. meat, fish, poultry, and shellfish
       b. milk, cheese, eggs

I. Vitamin relatives

    1. Inositol, choline, and lipoicinositol
       a. coenzymes in metabolism
       b. abundant in foods
    2. Lecithin can cause short term discomfort
    3. Other substances mistaken for essential nutrients

CHAPTER 9, THE WATER SOLUBLE VITAMINS: B VITAMINS AND VITAMIN C

IV. The B Vitamins - In Concert   TA68 Metabolic Pathways Involving B Vitamins

    A. B Vitamin interactions

        1. Riboflavin and Vitamin B_6
        2. Folate and Vitamin B_{12}

    B. B Vitamin deficiencies

        1. Seldom isolated
        2. Food vs pills
        3. Skin and tongue especially vulnerable

    C. B Vitamin toxicities

        1. Uncommon
        2. Occur with supplementation

    D. B Vitamin food sources

V. Vitamin C

    A. History of ships and scurvy

    B. Vitamin C roles   TA69 Vitamin C's Role in Hydroxyproline

        1. antioxident
        2. collagen formation
        3. stress hormones
        4. cancer research

    C. Vitamin C recommendations

        1. RDA 60 mg/day
        2. Tissue saturation   TA70 Vitamin C Intake
        3. Affected by smoking, stress and healing

    D. Vitamin C deficiency

        1. Capillary hemorrhages
        2. Scurvy symptoms

    E. Vitamin C toxicity

CHAPTER 9, THE WATER SOLUBLE VITAMINS: B VITAMINS AND VITAMIN C

        1. Nausea, abdominal cramps, and diarrhea
        2. Affects medical tests
        3. Kidney stones
        4. Dependency

F. Vitamin C food sources

        1. Fruits and vegetables
        2. Citrus fruits
        3. Potatoes

VI. Highlight: Vitamin C - Rumors and Research

Chapter 10
THE FAT-SOLUBLE VITAMINS: A, D, E, AND K

CHAPTER SUMMARY

The fat-soluble vitamins play different roles from the water-soluble vitamins. Vitamin A, Vitamin D, Vitamin E and Vitamin K are important in growth and maintenance of the body. Specific functions, deficiency and toxicity symptoms, intake recommendations, significant food sources, and unique characteristics are given. Interrelationships with other nutrients are explained.

Highlight 10 explores the controversy over the use of vitamin and mineral supplements. Arguments for and against are discussed. Guidelines for the selection of supplements are included.

CHAPTER 10, THE FAT-SOLUBLE VITAMINS: A, D, E, AND K

Learning Objectives

1. List the fat-soluble vitamins. What characteristics do they have in common? How do they differ from the water-soluble vitamins?
2. Summarize the roles of vitamin A and the symptoms of its deficiency.
3. What is meant by vitamin precursors? Name the precursors of vitamin A, and tell in what classes of foods they are located. Give examples of foods with high vitamin A activity.
4. How is vitamin D unique among the vitamins? What is its chief function? What are the richest sources of this vitamin?
5. Describe vitamin E's role as an antioxidant. What are the chief symptoms of vitamin E difficiency?
6. What is vitamin K's primary role in the body? What conditions may lead to vitamin K deficiency?

Chapter Outline   Acetates/Handouts

I. Introduction

    A. Found in the fat and oily parts of foods

    B. Insoluble in water

    C. Require bile for digestion

    D. Require chylomicrons for transport

    E. Absorbed and enter lymph system

    F. Stored in liver and adipose tissue

    G. Average daily intake is needed

    H. Risk of toxicity

II. Vitamin A

    A. Three forms

    B. Precursor   TA71 Three Forms of Vitamin A

    C. Vitamin A roles

        1. Vision

CHAPTER 10, THE FAT-SOLUBLE VITAMINS: A, D, E, AND K

      a. Retina of the eye transforms light energy into nerve impulses
      b. Transformers are molecules of pigment in the cells of the rods   TA72 Vision of the Retinol

  2. Cell differentiation
      a. Skin and linings
      b. Vitamin A helps maintain epithelial cells   TA73 Mucous Membrane Integrity

  3. Immunity
      a. Fight infection
      b. Immune system role

  4. Supports growth of bones

D. Vitamin A recommendations

  1. 1000 micrograms RE men
  2. 800 micrograms RE women

E. Vitamin A deficiency

  1. Night blindness is an early deficiency
  2. Blindness follows
  3. Diminished membrane integrity, affects digestion, absorption; infections are likely, affects skin and hair

F. Vitamin A toxicity

  1. Birth defects
  2. Not for acne
      a. Accutane is different
      b. Retin A caution   TA74 Vitamin A Deficiency and Toxicity
  3. Not for cancer

G. Vitamin A in foods   TA75 Vitamin A Compounds

  1. Preformed Vitamin A in animal products
  2. Provitamin A carotenoids in plant products
  3. International units is the old IU (international unit) of measure (1 RE = 3.33 IU)
  4. The colors of Vitamin A foods
      a. High Vitamin A activity in deep green, gold, red, and orange
      b. Chlorophyll masks carotene

CHAPTER 10, THE FAT-SOLUBLE VITAMINS: A, D, E, AND K

        c.   Xanthophyll is unrelated
        d.   White and colorless foods have no Vitamin A
    5.   Typical intakes
        a.   Half from fruits and vegetables
        b.   Half from dairy products
    6.   Vitamin A is poor in fast foods
    7.   Vitamin A is rich in liver

III.   Vitamin D

    A.   Introduction   TA76 Vitamin D Synthesis and Activation

        1.   Synthesized with the help of sunlight
        2.   Acts like a hormone

    B.   Vitamin D's bone formation role

        1.   Promotes bone mineralization
        2.   Raises blood concentration of calcium and phosphorus

    C.   Vitamin D deficiency
        1.   Rickets is characterized by bowed legs
        2.   Osteomalacia is adult rickets: a softening of the bone

    D.   Vitamin D toxicity

        1.   Increases calcium absorption
        2.   Produces high blood calcium
        3.   Promotes the return of bone calcium to the blood
        4.   Kidney stones

    E.   Vitamin D recommendations and sources

        1.   RDA 10 micrograms/day (19-25 year old)
             5 micrograms/day (25 and older)
        2.   Children need more
        3.   Fortified milk, fortified margarine
        4.   Egg yolk, liver and fatty fish
        5.   Sunlight

IV. Vitamin E

    A. Vitamin E's antioxidant role

        1. Fat-soluble
        2. Protects lipids
        3. Protects mitochondria and cell membranes
        4. Protects lungs
        5. Immune system

    B. Claims of vitamin E benefits have been discredited

    C. Vitamin E deficiency

        1. Neuralmuscular disfunction
        2. Nonmalignant breast disease
        3. Cramping in legs
        4. Breaking of red blood cells

    D. Vitamin E toxicity

        1. Not as common
        2. Not as detrimental

    E. Vitamin E recommendations

        1. RDA 10 mg α-TE/day men
           RDA 8 mg α-TE/day women

    F. Vitamin E in foods

        1. Plant oils
        2. Green leafy vegetables
        3. Wheat germ and whole grains
        4. Liver and egg yolks
        5. Nuts and seeds
        6. Fresh and lightly processed

V. Vitamin K

    A. Introduction

        1. Functions in blood clotting   TA77 Blood Clotting
        2. Synthesis of bone protein   Process
        3. Synthesized by bacteria in the GI tract

CHAPTER 10, THE FAT-SOLUBLE VITAMINS: A, D, E, AND K

          4. RDA 65 micrograms/day women
              RDA 80 micrograms/day men

    B. Vitamin K deficiency and toxicity

        1. Hemorrhagic disease
        2. Hemophilia
        3. Abnormal circumstances
        4. Newborns
        5. Toxicity uncommon

    C. Vitamin K from bacterial synthesis and foods

        1. Stored in liver
        2. Liver, green leafy vegetables, cabbage-type vegetables are good sources
        3. milk

VI. The Fat-Soluble Vitamins - In Summary

    A. Specific roles in growth and maintenance

    B. Functions depend on other fat-soluble vitamins

    C. Interact with minerals

    D. Toxicity with supplementation may be a problem

    E. Essential to life

VII. Highlight: Vitamin and Mineral Supplements

Chapter 11
THE BODY FLUIDS AND THE MAJOR MINERALS

CHAPTER SUMMARY

The chemical nature of minerals distinguishes them from other nutrients. Minerals are inorganic elements that can form compounds when in solution.

Body fluids are important in carrying nutrients and waste throughout the body. They actively participate in chemical reactions and help to form macromolecules. They act as lubricants, shock absorbers, solvents, and aid in temperature regulation.

Imbalances of fluids cause dehydration or water intoxication. The body has specific mechanisms for regulating water balance and excretion. The body uses minerals to help regulate the distribution of body fluids and electrolytes.

Sodium, potassium, calcium, phosphorus, magnesium, and sulfur are reviewed. Specific functions, deficiency and toxicity symptoms, intake recommendations, significant food sources, and unique characteristics are given. Interrelationships with other nutrients are explained.

Highlight 11 explores the relationship of osteoporosis and calcium. Factors such as age, physical activity, genetics, race, smoking, alcohol and nutrition are discussed. Guidelines for supplementation are included.

CHAPTER 11, THE BODY FLUIDS AND THE MAJOR MINERALS

Learning Objectives

1. What do the terms *major* and *trace* mean when describing the minerals in the body?
2. Describe some characteristics of minerals that distinguish them from vitamins.
3. List the roles of water in the body.
4. Name the organs, hormones, and major minerals responsible for regulating the constancy of body salts and water balance.
5. What is the major function of sodium in the body? Describe how the kidneys regulate blood sodium.
6. List calcium's role in the body. How does the body keep blood calcium constant regardless of intake?
7. List the roles of phosphorus in the body. Discuss the relationships between calcium and phosphorus.
8. State the major functions of chloride, potassium, magnesium, and sulfur in the body. Are deficiencies of these nutrients likely to occur in your own diet? Why?

Chapter Outline   Acetates/Handouts

I. The Minerals

    A. Inorganic elements or ions

    B. The body's handling of minerals   TA78 The Amounts of Minerals in a 60-Kilogram Human Body

    C. Variable bioavailability

II. The Body Fluids

    A. Water balance and recommended intakes

        1. Water intake regulation
            a. thirst mechanism
            b. response to thirst
        2. Water excretion regulation   TA79 How the Body Regulates Water Excretion

            a. hypothalamus responds
            b. kidneys responds
            c. low blood pressure

CHAPTER 11, THE BODY FLUIDS AND THE MAJOR MINERALS

                (1)   angiotensin restricts blood vessels
                (2)   ADH causes retention
                (3)   Aldosterone causes sodium retention
        d.   excrete minimum 500 ml/day average 2 1/2 liters/day
    3.   Water recommendations
        a.   1.0-1.5 ml/kcal expended for adults
        b.   1.5 ml/kcal expended for infants
        c.   variable
    4.   Water sources
        a.   liquids
        b.   foods
        c.   metabolic water

    B.   Fluid and electrolyte balance   TA80 Water Follows Salt
                                                                       H11-1 Osmotic Pressure

        1.   Dissociation of salts in water
        2.   Water's attraction to salt
        3.   Water follows electrolytes
        4.   Proteins regulate flow of fluids and ions
        5.   Maintenance of fluid and electrolyte balance
        6.   GI tract regulation
        7.   Renal regulation
        8.   Thirst regulation

    C.   Fluid and electrolyte imbalance

        1.   Sodium and chloride most easily lost
        2.   Different solutes lost by different routes

    D.   Acid-Base balance   TA82 pH's of Common Substances and Body Fluids pH

        1.   Regulation by buffers
        2.   Regulation by excretion
        3.   Renal regulation

III.   Sodium

    A.   Sodium roles in the body

1. Regulates volume of extracellular fluid
2. Maintains acid-base balance
3. Essential to nerves and muscles

B. Sodium recommendations

1. Estimated minimum requirement at 500 mg/day
2. Limit at 2000-3000 mg/day by various health groups

C. Sodium intakes

1. Vary widely
2. Consume more than needed

D. Sodium in foods

1. High in processed foods
2. Salted or smoked meats and fish
3. Canned and instant soups
4. Cheeses
5. Condiments

E. Restricting sodium

1. Avoid highly salted foods
2. Read labels
3. Avoid fast foods

F. Sodium and taste

1. Use sodium-free seasonings
2. Enjoy unsalted foods

G. Sodium deficiency

1. Low-sodium diets, vomiting, diarrhea, and heavy sweating can deplete sodium
2. Salt tablets, without water, can incur dehydration

H. Sodium toxicity

1. edema
2. hypertension

IV. Chloride

    A. Chloride roles in the body

        1. Anion in extracellular fluid
        2. Associates with potassium
        3. Part of HCL

    B. Chloride recommendations and intakes

        1. Estimated minimum requirement 750 mg/day
        2. Never lacking in the diet
        3. Found in processed foods

    C. Chloride deficiency and toxicity are generally not problems

V. Potassium

    A. Potassium roles in the body

        1. Maintains blood pressure
        2. Cation inside body cells
        3. Maintains fluid and electrolyte balance
        4. Nerve transmission and muscle contractions

    B. Potassium recommendations and food sources

        1. Estimated minimum requirements are 2000 mg/day
        2. Found in fresh fruits, vegetables, and legumes

    C. Potassium deficiency

        1. Unlikely but possible
        2. Excessive losses deplete potassium rather than deficient intakes
        3. Drugs may deplete

    D. Potassium toxicity

VI. Calcium

    A. Calcium in the body

        1. Calcium in bones   TA83 Calcium
        2. Control of blood calcium   Balance in Bones

CHAPTER 11, THE BODY FLUIDS AND THE MAJOR MINERALS

        3. Regulatory abnormalities
        4. Calcium absorption
        5. Calcium in the body fluids
        6. Calcium in bone

    B. Calcium recommendations

        1. Calcium sources
        2. Importance of milk products
        3. Other sources   H11-2 Choosing a Milk Substitute

    C. Calcium deficiency

VII. Phosphorus

    A. Phosphorus roles in the body

        1. Bones and teeth
        2. Genetic material
        3. Buffer

    B. Phosphorus recommendations: RDA 800 mg/day

    C. Phosphorus intakes from animal protein

VIII. Magnesium

    A. Magnesium functions in enzyme systems

    B. Magnesium intakes

        1. RDA 350 mg/day for men
        2. 280 mg/day for women
        3. Legumes, seeds and nuts

    C. Magnesium deficiency in disease

IX. Sulfur occurs with other nutrients

X. Highlight: Osteoporosis and Calcium

Chapter 12
THE TRACE MINERALS

CHAPTER SUMMARY

Each of the trace minerals provides a vital role in the body. A deficiency as well as an excess could be fatal. Diets normally supply just the right amount to maintain health.

Each of the following trace minerals are reviewed: iron, zinc, iodide, copper, manganese, fluoride, chromium, selenium, and molybdenum. Chief functions in the body, deficiency and toxicity symptoms, and significant food sources are studied.

Recommendations are listed for RDA's or Estimated Safe and Adequate Intakes. Factors affecting absorption and utilization are covered. Environmental contamination is examined. Supplementation and fortification are mentioned. Information is presented about interactions among the trace minerals.

Highlight 12 expands upon the problem of lead in the diets of children. Functions of lead in the body are reviewed with special emphasis on the problems of toxicity during periods of rapid growth. The connection between malnutrition and lead is significant. Environmental contamination of lead is outlined. Strategies to decrease lead poisoning are listed in detail.

CHAPTER 12, THE TRACE MINERALS

Learning Objectives

1. Distinguish between iron deficiency and iron-deficiency anemia. What are the symptoms of iron-deficiency anemia?
2. Distinguish between heme and nonheme iron. Discuss the factors that enhance iron absorption.
3. Discuss possible reasons for a low intake of zinc. What factors affect the bioavailability of zinc?
4. Describe the principle functions of iodide, copper, fluoride, chromium, and selenium in the body.
5. What public health measure has been used in preventing simple goiter? What measure has been recommended for protection against tooth decay?
6. Discuss the importance of balanced and varied diets in obtaining the essential minerals and avoiding toxicities.

Chapter Outline   Acetates/Handouts

I. Iron

    A. Iron roles in the body

        1. Involved in oxidation and reduction reactions
        2. Hemoglobin
        3. Myoglobin

    B. Iron absorption and metabolism   TA84 Iron Routes in the Body

        1. Iron absorption
            a. passes iron to blood
            b. holds iron in reserve
        2. Adjustability of absorption
            a. varies widely among individuals
            b. varies from time to time in an individual
        3. Iron transport and storage
            a. blood transferrin carries iron
            b. surplus iron stored in liver, bone marrow, and other organs
        4. Iron recycling
            a. body loses only tiny amounts
            b. salvaged iron is transported back to the bone marrow to be reused

    C. Iron deficiency

1. Blood losses
    a. regular menstrual cycles
    b. bleeding
    c. regular blood donators
2. Tests for iron deficiency
    a. red blood cell count
    b. transferrin concentration
    c. erythrocyte protoporphyrin
    d. hemoglobin concentration
3. Iron deficiency and anemia
    a. iron deficiency - depleted iron stores without regard to degree of depletion or the presence of anemia
    b. anemia - severe depletion of iron stores with low hemoglobin concentration
4. Prevalence of iron deficiency
    a. most common nutrient deficiency
    b. young children and women especially vulnerable
5. Nutritional and nonnutritional causes
    a. inadequate intake
    b. blood loss
6. Iron deficiency and behavior
    a. reduced work capacity
    b. reduced productivity
    c. mistaken for laziness
7. Iron deficiency and poor cold tolerance
8. Iron deficiency and pica
    a. appetite for clay, ice, paste and other unusual substances
    b. clay inhibits iron absorption

D. Iron Toxicity

1. Iron overload
    a. intestine absorbs excess iron
    b. tissue damage and infections
    c. fortification and supplementation does not contribute to iron overload
2. Iron poisoning
    a. massive amounts can cause death
    b. symptoms of intoxication

E. Iron recommendations and intakes

CHAPTER 12, THE TRACE MINERALS

   1. Recommended iron intakes
      a. RDA is 10 mg/day for adult man, easy to meet
      b. RDA is 15 mg/day for women of childbearing age, difficult to meet
   2. Iron in foods
      a. meat, fish and poultry provide 1/3 of needs
      b. milk, cheese and eggs provide 1/4 of needs
      c. enriched grains provide 1/4 of needs
      d. legumes, dark leafy vegetables and some fruits are high in iron
   3. Heme and nonheme ironheme
      a. heme iron is found in meat, fish and poultry and is absorbed better
      b. nonheme iron is found in vegetables, fruits, grains, eggs
   4. Absorption-enhancing factors
      a. MFP factor promotes absorption of nonheme iron
      b. Vitamin C enhances nonheme iron absorption when eaten at the same meal
   5. Absorption inhibitors
      a. phytates and fibers
      b. calcium and phosphorus in milk
      c. EDTA in food additives
      d. tannic acid
      e. polyphenols

   F. Contamination, supplement, and fortification of iron

      1. Contamination iron from cookware and soil
      2. Iron supplements
         a. needed by pregnant women
         b. ferrous sulfate
         c. consumed with meat or Vitamin C rich foods
      3. Breads and cereals are iron-enriched

II. Zinc

   A. Zinc roles in the body

1. supports functions of numerous metalloenzymes
   a. genetic materials
   b. digestive enzymes
   c. manufacture of heme
   d. essential fatty acid metabolism
   e. releases Vitamin A stores
   f. carbohydrate metabolism
   g. synthesis of protein
   h. metabolism of alcohol
   i. disposes free radicals

B. Zinc absorption and metabolism TA85 Zinc Routes in the Body

   1. Enteropancreatic circulation of zinc
      a. pancreas to intestine to pancreas
      b. can be bound in intestinal cells
      c. involved in metabolic functions in the cell
   2. Metallothionein, the zinc-binding protein regulates zinc absorption
   3. Zinc's interaction with copper
      a. intestinal zinc-binding protein also binds copper
      b. impairs copper absorption
   4. Factors affecting absorption
      a. absorbed at rate of 15-40% depending upon needs
      b. fiber and phytate inhibit absorption
      c. histidine enhances absorption
   5. Zinc is transported by albumin therefore lower blood concentrations of albumin affect zinc absorption
   6. Zinc interactions with iron
      a. binds with transferrin
      b. large doses of iron impair zinc absorption
   7. Zinc losses
      a. feces and urine
      b. tissue losses

C. Zinc deficiency

   1. Phytate inhibition of zinc absorption common in populations who consume unleavened bread
   2. Zinc-deficiency symptoms

6   CHAPTER 12, THE TRACE MINERALS

                a. growth retardation
                b. arrested sexual maturation
                c. alters digestive function
                d. impairs immune response
                e. central nervous system and brain function affected
                f. affects Vitamin A function
                g. disturbs thyroid function and metabolic rate
                h. alters taste
                i. slows wound healing

        D. Zinc toxicity

            1. Large doses may affect heart
            2. Small doses cause diarrhea, vomiting, fever, exhaustion
            3. Acidic foods stored in galvanized containers may be dangerous

        E. Zinc recommendations and intakes

            1. RDA is 15 mg/day (men) and 12 mg/day (women)
            2. Requirements for infants and children are high
            3. Foods high in zinc include shellfish, meats, and liver

        F. Contamination and supplement zinc

            1. Soil and water content may vary
            2. Galvanized pipes and pots not significant
            3. Supplements seldom appropriate

III. Iodide

        A. Iodide roles in the body involve thyroid hormones

        B. Iodide deficiency

            1. Goiter
            2. Goitrogen - a thyroid antagonist
            3. Causes sluggishness and weight gain
            4. Cretinism

        C. Iodide toxicity may enlarge the thyroid gland

D. Iodide sources

1. Coastal areas, seafood, and water
2. Variable in the soil
3. Iodized salt

E. Iodide intakes

1. 200-500 micrograms per day
2. 2000 micrograms is toxic
3. Excess from fast foods and dough conditioners, also medications

F. Iodide recommendations

1. 150 micrograms per day
2. Easily met

IV. Copper

A. Copper roles in the body

1. Constituent of enzymes
2. Absorption and use of iron

B. Copper deficiency

1. Rare
2. Disturbed growth and metabolism

C. Copper toxicity

1. Unlikely with food
2. Vomiting and diarrhea

D. Copper recommendations and intakes

1. Estimated safe and adequate intake is 1.5-3.0 mg/day
2. High in legumes, grains, nuts, organs meats, and seeds

V. Manganese

A. Manganese deficiencies rare

CHAPTER 12, THE TRACE MINERALS

    B.   Manganese toxicity

        1.   Environmental contaminants
        2.   Nervous system disorders

VI.   Fluoride

    A.   Fluoride roles in the body

    B.   Fluoridation and dental caries

    C.   Fluoride and osteoporosis

    D.   Fluoride deficiency

    E.   Fluoride toxicity

        1.   Symptoms with very high doses only
        2.   Fluorosis, nausea, diarrhea, chest pain, itching, and vomiting

    F.   Fluoride intakes

        1.   Estimated safe and adequate intake 1.5-4.0 mg/day
        2.   Best source is drinking water

VII.   Chromium

    A.   Chromium roles in the body

    B.   Chromium recommendations and intake

        1.   Estimated safe and adequate intake, 50-200 micrograms/day
        2.   Liver, brewer's yeast, whole grains, nuts and cheese

    C.   Chromium supplements

VIII.   Selenium

    A.   Selenium deficiency

B. Selenium and cancer

1. Selenium poor soil correlates with high incidence of cancer
2. Research is inconclusive

C. Selenium intakes

1. RDA 70 micrograms/day (men)
   55 micrograms/day (women)
2. Meats and other animal products

D. Selenium toxicity

1. High intakes are toxic
2. Vomiting, diarrhea, loss of hair and nails, skin lesions, and nervous system problems

IX. Molybdenum

A. Functions as facilitator of many cell processes

B. Goutlike symptoms with toxicity

C. Estimated safe and adequate intake at 75-250 micrograms/day

D. Sources include legumes, cereals, and organ meats

X. Other Trace Minerals

A. Nickel

B. Silicon

C. Tin

D. Vanadium

E. Cobalt   TA86 Cobalt with Vitamin B12

F. Boron

G. Others

CHAPTER 12, THE TRACE MINERALS

XI. The Trace Minerals - In Summary

　　A. Food sources

　　　　1. Content is unpredictable due to soil and water variability
　　　　2. Food processing factors
　　　　3. Absorption and availability affected
　　　　4. Wide variety of sources

　　B. Deficiencies

　　　　1. Severe deficiencies of well-known minerals are easy to recognize
　　　　2. Deficiencies of other minerals are less easy to diagnose
　　　　3. Cause failure to grow and thrive

　　C. Excess intakes and supplements

　　　　1. Toxic levels are not much greater than estimated requirements
　　　　2. Supplements may cause problems with toxicity

　　D. Interactions

XII. Meal Selections Revisited

XIII. Highlight: Our Children's Daily Lead

Chapter 13
FITNESS: PHYSICAL ACTIVITY, NUTRIENTS, AND BODY ADAPTATIONS

CHAPTER SUMMARY

Regular physical activity improves fitness and provides many health benefits. Flexibility, muscle strength and muscle endurance are components of fitness.

Training conditions the human body to be more fit. Muscle cells adapt in size and work capacity in response to demands. Cardiovascular conditioning improves heart and lung function to bring more oxygen to the cells. Both strength and endurance activities need to be included in a balanced fitness program.

Physical activity demands carbohydrate and fat for fuel. Protein is needed to build and maintain body lean tissues. Vitamins and minerals must be provided to support energy metabolism and tissue building. Water helps to distribute the fuels and eliminate waste.

The most common nutrition related problems of athletes include iron deficiency and amenorrhea. High incidence of eating disorders has also been noted. A suggested diet for physically active people differs very little from the diet of a sedentary person. The diet must provide ample fluids and a variety of nutrient-dense foods in quantities to meet energy needs.

A healthful diet surpasses the need for pills and powders to enhance athletic performance. Highlight 13 addresses the issues of supplements and ergogenic aids.

CHAPTER 13, FITNESS: PHYSICAL ACTIVITY, NUTRIENTS, AND BODY ADAPTATIONS

Learning Objectives

1. Define fitness, and list its benefits.
2. Describe the relationships between muscle fibers, energy production, type of activity, and oxygen use.
3. What types of exercise are aerobic? Which are anaerobic?
4. What factors influence the body's use of glucose during physical activity? How?
5. What factors influence the body's use of fat during physical activity? How?
6. What factors influence the body's use of protein during physical activity? How?
7. Discuss the importance of hydration during training, and list recommendations to maintain fluid blance.
8. Why are some athletes likely to develop iron-deficiency anemia? Compare iron-deficiency anemia and sports anemia, explaining the differences.
9. What special problems do female athletes face? How do these problems interrelate with each other?
10. Describe the components of a healthy diet for athletic performance.

Chapter Outline
Acetates/Handouts

I. Fitness and its Benefits

    A. Physical activity and fitness benefits

        1. Restful sleep
        2. Nutritional health
        3. Optimal body composition
        4. Optimal bone density
        5. Resistance to colds and other infectious diseases
        6. Low risk of some cancers
        7. Strong circulation and lung function
        8. Low risk of diabetes
        9. Low incidence and severity of anxiety and depression
        10. Strong self-image
        11. Long life and high quality of life in the later years

H13-1 Ways to Include Exercise in a Day

    B. Physical activity begets fitness

        1. The lack of fitness affects as many as 60% of people in the United States

CHAPTER 13, FITNESS: PHYSICAL ACTIVITY, NUTRIENTS, AND BODY ADAPTATIONS

2. The components of fitness
   a. flexibility
   b. muscle strength
   c. muscle endurance
3. Conditioning by training
   a. progressive overload principle
   b. increase intensity
   c. increase duration
   d. increase frequency

C. Muscle fibers and work

1. Types of muscle fibers may be set by heredity
2. Fast-twitch fibers and anaerobic work
   a. high-intensity exercise
   b. short-duration activity
3. Slow-twitch muscles and aerobic work
   a. low-intensity exercise
   b. long-duration activity

D. Cardiovascular endurance

1. Training requires oxygen
2. Rewards   TA87 Delivery of Oxygen by the Heart
   a. increases blood volume and oxygen delivery
   b. increases heart strength stroke volume
   c. slows resting pulse
   d. increases breathing efficiency
   e. improves circulation
   f. reduces blood pressure
3. Achieving and maintaining cardiovascular and muscular fitness
   a. frequency - three to five days per week
   b. intensity - 50-85% maximum heart rate
   c. duration - 20-60 minutes of continuous activity
   d. mode - use large muscle groups
   e. resistance training - moderate strength training two times per week

E. A safe, balanced fitness program

1. Safety
   a. include warm-up and cool-down exercises

CHAPTER 13, FITNESS: PHYSICAL ACTIVITY, NUTRIENTS, AND BODY ADAPTATIONS

        b. slow and steady progress
        c. notice body symptoms of problems
        d. be active throughout the week
        e. use proper equipment and attire
        f. perform exercise properly

2. A balanced program   H13-2 How to Evaluate a Fitness Program
    a. flexibility
    b. muscle strength and endurance
    c. aerobic activity
    d. nutritious diet

II. Fuels and Nutrients to Support Activity

    A. First fuels of exercise - ATP and PC

        1. ATP (adenosine triphosphate) provides the energy for muscle contraction
        2. PC (creatine phosphate) provides energy for short bursts of energy
        3. Energy-yielding nutrients (glucose, fat, carbohydrate) provide fuels for ongoing physical activity

    B. Glucose use during physical activity

        1. Storage of glycogen in the liver and muscle cells depends on dietary carbohydrate   TA88 The Effect of Diet on Physical Endurance
        2. Intensity of the physical activity affects the extent of glycogen used
            a. intense exercise uses glycogen quickly
            b. moderate exercise conserves glycogen
        3. Oxygen debt   TA89 Incomplete Breakdown of Glucose
        4. Lactic acid
            a. builds up with high-intensity exercise
            b. Cori cycle
        5. Duration of activity
            a. during first 20 minutes of exercise the body uses glycogen for fuel
            b. after 20 minutes the body uses less glycogen and more body fat for fuel

CHAPTER 13, FITNESS: PHYSICAL ACTIVITY, NUTRIENTS, AND BODY ADAPTATIONS

      6. Glucose depletion
- a. 2 hours of strenuous activity depletes glucose
- b. maximize glucose debilitation
  - (1) eat high-carbohydrate diet
  - (2) take some glucose during exercise lasting more than one hour
  - (3) train muscles to store glycogen

      7. Training
- a. muscles trained at high-intensity work store more glycogen
- b. conditioned muscles rely more on fat for energy

C. Fat use during physical activity

1. Duration of activity
   - a. blood fatty acids are used first
   - b. stored triglycerides are used second
2. Intensity of activity
   - a. high intensity exercise uses less fat
   - b. oxygen must be available
3. Training
   - a. repeated aerobic exercise allows the body to use fat for fuel
   - b. increased oxygen delivery
4. Recommended intensities and durations
   - a. activities of long duration and slow to moderate intensity help to lose body fat
   - b. stimulated metabolism after exercise
   - c. strength training improves muscle tightness

D. Protein use during physical activity and between times

1. RDA protein recommendations are appropriate for athletes
2. Protein use during muscle building
   - a. repeated exercise helps muscle cells to adapt
   - b. during active muscle building 7-28 grams of protein may be added to existing muscle mass
3. Protein use as fuel: 10% of total fuel used is protein
4. Effects of diet on protein use

CHAPTER 13, FITNESS: PHYSICAL ACTIVITY, NUTRIENTS, AND BODY ADAPTATIONS

                        a. high carbohydrate diets use less protein for fuel
                        b. carbohydrates spare protein
            5. Effects of intensity and duration of exercise
            6. Effects of training
            7. Recommended protein intakes for active people
                      a. 1 gram per kilogram body weight
                      b. slightly higher than sedentary individuals and backed up with carbohydrate
                      c. endurance athletes when training may need 1.5 grams per kilogram body weight
                      d. power athletes building muscle may need 1.1 grams per kilogram body weight

    E. Vitamins and minerals to support activity

        1. RDA recommendations are sufficient
        2. Supplements do not improve performance

    F. Fluids and electrolytes to support activity

        1. Fluid losses via sweat
        2. Hyperthermia
            a. prevent heat stroke
            b. drink fluids before and during exercise
            c. promote sweat evaporation
        3. Hypothermia
        4. Fluid replacement via hydration
            a. hydrate before activity
            b. rehydrate during and after activity
            c. water needed at 1.0-1.5 ml/kcal expended or 1/2 cup per 100 kcal
            d. sports drinks may have a slight advantage for endurance athletes
            e. water is the best fluid
        5. Electrolyte losses and replacement
            a. sodium, potassium, chloride and magnesium are lost
            b. eat regular diet to replenish

III. Special Nutrition-Related Problems of Athletes

    A. Iron-deficiency states

CHAPTER 13, FITNESS: PHYSICAL ACTIVITY, NUTRIENTS, AND BODY ADAPTATIONS

       1. Iron deficiency is especially prevalent in young female athletes
       2. Iron-deficiency anemia impairs physical performance
       3. Sports anemia is an adaptive, temporary response to endurance training
       4. Iron recommendation for athletes are individualistic
       5. Medical testing should determine the need for iron supplements

   B. Special problems of female athletes

       1. Athletic amenorrhea
          a. associated with strenuous activity
          b. low estrogen concentrations
          c. infertility
          d. increased bone mineral loss
       2. Exercise and bone loss
          a. low estrogen leads to diminished bone loss
          b. excessive exercise may impair bone health
       3. Eating disorders in athletes
          a. high incidence
          b. weight-height charts are not appropriate for athletes

IV. Diets for Physically Active People

   A. Choosing a diet to support fitness

       1. Water - replace losses
       2. Nutrient dense foods
       3. Carbohydrate
       4. Glucose during exercise
       5. Protein
       6. A performance diet is similar to a diet recommended for most people
       7. Caffeine and alcohol
          a. Caffeine used to stimulate performance
          b. Alcohol
              (1) diuretic effect
              (2) impairs temperature regulation
              (3) impairs performance

CHAPTER 13, FITNESS: PHYSICAL ACTIVITY, NUTRIENTS, AND BODY ADAPTATIONS

    B. Meals before competition

1. fluids
2. easy to digest foods
3. high carbohydrate
4. low fat
5. low protein
6. low fiber

V. Highlight: Supplements and Ergogenic Aids Athletes Use

Chapter 14
CONSUMER CONCERNS ABOUT FOODS

CHAPTER SUMMARY

Food-borne illness refers to both food infections and food intoxications. Food-borne illness symptoms include nausea, vomiting, abdominal cramps, diarrhea, and possible fever. Episodes of food-borne illness far outnumber other types of food contamination.

The potentially harmful effects of environmental contaminants depend on many factors. Methylmercury and PBB have been identified as potentially harmful. Natural toxicants also show potential for harm.

Pesticides kill pests' natural predators, accumulate in the food chain and can pollute the air, water and soil. Residues and tolerance levels are regulated.

Benefits of direct additive use include reducing the risk of food-borne illness, enhancing nutritional quality, preventing spoilage, stabilizing foods, and enhancing the taste and appearance of food. The GRAS List and the Delaney clause are subject to reevaluation. Irradiation is under current scrutiny. Indirect food additives, those that find their way into foods during harvesting, production, processing, storage, and packaging, include microwave packaging materials, dioxins, and hormones.

The safety of the public water supply has been questioned. Both surface water and ground water sources are being tested for safety. Drinking water can be contaminated from heavy metals, pathogenic microorganisms and organic compounds.

Highlight 14 discusses environmentally conscious foodways.

CHAPTER 14, CONSUMER CONCERNS ABOUT FOODS

Learning Objectives

1. Distinguish between the two types of food-borne illnesses and provide an example of each. Describe measures that help prevent food-borne illnesses.
2. Describe how contaminants get into foods and build up in the food chain.
3. What dangers do natural toxicants present?
4. How do pesticides become a hazard to the food supply, and how are they monitored?
5. What is the difference between a GRAS substance and a regulated food additive? Give examples of each. Name and describe the different classes of additives.

Chapter Outline   Acetates/Handouts

I. Food-Borne Illness

   A. Introduction
      1. Food-borne infections
      2. Food-borne intoxications

   B. Safety in the kitchen   H14-1 Safe Internal
                                                     Temperatures for
      1. Time/temperature principle   Meat and Poultry
      2. Meat and cross contamination
      3. Seafood
         a. raw
         b. environmental contamination
      4. Precautions and procedures
         a. check odors
         b. contact
         c. health experts

   C. Food safety while traveling
      1. Boil or sterilize water
      2. Drink only boiled, sterilized, canned or bottled beverages
      3. No ice
      4. Eat cooked foods only

II. Nutritional Adequacy of Foods and Diet

CHAPTER 14, CONSUMER CONCERNS ABOUT FOODS

- A. Many new foods
- B. Nutritional labeling

III. Environmental Contaminants

- A. Contaminants that resist breakdown are of concern
- B. Methylmercury
- C. PBB

IV. Natural toxicants in Foods

- A. goitrogens
- B. cyanogens
- C. solanine

V. Pesticides

- A. EPA and FDA regulate pesticides and their use
- B. Some are hazardous
- C. Residue testing
- D. Total Diet Study
- E. Pesticide free produce

VI. Food Additives

- A. Regulations governing additives
    1. Effective
    2. Detectable and measurable in the final food product
    3. Safe
    4. Toxicity versus hazard
    5. Margin of safety
    6. Additive regulation
        a. cannot disguise faulty or inferior products
        b. cannot deceive the consumer
        c. cannot significantly destroy nutrients

4 CHAPTER 14, CONSUMER CONCERNS ABOUT FOODS

        d. cannot be used when the effects can be achieved through manufacturing

  B. Intentional food additives

    1. Antimicrobial agents
       a. salt and sugar
       b. nitrites and nitrates
    2. Antioxidants
       a. Vitamins C and E
       b. sulfites
       c. BHT and BHA
    3. Artificial colors
       a. extensively research
       b. seven allowed
    4. Artificial flavors and flavor enhancers
    5. Nutrient additives
       a. correct dietary deficiency
       b. restore nutrients lost during processing
       c. balance nutrient/energy content
       d. correct nutritional inferiority
    6. Radiation
       a. destroys living cells and sterilizes food
       b. chemical changes in food
       c. strong negative consumer emotion
       d. international symbol

  C. Indirect food additives

    1. Microwave packaging
    2. Dioxins
    3. Hormones

  D. Food Biotechnology

VII. The Public Water Supply

  A. Sources of drinking water

    1. Surface water
    2. Groundwater
    3. The cleaning process

  B. Drinking water contamination

1. Heavy metals
2. Pathogenic microorganisms
3. Organic compounds

C. Water systems and regulations

1. Home water treatments
2. Bottled water

VIII. Highlight: Environmentally Conscious Foodways

CHAPTER 15
NUTRITION ASSESSMENT

Scope

The purpose of this chapter is to describe the process of nutrition assessment. The data collection consists of historical information; including dietary history, anthropometric measurements, physical examination and biochemical analysis. Nutritional anemias and protein energy malnutrition illustrate the importance of data collection in the nutritional assessment process. Laboratory tests of hemoglobin, hematocrit, serum ferritin, transferrin saturation, erythrocyte protoporphyrin and mean corpuscular volume are essential in defining and distinguishing between the types of nutritional anemias. Protein energy malnutrition is a general term defined according to its subtype: kwashiorkor, marasmus, or kwashiorkor-marasmus mix. Kwashiorkor is caused by physiological stress or protein deficiency. Marasmus is a deficiency of calories and protein resulting in starvation. The mixed form generally occurs in a marasmic individual with superimposed physiological stress. In this example, the nutritional assessment process is useful in determining the extent and type of malnutrition protein calorie malnutrition. The nutritional assessment process also assists in determining an individuals nutrient needs. Assessment data to determine calorie and protein requirements are described.

Objectives

1. Describe the components of the nutritional assessment process.
2. Compare and contrast the four different methods of obtaining a diet history.
3. Describe the relationship between anthropometric data and body composition and development.
4. Analyze physical changes associated with nutrient deficiencies and toxicity.
5. Identify the laboratory tests that reflect nutritional status.
6. Define and distinguish between the types of nutritional anemias.
7. Classify the types of protein energy malnutrition using the nutrition assessment process.

2   Chapter 15   Nutrition Assessment

8. Characterize candidates for nutritional screening.
9. Use the nutritional assessment process to calculate protein and kcal requirements for adults.

OUTLINE

TA

I. Nutritional Status

    A. Historical Information   90 Information Gathered During Nutrition Assessment Helps Determine a Person's Nutrition Status
        1. Health History
        2. Socioeconomic History
        3. Drug History
        4. Diet History
            a. 24-hour Recall
            b. Food Frequency Checklist
            c. Food Records
    B. Anthropometric Measurements
        1. Measures of Growth and Development   99 Examples of Growth Charts
            a. Height
            b. Weight
            c. Head Circumference
            d. Analysis of Measures for Infants and Children
        2. Measures for Adults
            a. Height
            b. Weight
            c. Ideal Body Weight
            d. Usual Body Weight
            e. Pregnancy
        3. Measures of Body Fat and Lean Body Mass   91 How to Measure Triceps Fat Fold
            a. Fat-Fold Measures   92 How to Measure Midarm Circumference
            b. Midarm Circumferences
            c. Waist-to-hip Ratio
            d. Hydrodensitometry
            e. Bioelectrical impedance
            f. Analysis and interpretation of the Measures
            g. Other
    C. Physical Examinations
        1. Nutrient Deficiencies
        2. Nutrient Toxicities
    D. Biochemical Analyses
        1. Internal Assessment
        2. Blood and Urine Samples
        3. Disease Related
        4. Potential Errors/limitations

Chapter 15   Nutrition Assessment   3

II. Nutritional Anemias

    A. Iron Deficiency
        1. Hemoglobin
        2. Hematocrit
        3. Serum Ferritin
        4. Total Iron Binding Capacity
        5. Serum Iron
        6. Transferrin Saturation
        7. Erythrocyte Protoporphyrin
        8. Mean Corpuscular Volume/microcytic
    B. Folic Acid and B_{12}
        1. Mean Corpuscular Volume/megaloblastic
        2. Folate Levels
        3. B_{12}

III. Protein - Energy malnutrition (PEM)

    A. Assessment of PEM/Lab Data
        1. Albumin
        2. Transferrin
        3. Prealbumin
        4. Retinol Binding Protein
        5. Total Lymphocyte Count
        6. Urinary Creatinine Excretion
    B. Classification of PEM
        1. Kwashiorkor
        2. Marasmus
        3. Mixed Form

IV. Nutrition Screening

    A. Abbreviated Nutritional Assessment
    B. Components
        1. Historical Review
        2. Serial Weights
        3. Available Labs
        4. Visual Observation

V. Estimation of Nutrient Needs

    A. Energy Requirements
        1. Basal Metabolic Rate
        2. Harris Benedict Equation
        3. Indirect Calorimetry
    B. Protein Requirements
        1. Nitrogen Balance
        2. RDAs and Disease States

Chapter 15 Nutrition Assessment
KEY TO CLINICAL APPLICATION QUESTIONS

1. Percent ideal body weight

    160/166 = 96%   % ideal body weight = actual weight/ideal weight

    160/180 = 88%   % usual body weight = actual weight/usual weight

    According to Table 15-5, this client is 88% of usual body weight and may be considered mildly undernourished. This is more significant than his percent usual weight at 96%. It would be important to discover if this was an intentional weight loss and if so, how was it accomplished (i.e., a popular weight loss program vs fasting). Another critical piece of information would be the time frame over which this weight was lost, and any possible physical or psychosocial causes for the weight loss.

2. The nutritional implications of these findings begin with the suspicion of an iron deficiency anemia. This is evidenced by the elevated transferrin (inversely correlated with iron status) and manifested by pale skin and lack of energy. Nutritional repletion will need to include assessment of this client's ability to shop for, cook, prepare, and chew iron rich food. If finances are limited, iron rich dried beans and peas would be a possibility. Soft cooked meats such as hamburger, or roast in a tomato sauce to moisten it would also provide valuable sources of heme iron. Vitamin C rich fruits or juices would increase the bioavailability. The unintentional weight loss is a concern. Exploring root causes such as disease, loss of appetite secondary to drug therapy, or depression should be examined. The student should note that although the albumin is normal that this doesn't rule out the possibility of marasmus: a form of protein energy malnutrition. This information indicates the need for a comprehensive nutrition assessment.

3. The energy needs of a 48 year old woman who is 5'6" and weighs 133 lbs.

    BMR method
    .9 kcal/kg/hr
    .9 kcal/60.45/24° = 1306

    BEE method
    655 + (9.6 x 60.45) + (1.7 x 165.1) - (4.7 x 48) =

    655 = 580.32 + 280.67 - 225.6 = 1290.4

    Protein requirements
    RDA = .8 gm kg IBW = 48.36 grams

CASE STUDY - NUTRITION ASSESSMENT

Mrs. Green's ideal body weight is approximately 135 lbs. using the Hamwi equation provided in Table 15-4. Her percent ideal body is 150/135 x 100 = 111%, however, her percent usual body weight is 150/175 x 100 = 86%. The percent usual body weight puts her at nutritional risk. She has been intentionally attempting to lose weight, however a very low kcal, low carbohydrate is not considered well-balanced. These diets are often designed to promote ketosis and are sodium and potassium wasting. Therefore, the method by which she lost weight increases her risk of malnutrition.

Mrs. Green's lab values suggest mild to moderate protein depletion. Low albumin generally suggests malnutrition of a chronic nature although albumin decreases in stress independent of intake. She is more likely to develop infections and decubitus ulcers. Her lifestyle, particularly relying on fast foods, would raise suspicion concerning the adequacy of vitamins A & C. Both nutrients are important in wound healing and immunocompetence. Although Mrs. Green takes a multivitamin/mineral preparation, these supplements do not provide adequate calcium. Her hair which is dull and easily plucked is also suggestive of PEM which is chronic in nature.

Calorie and protein requirements can be calculated by a variety of means. Using the Harris Benedict equation her BEE would be:

$$655 + (9.6 \times 68) + (1.8 \times 170.18) - (4.7 \times 38) =$$

$$655 + 652.8 + 306.32 = 1614 - 178.6 = 1435.4$$

Protein requirements using Table 15-14 can be estimated at 102-136 g.

TEACHING STRATEGIES

Have the students keep a food record for two weeks. From this data base have them analyze the adequacy of their diet using the West Computer Software or the Food Pyramid.

In a laboratory setting have the students measure/calculate:

Height, weight and head circumference on an infant or young child.

Height and weight on an adult.

Fat-fold measures, midarm circumferences and waist-to-hip ratios.

Have the students collect a nutritional assessment.

ADDITIONAL RESOURCES (available through Ross Products, Division of Abbott Laboratories, 625 Cleveland Ave., Columbus OH 43215)

1. Height and weight charts for infants through adults

2. Skinfold calipers

3. Nutrition assessment kits

CHAPTER 16
NUTRITION CARE STRATEGIES

Scope

The purpose of this chapter is to emphasize the nutrition care process and the vital role communication plays in achieving nutritional health in clients. The nutrition care process is described as logical and systematic. The steps of the nutrition care process and the development of care plans are detailed. Comparisons are made between the nursing and nutrition care processes and then nutrition related nursing diagnoses are introduced. Diet therapy, orders, and manuals are reviewed. Examples of effective communication techniques and barriers to communication and learning are explored. The need for intradisciplinary communication by health care professionals such as dietitians, nurses, and physicians is illustrated in examples of unclear diet orders, nutritional assessments, and recording dietary information and assessment on the client's chart.

Objectives

1. Define the objectives of the nutrition care plan.
2. Formulate a nutrition care plan.
3. Identify strategies needed in the evaluation of nutrition care plans.
4. Discuss the use of nursing diagnoses in the nutrition assessment process.
5. Compare and contrast the nutrition care process to nutrition nursing diagnoses.
6. Outline the goals of diet therapy.
7. Describe the use of diet manuals in patient care activities.
8. Identify communication skills necessary for implementing the steps in the nutrition care process.
9. Identify factors that can affect communication.
10. Characterize the methods by which health care professional communicate the nutritional needs of clients.

Chapter 16 Nutrition Care Strategies

OUTLINE

I. Nutrition Care Process

    A. Assess Nutrition Status
    B. Determine Nutrient Requirements
    C. Develop Nutrition Care Plan
    D. Implementation
    E. Evaluation

II. Nutrition Care Plans

    A. Achievement of Nutrition Needs
    B. Education of Client
    C. Evaluation

III. Nutrition in the Nursing Process

    A. Nursing Diagnoses
        1. High Risk for more than Body Requirements
        2. More than Body Requirement
        3. Less than Body Requirement
    B. Congruent with Nutrition Care Plans

IV. Diet Therapy

    A. Delivery of Needed Nutrients in Usable Form for the Client
    B. Standard vs Modified Diets

V. Food Service in Health Care Facilities

    A. Personnel
    B. Menus
    C. Institutional Procedures
    D. Diet Manuals and Diet Orders

VI. Communication and Nutrition Care   93 Communications Channels

    A. Principles
        1. Verbal
        2. Non-verbal
        3. Miscommunications
        4. Clear Communications

B. Client Communications
1. Interview
2. Counseling
   a. Readiness
   b. Emotions
   c. Empathy and Rapport
   d. Background
   e. Learning Styles
C. Professional Communications
1. Medical Record
2. Other Channels

KEY TO CLINICAL APPLICATION QUESTIONS

1. Clients who cannot mark their menus may receive foods they do not like or do not tolerate. For example, an elderly woman who is lactose intolerant may receive milk and pudding on her tray. Ways to prevent errors are to assist clients unable to mark their menus or provide large print menus for the visually impaired. There is also potential for error in menu collection and delivery to the dietary office. Often the menus are delivered with trays or laid on the bedside table when the client is not in the room, so it is easy to misplace the menu. One solution would be not to deliver menus with trays. They could be delivered separately. The nursing staff could be alerted that a menu was left for the client. Assembling of the food tray and insuring that the proper food and portion is on the tray are problems in the hospital. Often the food service manager is responsible for checking the trays, an overwhelming task for a large institution. Realizing that mistakes can occur is the first step in solving that problem. Dietitian and nurses can be responsible for detecting and correcting problems. Modified diets, such as a diabetic diet, should be doubled checked. If an obvious error, such as chocolate cake, is delivered on a diabetic tray. The nurse can use this as a teaching opportunity to reinforce the basic principles of this diet therapy.

    When new procedures are implemented there is often the need to provide in-service instruction. This requires an outlay of time and resources. Additionally, any permanent changes should be outlined in an updated diet manual.

2. In an effort to provide comprehensive education, health care professionals often attempt to instruct clients on all aspects of disease management. Hospitalized clients may not view diet therapy as a priority item. Pain, medications, and acceptance of the disease process are all complicating factors. Prioritizing the most critical elements of the diet, in a single concept format, helps to facilitate learning. If the client is obese and has elevated cholesterol, the concept may be "eat less fat" rather than the complexities of saturated, monounsaturated and polyunsaturated fat.

    A common nursing diagnosis for this client would be "knowledge deficit related to unfamiliarity with diet". But consider also ineffectual individual coping related to a situational crisis (myocardial infarction). Readiness to learn must be taken into account. This client has just suffered a myocardial infarction which is a life threatening illness. The grief process explains how an individual copes with such events. In the first stages of the grief process an individual experiences denial, resistance, and/or anger. None of

Chapter 16 Nutrition Care Strategies

these stages would have a positive influence on learning. In order for him to be ready to learn, he must have the motivation to do so, which means that he perceives the severity of his condition and the necessity of make lifestyles changes. A referral to a community based agency, i.e., home health or cardiac rehabilitation, would be appropriate to help him learn about and adhere to his diet and other necessary lifestyle changes.

CASE STUDY - NUTRITION CARE

A comprehensive nutrition assessment is the first step in developing a nutrition care plan. Problems that will need to be addressed include but are not limited to: analysis of the assessment data in order to determine nutrient/nutrition requirements needs. Sam and his family have extensive educational needs. The health care team needs a coordinated system to meet his needs. Team meetings and rounds are effective methods to ensure that Sam and his family are getting consistent and systematic education. There is a temptation to provide Sam with all the knowledge he needs to know to manage his disease. However, setting a priority system of critical knowledge is a must.

LEARNING ACTIVITIES

Have the students complete the following case studies:

1. Mrs. Cartwright is a 48 year old woman. She is 5'6" tall and weights 152 lbs. She is admitted to the hospital for a hysterectomy.

Her pre-op lab reports are:
  Serum Albumin 3.5 gms/dl
  Prealbumin 15 mg/dl

No abnormal physical nutrition assessment signs noted.

Her diet history is as follows:
  Breakfast: 3 oz apple juice
                     2 slices of toast with butter/jelly
                     2 scrambled eggs
                     1 strip bacon
                     4 oz whole milk
                     black coffee
  Snack: peanut M&M's
  Lunch: tuna sandwich on whole wheat
                     1 oz bag potato chips
                     Coke
  Dinner: 5 oz meatloaf
                     1 c mashed potatoes
                     1 dinner roll
                     2 chocolate chip cookies

Evaluate her diet using the food pyramid.

What is the most likely nutrition nursing diagnosis?

Rationale:

2. Mr. Trump is a 52 year old man. He is 5'1"" tall and weighs 192 lbs. He is admitted to the hospital for a hernia repair.

His pre-op lab results are:
   Albumin 3.7 grams/dl
   Prealbumin 15 mg/dl (normal)

No abnormal physical nutrition assessment signs are noted.

His diet history is as follows:

Breakfast	4 oz. orange juice
	2 slices toast with butter/jelly
	2 scrambled eggs
	1 strip of bacon
	4 oz. milk
	coffee
Snack	1 glazed doughnut
	4 oz. milk
Lunch	Burger King Whopper
	french fries
	1 chocolate milkshake
Dinner	5 oz. meatloaf
	1 cup mashed potatoes with gravy
	½ cup buttered corn
	1 dinner role with butter
	1 cup chocolate ice cream
Snack	3 cups buttered popcorn

Evaluate his diet using the Food Pyramid.

What is the most likely nutrition nursing diagnosis?

Rationale:

ADDITIONAL RESOURCES

Nursing Diagnoses Guides

Gordon, M. (1993). Manual of nursing diagnoses. St. Louis: Mosby.

Kim, M., McFarland, G., & McLane, A. (1993). Pocket guide to nursing diagnoses (5th ed.). St. Louis: Mosby.

Chapter 17
LIFE CYCLE NUTRITION: PREGNANCY, LACTATION AND INFANCY

CHAPTER SUMMARY

Normal placenta development is important for fetal development. Nutrition is important, especially during the critical periods of fetal development. A woman's nutritional health determines the course of a pregnancy, even before conception. Energy needs increase during pregnancy, especially during the second and third trimester. Needs for protein, thiamin, riboflavin, niacin, Vitamin B_6, folate, Vitamin B_{12}, Vitamin D, iron, and zinc increase as well.

High risk pregnancies result from various conditions. The most common outcome of high risk pregnancy is a low birth weight infant.

Nutrient needs of the mother during breastfeeding include increased need for energy, vitamins and minerals, and water. Iron supplements may be necessary.

An infant's rapid weight gain during the first year of life requires an ample supply of all nutrients. Breast milk provides all nutrients needed for the first four to six months and immunological protection. Infant formulas closely resemble human milk and are appropriate for feeding to infants. Cow's milk is not recommended during the first year of life.

Solid foods can be introduced when the infant gives indications for readiness. New foods should be introduced slowly. High Vitamin C and high iron foods are important. Mealtime should be a pleasant experience.

Highlight 17 describes the result of excess alcohol consumption during pregnancy.

CHAPTER 17, LIFE CYCLE NUTRITION: PREGNANCY, LACTATION AND INFANCY

Learning Objectives

1. Describe the placenta and its function.
2. Describe the normal events of fetal development. How does malnutrition impair fetal development?
3. Define the term critical period. Explain the significance to later health of adverse influences on critical periods.
4. How does nutrition prior to conception influence a pregnancy?
5. Which nutrients are needed in the greatest amounts during pregnancy? Why are they so imporant? Describe wise food choices for the pregnant woman.
6. What is the recommended pattern of weight gain during pregnancy?
7. What does a pregnant woman need to know about exercise?
8. Define low-risk and high-risk pregnancies. What is the significance of infant birthweight in terms of the child's future health?
9. Describe some of the special problems of the pregnant adolescent.
10. What practices should be avoided during pregnancy?
11. How do nutrient needs during lactation differ from nutrient needs during pregnancy?
12. Describe some of the nutrient and immunological attributes of breast milk.
13. What are the advantages of formula feeding? What criteria would you use in selecting an infant formula?
14. Why are solid foods not recommended for an infant during the first few months of life? When is an infant ready to start eating solid foods?

Chapter Outline   Acetates/Handouts

I. Growth and Development During Pregnancy

    A. The placenta   TA94 The Placenta

    B. The stages of fetal development

        1. The zygote
        2. The embryo
        3. The fetus   TA95 Stages of Embryonic and Fetal Development

    C. Critical periods   TA96 The Concept of Critical Periods

II. Nutrition Prior to Conception

    A. The risks of malnutrition

CHAPTER 17, LIFE CYCLE NUTRITION: PREGNANCY, LACTATION AND INFANCY

        1. Malnutrition and fertility
        2. Malnutrition and early pregnancy
        3. Overweight and underweight

    B. Establishing healthful habits

        1. Eat well and be active
        2. Abstain from alcohol/drugs

III. Nutrition During Pregnancy

    A. Energy and nutrient needs during pregnancy   TA97 Comparison of Nutrient RDA of Nonpregnant, Pregnant, and Lactating Women

        1. Energy nutrients
        2. Protein
        3. B Vitamins associated with energy intake
        4. Vitamin B_6 associated with protein intake
        5. Folate and Vitamin B_{12} for neural tube defects, blood cells, and growth
        6. Vitamin D and minerals for bone development
        7. Iron
        8. Zinc

H17-1 Effects of Nutrient Deficiencies During Pregnancy

    B. Food choices during pregnancy

        1. High nutrient density
        2. Avoid overeating
        3. Iron supplementation
        4. Servings from the food groups
            a. breads and cereals, 7-11 servings
            b. vegetables, 4-5 servings
            c. fruit, 3-4 servings
            d. meat, 3 servings
            e. milk, 3-4 servings

    C. Weight gain and exercise

        1. Recommended weight gain
        2. Components of weight gain
        3. Weight loss after pregnancy
        4. Exercise

    D. Nutrition related problems of pregnancy

CHAPTER 17, LIFE CYCLE NUTRITION: PREGNANCY, LACTATION AND INFANCY

        1. Nausea
        2. Constipation and hemorrhoids
        3. Heartburn

IV. High-Risk and Low-Risk Pregnancies

    A. The infant's birthweight

    B. The mother's health status

        1. Preexisting diabetes
        2. Gestational diabetes
        3. Preexisting hypertension
        4. Pregnancy-induced hypertension

    C. Adolescent pregnancy

        1. Maternal illness is common
        2. Iron-deficiency anemia is prevalent
        3. Prolonged labor
        4. Higher deaths rates in infants
        5. Weight gain of 35 pounds may be recommended

    D. Alcohol use and other practices incompatible with pregnancy

        1. Alcohol consumption
        2. Medicinal drugs
        3. Drugs of abuse
        4. Smoking and chewing tobacco
        5. Environmental contaminants
        6. Vitamin-Mineral megadoses
        7. Caffeine
        8. Weight-Loss Dieting

V. Breastfeeding - The mother's nutrient needs

    A. Food energy

        1. Extra 500 kcalories/day
        2. 1800 kcalorie minimum
        3. Severe kcalorie restriction hinders milk production

    B. Vitamins and minerals

CHAPTER 17, LIFE CYCLE NUTRITION: PREGNANCY, LACTATION AND INFANCY

- C. Water
    1. Protect from dehydration
    2. Extra water will not produce more milk

- D. Supplements
    1. Not needed if consuming a well-balanced diet
    2. May need iron

- E. Particular foods
    1. Strong and spicy foods may alter milk flavor
    2. Foods that present problems should be eliminated

VI. Nutrition and the Infant   TA98 Weight Gain of Human Infants

- A. Nutrient needs
    1. Nutrients to support growth
    2. Water
    3. Breast milk
    4. Energy nutrients
    5. Vitamins
    6. Minerals
    7. Supplements
    8. Immunological protection

    TA99 Examples of Growth Charts
    TA100 Nutrient RDA of a Five-Month Old Infant and An Adult Male

- B. Infant formula
    1. Infant formula composition
    2. Infant formula standards
    3. Special formulas
    4. Nursing bottle syndrome

- C. Special needs of the preterm infant
    1. Limited nutrient stores
    2. Metabolic immaturity
    3. High calcium and phosphorus requirements
    4. Combination of breast milk and formula is desired

- D. Introducing cow's milk
    1. Not recommended during first year

CHAPTER 17, LIFE CYCLE NUTRITION: PREGNANCY, LACTATION AND INFANCY

    2. Low in Vitamin C and iron
    3. High in sodium and protein

  E. Introducing first foods

    1. When to introduce solid foods
    2. The need for water
    3. Allergy-causing foods
    4. Choice of infant foods
    5. Foods to provide iron
    6. Foods to provide Vitamin C
    7. Foods to omit
    8. Foods at one year

  F. Mealtimes with infants should be a pleasant experience

VII. Highlight: Fetal Alcohol Syndrome

Chapter 18
LIFE CYCLE NUTRITION: CHILDHOOD, ADOLESCENCE AND AGING

CHAPTER SUMMARY

Nutrient needs of children vary widely, depending upon their physical activity and growth. Nutrients of particular concern are energy, protein, zinc, Vitamin A, and iron. Food intolerance and food allergies need to be specifically identified so nutrient deficiencies do not occur.

Many relationships exist between nutrition and behavior. Iron deficiency can affect mood, attention span, and learning ability. Lead poisoning can cause mental, behavioral, and other health problems. Malnutrition, in general, may account for many abnormalities in behavior.

Balanced meals to provide adequate nutrients while honoring children's preferences is important. Mealtime should be a pleasant experience, devoid of conflict. Healthful snacks need to be provided.

Nutrient needs during adolescence are greater than at any other time in life, except pregnancy and lactation. There are gender differences in growth and development. Energy intakes vary depending on activity levels. Iron and calcium are crucial at this age. For the older age group, water, declining energy needs, and regular physical activity need to be addressed. The vitamins and minerals of particular importance are Vitamin A, Vitamin D, zinc, iron, and calcium.

Highlight 18 discusses issues related to caffeine intake.

CHAPTER 18, LIFE CYCLE NUTRITION: CHILDHOOD, ADOLESCENCE AND AGING

Learning Objectives

1. What nutrition problems are common in children? What strategies can help prevent them?
2. How do food allergies influence nutrition status?
3. Describe the relationships between nutrition and behavior. How does television influence nutrition?
4. How can parents encourage children to enjoy nutritious foods? What impact do school meal programs have on the nutrition staus of children?
5. Describe the changes in nutrient needs from childhod to adolescence.
6. How do teen eating habits influence their nutrient intakes?
7. How do marijuana, cocaine, alcohol, and tobacco use influence nutrition status?
8. What are some of the physiological changes that occur in the body's system with aging? To what extent can aging be prevented?
9. What roles does nutrition play in aging, and what roles can it play in retarding aging?
10. Why does the risk of dehydration increase as people age?
11. Why do energy needs usually decline with advanced age?
12. Which vitamins and minerals need special consideration for the elderly? Explain why. Name some factors that complicate the task of setting nutrient standards for older adults.
13. How do drugs affect a person's nutrition status?
14. What characteristics contribute to malnutrition in older people?

Chapter Outline   Acetates/Handouts

I. Growth and Development During Childhood

   A. Growth charts

   B. Developmental changes

II. Energy and Nutrient Needs During Childhood

   A. Energy intake and activity

      1. Energy needs per kilogram body weight decline
      2. Vary widely

   B. Other nutrients

      1. RDA table
      2. Nutrient storage before adolescence
      3. Nutrient dense foods

CHAPTER 18, LIFE CYCLE NUTRITION: CHILDHOOD, ADOLESCENCE AND AGING

- C. Malnutrition in children

    1. Protein-energy, Vitamin A, and zinc deficiencies affect millions of children
    2. Iron deficiency
    3. Zinc deficiency

- D. Adverse reactions to foods

    1. Food intolerances involve symptoms
    2. Food allergies elicit an immunological response

III. Nutrition and Behavior

- A. Nutrient deficiencies and behavior syndrome

    1. Iron deficiencies affect mood, attention span, and learning
    2. Lead poisoning affects iron status
    3. Malnutrition affects behavior

- B. Hunger and behavior

    1. Breakfast affects learning
    2. Hypoglycemia
    3. Brain and nerves need glucose

- C. Nutrition and hyperactivity

    1. Drug therapy
    2. No research correlating sugar and hyperactive behavior

- D. Caffeine and other stimulants

    1. Overlooked as a source of hyper behavior
    2. Needs to be controlled

- E. The effects of television

    1. Prevalence of obesity increases as amount of television watching increases
    2. Effect of commercials

IV. Food Choices and Eating Habits of Children

CHAPTER 18, LIFE CYCLE NUTRITION: CHILDHOOD, ADOLESCENCE AND AGING

- A. Mealtimes at home

    1. Prevent obesity by eating slowly, stopping when full, serving self, never forcing the clean plate, and providing physical activity
    2. Deal with obesity through weight maintenance during growth
    3. Preventing cardiovascular disease
        a. Prevent and treat obesity
        b. Screening for cholesterol
        c. Use dietary guidelines
    4. Planning children's meals
    5. Honoring children's preferences
        a. Vegetables raw or crunchy
        b. Child-size portions and utensils
        c. Warm temperatures and mild flavors
    6. Child participation in planning and preparing meals
    7. Avoiding power struggles with a relaxed atmosphere
    8. Prevent choking with supervision at meals, sitting while eating, and avoiding dangerous foods
    9. Play before meals
    10. Provide healthful snacks
    11. Preventing dental caries
        a. Avoid sticky, sugary foods
        b. Sweets at mealtime
        c. Brush and floss teeth
        d. Eat crisp and fibrous foods
    12. Serve as role models

- B. Nutrition at school

    1. School meal participants show improvements in learning
    2. Nutrition education at school (NET Program)

V. Nutrition During Adolescence

- A. Growth and development

    1. Male and female growth spurts
    2. Wide variations among individuals

- B. Energy and nutrient needs

CHAPTER 18, LIFE CYCLE NUTRITION: CHILDHOOD, ADOLESCENCE
AND AGING   5

                1.   Energy intake and activity vary
                2.   Iron a problem for females
                3.   Calcium is crucial to attain peak bone mass

       C.   Food choices and health habits

                1.   Snacks provide 1/4 caloric intake
                2.   Eating away from home
                3.   Adult influence - adolescence must make own food choices
                4.   Problems of physical maturity and growing independence
                5.   Marijuana accumulates in body tissue and alters sense of taste
                6.   Cocaine affects appetite
                7.   Alcohol provides empty calories and displaces other nutrients
                8.   Tobacco influences hunger, body weight, and nutrient status

VI.   Adulthood and Later Years   H18-1 Changes with Age: Preventable Versus Unavoidable

       A.   Nutrition and longevity   TA101 The Aging of the US Population

                1.   Energy restriction in rats leads to prolonged life
                2.   Healthful practices in human beings
                        a.   moderate or no alcohol
                        b.   regularity of meals
                        c.   weight control

       B.   Genetics, fitness, and stress

                1.   Genetics
                        a.   indicator of the tendency to contract disease
                        b.   environmental factors influence tendency
                2.   Fitness
                        a.   strong influences in the risk of death
                        b.   many benefits
                3.   Stress
                        a.   physical
                        b.   psychological stress response

       C.   Nutrition, Cataracts, and Arthritis

CHAPTER 18, LIFE CYCLE NUTRITION: CHILDHOOD, ADOLESCENCE AND AGING

            1. Cataracts
            2. Arthritis

VII. Water, Energy, and Nutrients in Later Life

    A. Water

        1. 6-8 glasses per day
        2. 1-1 1/2 oz/kg body weight

    B. Energy needs and activity

        1. Energy needs decline
        2. Regular physical activity

    C. Vitamins and minerals

        1. Vitamin A needs may be lower
        2. Vitamin D from milk and sunlight
        3. Iron deficiency
        4. Zinc intake is commonly low
        5. Calcium intakes well below RDA

    D. Supplements for older adults

        1. Self prescribed and often inappropriate
        2. Prescribed supplement beneficial

    E. Interactions of drugs with nutrients

        1. Nicotine gum
        2. Aspirin

VIII. Food Choices and Eating Habits of Older Adults

    A. Extremely diverse group

    B. Food assistance programs

    C. Taste and health beliefs

IX. Highlight: Caffeine — The Brewing Controversy

CHAPTER 19
NUTRITION AND ILLNESS

Scope

This chapter lays the foundation for the successive chapters concerning nutrition and disease. The interrelationship between illness and nutrition is outlined. Illness often alters nutritional status by increasing metabolic need as well as altering the processes of nutrient utilization. Illness may also cause immobility which in and of itself may alter nutrient needs. Decubitus ulcers are highlighted to illustrate one possible consequence of immobility. Coupled with malnutrition, a hospitalized client is at high risk for developing pressure sores. This section provides the exciting opportunity to stress the importance of collaborative care. Although the physician may order the medical therapies, the nurse is responsible for recognizing that this client has the potential for altered nutrition. The dietitian is responsible for recommending and evaluating appropriate nutritional therapies. Should communications break down, the client suffers. Poor nutrition adversely affects all components of the immune system, especially the GI tract and T-cell function.

Drug therapy, including prescriptions and non-prescription drugs, can alter nutritional status by altering food intake and nutrition interactions. Health care professionals should recognize the impact of the presence or absence of food on drug absorption and use. This is particularly true in a client on a continuous tube feeding, who in essence, is never fasting. Foods and nutrients can alter drug metabolism and excretion. Non-prescription drugs are often overlooked as a source of drug nutrient interactions.

Objectives

1. Analyze the relationship between illness and nutritional status.
2. Assess the primary and secondary effects of illness on nutritional status.

Chapter 19 Nutrition and Illness

3. Describe how appropriate nutrition support and nutritional status can affect the outcome of an illness.
4. Discuss the synergistic cycle that can occur with illness, poor nutrition, and an impaired immune status.
5. Describe common drug-nutrient interactions.
6. Discuss the impact nonprescription drugs have on nutritional status.
7. Discuss the role health care professionals have in identifying and preventing drug nutrient interactions.
8. Plan interventions to alleviate eating problems associated with hospitalized adults and children.

OUTLINE

TA

I. Relationship Between Illness and Nutrition

    A. Illness and Nutritional Status   103 Interrelationships Between Malnutrition & Disease
        1. Primary Effects
            a. Alteration of Food Intake
            b. Changes in Digestion and Absorption
            c. Metabolic Changes
        2. Secondary Effects
            a. Immobility
            b. Decubitus Ulcers
                (1) Etiology
                (2) Malnutrition
                (3) Prevention and Treatment
            c. Psychological Stress
            d. Diagnostic Tests and Procedures
            e. Medical/Drug Therapy
    B. Nutrition: Effects on Illness
        1. Nutrient Deficiencies
            a. Stress to the Body
            b. Increased Likelihood of Infection
            c. Poor Wound Healing
    C. Nutrition and Immunity   104 Nutrition and Immunity
        1. Review of Immune System
            a. Cells of Immune System
            b. Non-specific Immunity
            c. Specific Immunity
        2. Role of Nutrients in Immunity   105 Two Antivitamins Used as Drugs
            a. Malnutrition
            b. Nutrition Therapy
    D. Nutrition and Drug Therapy
        1. Drug and Food Intake
        2. Absorption
        3. Metabolism
        4. Excretion
        5. Drug-Nutrient Interaction

                6.   Drugs and Restricted Diet
                7.   Non-prescription Drugs
                8.   The Role of Health Care Professionals
        E.   Food in the Hospital
                1.   Helping the Client Eat
                2.   Preparation for Meals
                3.   Checking Food Trays
                4.   Special Needs of Children

KEY TO CLINICAL APPLICATION QUESTIONS

1. Mrs. Gonzales should have a complete nutritional assessment including height, weight, fat fold measures, lab studies, physical exam and dietary evaluation. Her limited ability to stand and be weighed may interfere with data collection. If she is not able to stand, bed scales could be used and height can be estimated or measured with a knee height caliper. Physical exam and dietary history information should include evaluation of her ability to chew, and swallow and whether or not she wears dentures. Medications administered in the hospital, as well as those she took at home (including OTC) are important considerations. From these data, a nutritional care plan can be formulated. Calorie and protein requirements will be increased. The delivery of these nutrients will depend on many factors. If she wears dentures, soft foods may be more appropriate. The medical management of her diabetes may signal the need for dietary intervention or changes in the intensity of the diet. Her increased kcal requirements, along with physiological stress and its obligatory increase in blood glucose needs, to be evaluated. Her drug therapy, whether insulin or oral hypoglycemic agents (OHA), may need to be increased. The diet is planned according to the peak and duration of insulin or the duration of the OHA. Her heart disease may dictate the need for a low saturated fat, low cholesterol diet, or in the case of congestive heart failure, a sodium restriction. All of these factors are critical for development of an effective nutritional care plan.

    Before encouraging intake, Mrs. Gonzales should be assessed for her knowledge of the importance of nutrition in recovery and disease management. Also is she able to mark the menu? Is her vision affected by her diabetes? Can she read small print? Does she need help in preparing to eat or cut food? All are critical elements in the selection and mechanics of eating. However, because eating and food are more than nutrition, it would be useful to know favorite foods, any ethnic or religious preferences as well as psychosocial variables such as whether she eats alone at home or has company at meals.

    Drug-nutrient interactions are a potential problem for Mrs. Gonzales. Both chronic diseases, diabetes and heart disease require on going drug therapy. Her age may be a factor because decreasing liver and renal function with increasing age limit the body's ability to metabolize and excrete drugs and their metabolics.

2. A short duration illness is not a significant stress to a well nourished body. Although kcal requirements increased by 7% for each degree Fahrenheit, any weight loss Bennie experiences could be quickly corrected. However, with a longer duration of an illness, with no food intake significantly increases his risk of weight loss and malnutrition. Additionally, the special problems of children eating in the hospital adds to the complexity of delivery adequate nutrition.

Chapter 19 Nutrition and Illness

TEACHING STRATEGIES

1. Divide the class into two teams to debate the dual role, nutrients and drugs, of megadose vitamin therapy.

2. Invite a pharmacist to class to discuss food and drug interactions in enteral and parenteral nutrition.

3. Take a trip to the health food store to review labels and claims for herbal products. Discuss their use as food supplements as well as drugs.

SUPPLEMENTAL READING

Tyler, V. E. (1993). *The honest herbal: A sensible guide to the use of herbs and related remedies* (3rd ed.). New York City: Pharmaceutical Products Press.

CHAPTER 20
NUTRITION AND SEVERE STRESS

Scope

This chapter focuses on the effects of severe stress on the body's internal balance. When a person undergoes a period of stress from something such as an infection, heart attack, stroke, surgery, burn or fracture the body attempts to sustain life with a protective stress response. This response enables the body to borrow energy from one system to help keep another system functioning, at least for awhile. However, it does not take long for vital organs to deteriorate from the vicious cycle of borrowing and lending. Even if the heart and lungs continue to function at some level, the immune system is severely compromised and the person can develop an infection.

The nurse and dietitian work together to provide nutritional support to persons under severe stress. The challenge is to nourish adequately, without overfeeding, as overfeeding causes risk of further damage to the body. Therefore, careful assessment of nutritional needs and gradual progression from intravenous feeding to provision of regular food are essential. Methods of assessment and nutrition intervention are described in Chapter 20, along with the research findings to support their use.

Objectives

1. Compare and contrast the metabolic effects of starvation versus stress.
2. Discuss the effects of severe stress on an individual with protein-energy malnutrition.
3. Outline the nutritional needs during stress.

2   Chapter 20   Nutrition and Severe Stress

4.   Analyze the barriers associated with nutrient delivery during stress.
5.   Outline a nutrition strategy to prevent refeeding syndrome associated with PEM.
6.   Design a plan to meet the nutrient needs of clients experiencing the following stressors:
     Infection/Fever
     Trauma
     Organ Transplant
     Burn

OUTLINE

TA

I.   Metabolic effects of the stress response

     A.   Depletion of glycogen stores   106 Phases of a Stress Response
     B.   Mobilization of fatty acids
     C.   Compromise of vital organ function from protein depletion
     D.   Depletion of vitamins and minerals
     E.   Hypermetabolism

II. Relationships between protein-energy malnutrition (PEM) and severe stress

     A.   Vicious cycle in a malnourished person under stress
          1.   Use of skeletal muscle protein for energy
          2.   Lack of protein replacement due to anorexia
          3.   Derivation of amino acids from vital organs   108 Immune Cells and Intestinal Villi
          4.   Deterioration of immune system
          5.   Development of infection and more stress
     B.   Long term consequences
          1.   Loss of ability to absorb nutrients
          2.   Loss of ability to synthesize protein

III. Differences among types of PEM and their prognoses

     A.   Marasmus
     B.   Kwashiorkor
     C.   Marasmus-Kwashiorkor mix

IV. Providing the right balance of nutrition support

     A.   Assessing and maintaining fluid and electrolyte balance
     B.   Assessing and meeting energy needs
     C.   Assessing and meeting protein needs
     D.   Assessing and meeting fat needs

V.   Providing nutrients in a form the body can handle

     A.   Risks of under and overfeeding
     B.   Gradual progression from parenteral nutrition to regular food
     C.   Use of nutrition formulas
     D.   Ways to improve appetites

VI. Nutritional implications of specific types of stress
- A. Trauma and surgery
    1. Lifestyle of healthy eating as cushion
    2. Deprivation during pre-operative testing
    3. High energy, high protein nutrition in pre-and post-operative periods
    4. Fluid and electrolyte balance
    5. Vitamin supplementation
- B. Organ transplants
    1. Risk of organ rejection vs risk of infection
    2. Risk of overfeeding
    3. Prevention of food borne infections
    4. Promotion of healing
    5. Long term protection of transplanted organ
- C. Burns
    1. Interstitial fluid accumulation
    2. Shock
    3. Tissue death
    4. Kidney dysfunction
    5. Loss of body mass
    6. Overcoming obstacles to eating
    7. Minimization of negative nitrogen balance
    8. Support of growth needs of children
    9. Use of vitamin supplements

107 Different Degrees of Burn Wounds

KEY TO CLINICAL APPLICATION QUESTIONS

1. Energy needs of a 28 year old man who is 6 ft tall, weighs 180 lbs and has a fever of 103° F.

    BEE = 66 + (13.8 x 82) + (5 x 183) - 6.8 x 28 = 1922)

    Assuming sedentary activity
    1922 x .20 = 384

    Fever increases BEE by 7% for each °F
    1922 x (4.4 x .07) = 30.8%
    1922 x .308 = 592
    1922 + 384 + 592 = 2898

2. Susan's pain affects her ability to eat because of the anoretic effect pain imparts. Care must be taken not to over medicate Susan as pain medications may have a sedative effect. The use of a patient controlled analgesia (PCA) pump, if possible, may be a reasonable way of balancing pain and pain control. Susan's depression can impact her ability or desire to eat. Helping Susan to realize she does have some control over her recovery based on her ability to eat a well balanced diet may empower her to improve her appetite. If her intake remains poor, a psych-mental health specialist may be called in. If Susan is at x-ray or special diagnostic procedures when her tray arrives, it may be possible to synchronize her tests and meals. Also, late trays can be sent and sandwiches can often times be ordered and be waiting for her when she returns. If diagnostic tests interfere with her intake and the tests will be ordered often, Susan may be a candidate for peripheral parenteral nutrition. This type of nutrition support utilizes peripheral veins and is designed for short term support.

CASE STUDY - SURGERY

Nutritional assessment data for Sally reveals the following: There is no evidence of any chronic illness which could have an adverse effect on her health. Appendicitis is an acute condition with an usually speedy recovery. Sally does not have any noted history of medications or nutrient supplements which could affect nutritional status. From her brief diet history, Sally's schedule and course of study provide insight into possible risk for poor nutrition. Recent unplanned weight loss also places her at risk for poor nutritional status. But using the information on p. 535, her % UBW is 96% which indicates at present, she is adequately nourished. Other helpful information would include a 24° diet history and food frequency questionnaire to evaluate her actual eating habits. This information should also include her use of fast and convenience foods. If nutrition education had been possible prior to surgery, a diet adequate in protein and carbohydrates, particularly fresh fruits and vegetables would have been recommended. Sally's energy needs can be estimated by the use of the Harris Benedict equation.

$$655 + (9.6 \times 60) + (5 \times 170) - (6.8 \times 20)$$

BEE =   1945 x .20 = 389 (sedentary)
           1945 x .17 = 327 (fever)
           1945 x .15 = 291 (elective surgery)
kcal total   2952
Protein requirement 60 x 1.5 - 60 x 2.0 =
                     90   - 120 g

Immediately post surgery, Sally should be quickly advanced through clear and full liquids then possibly to a soft diet if indicated. Again, foods high in carbohydrate and protein such as milkshakes would provide needed calories as well as being a source of calories. As her diet progresses, salads, vegetables, fresh fruit and juices provide the needed vitamin C and vitamin A. Sally could benefit from nutrition education. Instruction on healthy snacks, nutritious quick meals and planning interesting yet healthy food with limited time. A dietitian is best trained to give this advice. This is particularly true if the dietitian conducted the interview and obtained the needed health history data.

CASE STUDY - BURNS

Mr. Sampson's immediate post-burn needs include resuscitation, fluid and electrolyte stabilization, preservation of vital organ function, early closure of the wound and nutrition support. Research indicates that early aggressive enteral support minimizes the hypermetabolism associated with stress. The prevention of shock includes adequate delivery of fluids IV to maintain an urinary output of 50 ml/hr. Nursing staff should maintain strict input/output records.

To determine Mr. Sampson's preinjury nutrition a health history could provide data on any previous history of illness, such as diabetes or heart disease, medication usage and typical intake. All of this data can be used to formulate short term and long term nutritional goals.

Mr. Sampson's energy requirements ideally should be determined by indirect calorimetry. If this is not available, the Harris Benedict equation can be used.

Using the Harris Benedict equation, Mr. Sampson would need:

$$BEE = 66 + (13.8 \times 79.5) + (5 \times 183) - (6.8 \times 48) = 1752$$

A major burn would add additional calories of approximately 75%. Therefore:

$$1752 \times .75 = 1314 \qquad \text{Total calories} = 3066$$

His protein requirements can be estimated based on the general guideline that the range of protein needed in burns is 1.5-3 g pro/kg body weight.

$$1.5 \text{ g} \times 175 \text{ lbs}/2.2 \text{ lbs/kg} = 119 \text{ g}$$

$$3 \text{ g} \times 175 \text{ lbs}/2.2 \text{ lbs/kg} = 238 \text{ g}$$

In addition to kcal & protein, increases in vitamin C & A are needed. However, individual assessment is warranted particularly if Mr. Sampson had other diseases known to affect specific nutrients. Alcoholism would be an example of a pre-existing disease which would necessitate vitamin and mineral supplements.

Oral intake should be encouraged as soon as possible; however, depending on the location of the burn, oral intake may not be possible or kcal goals may not be met. If assessment reveals this is the case, nutritional support should be instituted without delay. A trend in clinical practice is to place feeding tubes immediately after stabilization and introduce small amounts of an enteral feeding and gradually increase the volume. McArdle, Palmason, & Brown (1984) have demonstrated increased survival with immediate post-burn enteral support. If oral intake is possible, consultations from occupational therapy and physical therapy are beneficial. Adaptive feeding devices promote self feeding and exercise may promote regeneration of lean body mass and increase appetite. Emotional factors, such as depression, can significantly alter intake. Health care professionals should offer emotional support. However, a mental health professional such as a psychologist, psych/mental health nurse practitioner or psychiatrist should be a member of the burn care team.

If Mr. Sampson can not eat orally, tube feedings should be started. He may still be allowed to eat by mouth for the pleasure food brings but the tube feeding is there as a safety net. Because of the high volume of enteral product required to meet kcal needs, he may not be able to tolerate the volume of product. For example, if a one cal/ml product is chosen, Mr. Sampson would require approximately 3 liters. Therefore, TPN could be used in combination with an enteral feeding. If he developed Curling's ulcer and major GI bleeding, then TPN is the preferred mode of nutrition support.

Therefore physical therapy and exercise are important. As the burn wound heals, and the new skin is tight, contractures may develop. Exercise may also increase appetite. Additionally, if Mr. Sampson sees exercise and movement as steps in the recovery process they may boost his morale.

McArdle, A. H., Palmason, C., & Brown, R. A. (1984). Early enteral feeding in patients with major burns: Prevention of catabolism. Annuals of Plastic Surgery, 13, 396.

TEACHING STRATEGIES

Let the students experience what it is like to be on different diets. Start them off on a clear liquid diet and give them a schedule for progression. Have the students keep a diary about their tolerance to the diet.

Develop a teaching scenario for a client who does not understand their liquid diet restrictions. This is evidenced by their questions concerning why they can have a popsicle when it is not clear but can not have ice cream.

Videotapes available from Ross Products, Division of Abbott Laboratories	Running Time
Clinical Decision: Parenteral or Enteral Nutrition Support	26 min
The Malnourished Patient: Hypermetabolic States versus Inadequate Intake	27 min
Slides Series	
Pressure Ulcers: Causes and Prevention	18 min

Chapter 21
ENTERAL NUTRITION

Scope

Balanced nutrition for healthy people is best achieved through oral ingestion of solid foods using the Food Pyramid as a guide. However, during illness eating may become difficult. At the same time, the body draws upon its stores of protein and fat for energy and there is a subsequent compromise to vital organs. Chapter 20 described the effects of this process on the gastrointestinal tract, namely a decrease in motility and destruction of it's absorbing surface. These conditions can be reversed with carefully orchestrated nutritional therapy.

Chapter 21 analyzes the available options and the conditions under which each one is appropriate. For example, a liquid formula may be selected to meet the specific protein, fat and carbohydrate needs of an individual. If that person has an absorption problem, the route of administration may have to be enteral rather than oral.

Each route of administration and each form of nutritional support carries with it certain risks. Chapter 21 discusses these risks in detail and offers nurses and nutritionists some ways to prevent complications from occurring. The authors also suggest ways to help clients progress to eating table foods again. The special focus of this chapter is on enteral feeding while Chapter 22 will focus on parenteral feeding.

Objectives
1. Compare and contrast the following nutritional formulas and their indications for use:
   blenderized
   complete
   hydrolyzed
   intact
   modular
2. Identify the indications and contraindications for enteral tube feeding.
3. Describe the selection criteria for a feeding tube.
4. Explain and interpret the assessment data that would be collected on a client on a tube feeding.
5. Describe ways to identify and alleviate the complications of tube feedings and feeding tubes.
6. Describe how age and development influence the enteral feeding process.
7. Describe the steps associated with formula preparation and administration.
8. Describe the administration of medications via a feeding tube.

OUTLINE

TA

I. Feeding strategies for clients under prolonged stress

    A. Selecting the appropriate route   109 Selection of the Feeding Method
         1. Oral
         2. Enteral
         3. Intravenous
    B. Estimating energy needs and planning feeding schedule
    C. Selecting the appropriate nutritional supplement
         1. Fortified beverages
         2. Liquid formulas
    D. Facilitating intake   111 Selection of Formulas
         1. Variety
         2. Palatability
         3. Minimization of trauma and discomfort
    E. Preventing complications   110 Feeding Tube Placement Sites
         1. Aseptic precautions
         2. Control of rate of administration
         3. Attention to indicators of problems
         4. Maintenance of mobility
         5. Provision for normal growth and development

II. Drug administration for clients with feeding tubes

    A. Selecting the route
    B. Preventing a clogged tube
    C. Preventing formula-drug incompatibility
    D. Preventing drug-drug interactions
    E. Preventing gastrointestinal irritation

III. Progression from enteral feeding to table food

    A. Indicators of readiness
    B. Transitional trial feedings

KEY TO CLINICAL APPLICATION QUESTIONS

Clients who require transnasal tubes often focus on areas of concern frequently neglected by the health care team. Clients are concerned about the cosmetic effects of the tube. How will others perceive the tube? What comments will be raised? Other clients may experience a loss of control. Food and the ability to ingest it is a basic need and the loss of this function triggers a grief response or process. Anger, resentment, and depression are often expressed. The insertion procedure can be a frightening experience without appropriate education. Each step in the procedure should be carefully explained to minimize anxiety. Clients often miss favorite home cooked meals and frequently miss chewing the food. Meal times are also a gathering time for families and the loss or change in social aspect of eating is a concern as well. Talking about these losses is often helpful and should be encouraged or fostered.

The nutrition support team is a group of specially trained health professionals equipped to institute and manage nutrition support. This team often consists of a physician, nurse, dietitian, pharmacist and a social worker. This team can quickly identify and treat complications that develop thereby reducing the time clients receive less than adequate nutrition support. Nontraditional members of this team include but are not limited to, speech therapists, occupational therapists, and physical therapists. Speech therapists are invaluable members whose expertise can pinpoint and help manage swallowing disorders. By identifying the appropriate viscosity needed to prevent aspiration, clients can often return to some oral intake. Occupational therapists can identify which activities of daily living clients need assistance with and can often tailor assist devices for eating which allow control and dignity of the eating process. Physical therapy can promote physical activity tailored to the level of disability and this physical activity often stimulates regeneration of lean body mass, physical strength and appetite.

CASE STUDY - ENTERAL NUTRITION

Mrs. Innis should be informed of the need for tube feeding, rationale and the mechanics of the procedure. She will be awake during the procedure and her cooperation will be needed. If possible, Mrs. Innis should be allowed to continue to eat so she may still experience the satisfaction and pleasure from eating food. Nasoduodenal feeding placement decreases the risk of aspiration. This is important for Mrs. Innis as she is immobilized. Mrs. Innis was adequately nourished and has no prior history of GI pathology so an intact formula may be appropriate. However, because the feeding tube is place directly into the small intestine, a hydrolyzed product may be better tolerated. Therefore, Mrs. Innis should be started on an intact or polymeric formula. On an intermittent schedule she would receive 2500/6 = 417 ml/6 times per day. Hydration status can be monitored by weighing clients. However, this may not be possible due to the extent and nature of her injuries. Mrs. Innis can communicate her desire for water and thirst should be assessed. Additionally, monitoring electrolytes and blood urea nitrogen can also provide insight into hydration status. Urine output declines with dehydration. Additional fluids can be administered through the feeding tube after the formula is given. Flushing the tube after feeding provides needed fluids and helps prevents clogging. If medications are given via the tube, a liquid medication should be given if possible. Liquid medications however are often diluted in a sorbitol base which can cause osmotic diarrhea. Liquid medications, particularly electrolyte solutions, have very high osmolarities as well. Tablets that can be crushed, should be finely ground and mixed with water prior to administration. Enterically coated and time released tablets/capsules should not be crushed. The tube should always be flushed before and after medication delivery. Other issues include the pH needed for optimum absorption and the compatibility of the medication with the tube feeding product. The causes of diarrhea are multifactorial. Investigation of the most likely causes in this client would include: 1) drug therapy is a likely cause and medication change, if possible, may be helpful. and 2) the delivery of intact or hydrolyzed product directly into the small intestine. Feeding directly into the small intestine generally requires the use of a pump with continuous infusion

Documentation regarding the tube feeding would include the use of a nasoduodenal tube feeding of intact lactose free formula providing 2500 kcal/day. The product is being administered via six intermittent feedings scheduled for 417 ml/feeding. Mrs. Innis' development of diarrhea should be charted along with the change to a feeding pump on a continuous drip schedule. Before the tube feeding is discontinued, Mrs. Innis should be able to consume about 75% of her calories orally. She could begin on a full liquid diet. She should be assessed for lactose intolerance, a lactose free full liquid or even possibly a soft diet. Calorie counts are a useful tool to chart her progress.

TEACHING STRATEGIES

Have students taste a variety of enteral products under different servings conditions, i.e., cold, with a straw, covered with plastic wrap. Discuss the methods that enhance palpability.

Videotapes available through Ross Products, Division of Abbott Laboratories, 625 Cleveland Ave., Columbus, OH 43215

	Running Time
Caring for the Tube-Fed Patient	28 min.
Fiber; Managing Enteral Nutrition Gastrointestinal Problems	13 min.
Insertion of an Infant Gavage Feeding Tube	11 min.
Nasal Intubation of Feeding Tubes	20 min.
Enteral Nutrition Support: Strategies for Use in Clinical Practice	25 min.
Clinical Decisions: Parenteral or Enteral Nutrition Support	26 min..

Chapter 22
PARENTERAL NUTRITION

Scope

Chapter 21 addressed different methods of providing enteral nutrition for persons whose GI tracts function but who, for some reason, cannot ingest food orally for long periods of time. Since enteral tube feedings are introduced into the GI tract, its integrity and mobility are maintained until a person can resume eating and drinking.

Enteral feedings involve some risks and discomforts which outweigh their benefits under certain circumstances; for example, a well nourished person undergoing uncomplicated surgery and likely to eat solid food in the very near future will not lose GI tract integrity. The individual needs short term nutritional support without irritation from a nasogastric tube or the risk of vomiting and aspirating tube feedings. Simple intravenous fluid-electrolyte solutions serve this purpose very well. Then there are people who are gravely ill from the stress of extensive mechanical injuries or burns. Others have had major surgery on the GI tract or organ transplantation. The severe stress responses described in Chapter 20 have dire consequences which can be offset only by intravenous solutions composed of all the essential nutrients. These solutions are designed differently for each individual based on the results of data from frequent laboratory tests.

Intravenous feedings have their own set of risks. Chapter 22 analyzes these risks and the ways to prevent them. As with enteral nutrition the ultimate goal is for clients to resume eating regular food. Ways to assist them to accomplish this goal are also discussed. Finally Chapter 22 analyzes some of the ethical dilemmas which evolve from efforts to restore people with complicated illnesses to health.

Chapter 22 Parenteral Nutrition

Objectives

1. Identify the components of a parenteral nutrition solution
2. Describe the selection criteria for using simple IV solutions versus total parenteral nutrition
3. Compare and contrast the indications for use of peripheral vs. central parenteral nutrition
4. Calculate the kcal and protein content of IV solutions
5. Explain the possible TPN complications and related interventions
6. Review the special concerns associated with the administration of parenteral nutrition in infants and children
7. Explain the transition process associated with the discontinuation of TPN
8. Discuss the unique challenge of delivering and monitoring parenteral nutrition in the community setting

OUTLINE

TA

I. Essential nutrients which can be given in IV solutions

    A. Amino acids, dipeptides and tripeptides   32 Amino Acid Structure
    B. Carbohydrates   27 Structural Formulas for Omega-3 and Omega-6 Fatty Acids
    C. Fat
    D. Vitamins and minerals

II. Factors to consider in selection of intravenous nutrients

    A. Client's nutrition status and caloric needs   112 Possible Indicators for TPN by Central Vein
    B. Client's medical condition
    C. Client's inability to tolerate the usual form of the nutrient
    D. Stability of the nutrient in solution
    E. Solubility of the nutrient
    F. Anticipated length of client's time on IVs
    G. Effect of nutrient product on venous integrity

III. Intravenous feeding methods

    A. Dextrose - water - electrolyte solutions
    B. Peripheral total parenteral nutrition
    C. Total parenteral nutrition by central vein

IV. Minimization of risks surrounding IV feedings

    A. Prevention of infection
    B. Regulation of flow rate
    C. Cyclic vs continuous administration
    D. Careful monitoring

V. Special needs of infants and children receiving IV nutrition

   A. Determination of nutrient needs
   B. Prevention of overload and dehydration
   C. Prevention of hyper and hypoglycemia
   D. Support from parents
   E. Promotion of growth and development

VI. Promoting progress to an oral diet

   A. Combining oral and IV nutrition
   B. Preventing malabsorption
   C. Providing emotional support during the transition

VII. Nutritional support at home

   A. Advantages of home care
   B. Ways to promote client independence

KEY TO CLINICAL APPLICATION QUESTIONS

1. One liter of 500 ml of $D_{50}W$ and 500 ml of 8.5% amino acid contains

   50 g/100 ml   x/500 ml   x = 250 g

   250 g x 3.4 kcal/gm = 850 kcal

   8.5 g/100 = x/500 ml   x = 42.5 g

   42.5 x 4 kcal/gm = 170 kcal

   Total for dextrose and amino acids = 1020 g
   A lipid emulsion of 20% provides 2 kcal/ml x 500 ml = 1000 kcal
   Over a week's time this represents 3 times/wk x 1000 kcal = 3000 kcal/week or 429 kcal per day
   Add this to kcal from dextrose and amino acids for a total of

   ```
         850
         170
   +     429
        1449 kcal
   ```

2. A home TPN program becomes a way of life for a client unable to tolerate food by mouth. Advantages to being at home include first and foremost having the comfort and security of being in familiar surroundings. Also, clients in home programs are trained to provide as much of the care of the solution and equipment as they are able to handle. As opposed to a typical hospital environment, the control and responsibility for the management is given to the patient. This empowerment fosters independence and self-esteem. Home health care teams often assist patients and their families to manage the feedings, and many have "hot lines" to handle emergencies as they arise. Although the

client is autonomous, he/she is not abandoned. This also aids the client in feeling secure. The time, cost and commitment are real issues. Eating and nutrition have taken on a new meaning and level of complexity. The loss of eating often has emotional implications. Some clients take satisfaction in smelling foods and enjoy sharing the companionship of meal times. Others don't. One helpful tip is to find some outlet for oral stimulation. some clients enjoy "just tasting" the food and then spitting it out to have the taste gratification. Others enjoy chewing gum. The health care team should discuss these options if they are appropriate for the particular individual. Holidays and special occasions that have a "food focus" often exacerbate the feeling of loss experienced by clients receiving TPN. Other non-food traditions should be highlighted so the client receiving TPN can feel like a true participant.

CASE STUDY - PARENTERAL AND TRANSITIONAL NUTRITION

Mr. Rossi is a candidate for central TPN due to the following factors. He has a chronic disorder of the small intestine. According to the A.S.P.E.N. criteria, clients with inflammatory bowel disease will most likely not have adequate enteral nutrition established within 7-10 days. He also has protein energy malnutrition upon admission. These factors all indicate the need for parenteral nutrition support. Mr. Rossi will need educational and emotional support. Educational instruction should include the goals of TPN, i.e., weight restoration, increased strength and endurance as well as improved appearance. Also as part of informed consent, he should be aware of the risks associated with TPN, and he should be guided through the insertion procedure. Emotional support is critical for Mr. Rossi as he experiences dependence on the mechanics of TPN for a basic need.

He should be encouraged to discuss his feelings and sense of loss and be involved in his care. The components of a typical TPN solution would consist of dextrose, amino acids, lipids, electrolytes and a multivitamin infusion. Minerals supplementation is also a necessity. Mr. Rossi, given his diagnosis, more than likely does not need fluid restriction. Therefore, the final volume of his solution could be as much as three liters using standard $D_{50}W$ and 10% amino acid solution and a lipid emulsion hung piggyback 2-3 times per week. The calorie value of one liter of this solution would be:

$D_{50}W$/100 ml = 250/500 ml   10 gm/100 ml = 50 gm/500 ml

250 gm x 3.4 kcal/gram = 850 kcal
50 gm x 4 kcal/gram = 200 kcal

NOTE: One liter would not meet his caloric or protein needs.

TEACHING STRATEGIES

Contact a local home health care organization and invite a nurse and/or a dietitian who provides care to clients receiving nutrition support at home. Discuss the unique challenges of providing nutrition support to the population.

Evans, M. A., Liffrig, R. D., Nelson, J. K., Compher, C. C. (1993). Home nutrition support education materials. Nutrition Clinical Practice, 8, 43-47. This article provides information on companies that have educational materials designed for clients receiving nutrition support at home.

CHAPTER 23
NUTRITION AND DISORDERS OF THE UPPER GI TRACT

Scope

This chapter focuses on diseases of the upper gastrointestinal tract and the dietary interventions included in their comprehensive management. Clients with difficulties in chewing and swallowing often need modifications in food texture and consistency. Strategies for these modifications are outlined as well as precautions. The role of medications, alcohol and caffeine in the etiology of gastritis ulcer disease is explored. Surgical options for ulcers and GI disorders are included, and common complications such as dumping syndrome and malabsorption are presented. Chronic and residual nutritional complications are emphasized here, as these disorders often have lasting effects.

Objectives

1. Describe, with rationale, the dietary therapy required for clients with chewing difficulties.
2. Discuss the conditions commonly associated with dysphagia and the appropriate dietary therapy.
3. Describe the role diet plays in the prevention and treatment of reflux esophagitis.
4. Outline dietary and pharmacological interventions needed for management of:
    indigestion
    nausea and vomiting
    gastritis
    peptic ulcer disease
5. Outline common nutritional problems and related therapies associated with gastric surgery.

Chapter 23 Nutrition & Disorders of the Upper GI Tract

OUTLINE

I. Disorders of mouth and esophagus

    A. Chewing difficulties
        1. Individual diets
        2. Pureed foods
        3. Importance of fluids
        4. Mouth ulcers
        5. Reduced flow of saliva
    B. Dysphagia
        1. Dietary interventions
        2. Tube feedings
    C. Reflux esophagitis   113 Effect of Gastric Press on Reflux
        1. Role of cardiac sphincter pressure   114 Relationship of the Upper GI Tract to the Diaphragm
        2. Dietary interventions
        3. Patient education

II. Disorders of the Stomach

    A. Indigestion
        1. Dietary interventions
        2. Antacids
    B. Nausea and vomiting
    C. Gastritis
        1. Acute
        2. Chronic
    D. Peptic ulcers
        1. Etiology
            a. Bacterial infection
            b. Antiinflammatory drugs
            c. Excessive gastric acid secretion
            d. Evolution of changes in therapy
        2. Liberal bland diet
    E. Gastric Surgery
        1. Complications   115 Typical Gastric Surgery Restrictions
            a. Dumping syndrome   116 Dumping Syndrome
            b. Anemia
            c. Blind loop syndrome
            d. Malabsorption
        2. Post-gastrectomy diet
        3. Gastric partitioning   118 Surgical Procedures to Control Obesity
            a. Therapy for obesity
            b. Diet following surgery
            c. Long term diet therapy

III. Nutrition assessment

   A. Diet history
   B. Monitor body weight
   C. Laboratory values

KEY TO CLINICAL APPLICATION QUESTIONS

1. Clients following a mechanical soft diet for years require different education from clients recently started on this form of diet. However, the process begins with assessment. Clients on a soft diet may avoid foods they could tolerate, because it was on a preprinted sheet given to them by a health care professional. Conversely, clients may include foods they should avoid for the same reason. For example; a client with coronary artery disease, who happens to be on a soft diet, adds gravy to soften the food because its on the diet sheet. Other clients on a soft diet may have learned to "expand their horizons" by adding foods not on the list but which they can tolerate. For example, an elderly client with few teeth can "chew" a green salad because he/she enjoys it and has adapted his/her chewing style. One consequence of a long term diet therapy for these clients may be constipation due to a lack of fiber. Others are deficiencies of folate, vitamin C or vitamin A due to limited intake of fruits/vegetables or lack of variety. Realizing that these consequences are a real possibility, the health care provider focuses in on these areas as potential sources of education.

   A client recently beginning to eat after mouth surgery has a different set of needs. These clients need basic instruction on the rationale for the modification as well as explanation of the allowed foods. However, this diet is more than likely to be used for a short duration so nutrient deficiencies are rare.

   The time required for both clients depends on their individual needs. However, when a modification is new, the educational effort is usually more intense.

2. Food intolerances can be tracked by the use of a journal or a log book. As new foods are gradually added, one at a time, the client could record the date the food was added, the amount and any adverse reactions. Adverse reactions would depend on the nature and extent of the gastrointestinal disorder. The reaction might be pain with ulcer disease, return of indigestion, or diarrhea post-gastrectomy. If an adverse reaction occurs, the suspected dietary culprit is removed and tolerance is reassessed. By actually recording the food and reintroducing foods slowly, the client becomes an active participant in disease management and symptom control.

CASE STUDY - HIATAL HERNIA

A sliding hiatal hernia is a condition where a portion of the stomach "slides" through the esophageal hiatus of the diaphragm. For explaining this process to Mrs. Herrera, diagrams or pictures are helpful because the volume or capacity of the stomach is reduced to the portion of the stomach remaining below the diaphragm. The reduced residual capacity, as a rationale for smaller meals becomes evident as does the avoidance of eating before bedtime. A comprehensive care plan for Mrs. Herrera would include:

1. weight reduction (40 lbs. overweight)
2. smoking cessation
3. exercise as a tool to relieve stress and promote weight loss
4. dietary intervention for symptom relief

Since it is tax time, symptom relief would be the first priority. To provide symptom relief through diet she would need to eat more frequently and avoid large meals. Discussion should focus on quick, simple meals that are easy to fix. A convenient breakfast might be a bagel and juice, a morning snack of fresh fruit and a low fat sandwich at lunch. Liquids should not be consumed with meals, rather an hour before or after meals. Coffee and alcohol are two beverages that lower cardiac sphincter pressure and aggravate heart burn. Switching to decaffeinated coffee is not an alternative as this beverage also lowers cardiac sphincter pressure. Although it is advisable for Mrs. Herrera to switch to a non-caffeinated beverage, such as herbal tea and avoid alcohol, she may not consider them practical alternatives. Moderation at this point may be the key, and abstinence from caffeine may indeed cause withdrawal symptoms such as headache. Long term goals may include time and stress management to reduce the need for stimulants such as caffeine and nicotine.

Other appropriate interventions include elevating the head of the bed 30° to reduce reflux, refraining from bending over at the waist particularly after eating and avoiding tight fitting clothes. As individuals gain weight, many attempt to fit into clothes sizes too small to avoid investing in a new wardrobe. Avoiding tight fitting belts and pantyhose may be specific helpful suggestions for Mrs. Herrera.

CASE STUDY - GASTRIC SURGERY

After gastric surgery nutritional problems may develop. In the case of Mrs. Grayson, a portion of the stomach was removed and the remaining portion reanastomized to the jejunum. In the medical record, this procedure is referred to as a Billroth II. Dumping syndrome occurs when the function of the pylorus is lost and the stomach no longer serves as a reservoir for food. Rather than delivering "spurts" of food into the small intestine, the food is dumped. Dumping can occur "early" or "late". Early dumping syndrome generally occurs within 30 minutes after eating. As hypertonic foods and fluids are dumped into the small intestine, fluid is drawn from the plasma to dilute the concentration and diarrhea results. Hypovolemia causes a rapid heart rate. Late dumping syndrome generally occurs 90 minutes after a meal rich in simple sugars. The rapid dumping of glucose into the small intestine and its absorption causes a rapid rise in blood glucose and subsequent release of excess insulin. Clients often exhibit clinical findings of a hypoglycemic reaction. In the Billroth II procedure, a blind loop is created. Serum levels of B_{12} and folate can be affected by the overgrowth of bacteria. Vitamin B_{12} status may be further compromised by the loss of intrinsic factor caused by the partial gastrectomy. Bypassing the duodenum may also compromise the ability to absorb calcium and iron. Some of these nutrient deficiencies can be overcome by oral supplements. However, vitamin B_{12} must be given by injection. The overgrowth of bacteria can also decrease the effectiveness of bile salts resulting in fat malabsorption. After Mrs. Grayson begins an oral diet, she will initially be placed on a diet to prevent the dumping syndrome. It is restricted in carbohydrates, particularly simple sugar. This diet is moderate in protein and fat as these nutrients have a slower gastric emptying time. Fluids are given between meals to avoid overdistention of the small intestine. Many people gradually adapt to the reduced stomach capacity and the diet may be liberalized somewhat. Conversely, some clients may develop lactose intolerance or steatorrhea and need further restriction. In explaining the diet restriction to Mrs. Grayson, diagrams and analogies may be helpful. Stress to Mrs. Grayson that the diet is designed to minimize the dumping of food. The pylorus of the stomach normally releases small amounts of food into the small intestine in a manner similar to the way a dam releases or controls the amount of water into a river. When the dam is broken or damaged the control of the water flow is lost.

TEACHING STRATEGIES

Have the students complete a nutritional assessment on someone who has had gastric surgery.

Discuss the research regarding causative organisms associated with ulcer disease.

Experiment with adding cornstarch, tapioca, pectin to clear and full liquids. Discuss the thickening of each of these agents and the effects on taste.

CHAPTER 24
NUTRITION AND DISORDERS OF THE LOWER GI TRACT

Scope

Chapter 24 focuses on the nutritional management of lower GI disorders. The common characteristic of most of these disorders is diarrhea resulting from malabsorption of food or fluids. However, the causes of the malabsorption vary and some are unknown.

Ideally, treatment of the client is directed at the cause. For example, if the cause of the diarrhea is a bacterial infection an antibiotic can be used. The integrity of the bowel recovers and malabsorption will no longer occur. Another client may not absorb food because he does not produce an essential digestive enzyme. Ingestion of the enzyme will improve absorption and the diarrhea will subside. On the other hand, many people have chronic diarrhea when the large intestine, for some unknown reason, moves it contents along so fast that it cannot reabsorb water as it should. Dehydration and loss of electrolytes result. Even though the cause is not known, nutrition therapy can be directed toward preventing irritation in the bowel so that peristalsis is not overstimulated further.

In all three of the examples above, clients can benefit from some type of nutrition therapy if only to keep them in good condition until their particular problem is under control. Recall also from Chapters 20-22 how untreated conditions interfering with nutrition will eventually cause structural damage to the GI tract, hence further malnutrition.

For each condition, the present chapter explains the pathophysiological processes that propel food from the GI tract before it can be absorbed. It discusses the structural damage that can occur over time and how nutrition therapy can interrupt a vicious cycle, thereby promoting normal structure and function.

Chapter 24 Nutrition & Disorders of the Lower GI Tract

Objectives

1. Delineate the nutritional management of motility disorders such as diarrhea and irritable bowel syndrome.
2. Describe the nutritional management of fat malabsorption.
3. Analyze, with rationale, the appropriate management of conditions associated with malabsorption syndrome.
4. Describe the nutritional management of diverticular disease.

OUTLINE

TA

I. Diarrhea

120 Nutrient Absorption in the GI Tract

    A. Basic processes involved
    B. Causes
    C. Nutritional consequences
    D. Methods of nutrition therapy and how they accomplish their purpose

II. Irritable bowel syndrome

    A. Consequences of steatorrhea due to malabsorption   117 Steatorrhea
        1. Energy loss   118 Surgical Procedures to Control Obesity
        2. Calcium loss
        3. Vitamin D loss
        4. Oxalate absorption
    B. Nutrition therapy for steatorrhea
        1. Dietary control of symptoms
        2. Replacement of losses
        3. Fat restriction

III. Pancreatitis

    A. Causes
    B. Nutrition consequences
    C. Long term effects on the pancreas
    D. Nutrition therapy
        1. TPN
        2. Hydrolyzed formula
        3. Pacing progression to regular diet

IV. Cystic fibrosis

    A. Characteristics and underlying processes
    B. Energy needs
    C. Enzyme replacement
    D. Vitamin and mineral supplementation
    E. Indications for enteral and parenteral nutrition
    F. Home nutrition programs

V. Crohn's disease

   A. Consequences of inflammation of the bowel
   B. Role of nutrition therapy
   C. Hydrolyzed formulas
   D. Bowel rest
   E. Characteristics of oral diets

VI. Ulcerative colitis

   A. Characteristics and consequences of inflammation of the large bowel
   B. Similarities and differences from Crohn's disease
   C. Characteristics of diets and nutrition support

VII. The nutritional impact of intestinal surgery

   A. Factors affecting absorption
      1. Extent and location of resection
      2. Preservation of ileocecal valve
      3. Adaptability of the bowel
   B. Nutrition support
      1. For persons with bowel resections
      2. For ostomates

   121 Ileostomy and Colostomy

VIII. Celiac disease

   A. Pathophysiological processes
   B. Gluten restricted diets

IX. Diverticular disorders

   A. Diverticulitis
   B. Diverticulosis
   C. Characteristics of diet therapy

X. Nutrition assessment

   A. History taking
   B. Use of anthropometric measures

Chapter 24 Nutrition & Disorders of the Lower GI Tract

KEY TO CLINICAL APPLICATION QUESTIONS

1. A 24-hour diet with less than 50 grams of fat would include:

	Fat grams
Breakfast	
toasted oat cereal	.5
banana	0
skim milk	0
coffee (with sugar and skim milk)	0
Lunch	
lean roast beef sandwich (2 oz. meat)	10
French bread	0
apple	0
angel food cake with fresh strawberries	0
Dinner	
3 oz broiled fish	9
baked potato with 1 tsp margarine and chives	5
steamed asparagus	0
green salad with 1T Italian dressing	7
popsicle	0
	31.5

To increase the acceptability of this diet, known favorites such as ½ c. ice cream (10 grams), apple pie (11 grams) or 2 oz reduced fat cheese (10 grams) and crackers (2 grams) could be introduced. Popsicles, fruit bars, licorice, jelly beans and gumdrops are fat free desserts or treats that may increase the acceptance. Additionally, fruit sauces or chutney can be served with lean meats to enhance the flavor and reduce the dryness of these foods.

2. Crohn's disease is a disorder of the lower GI, generally occurring in the small intestine, with recurring nutritional problems. Crohn's disease has no cure and is usually managed by a combination of diet, medications, and surgery. Clients may be malnourished due to pain, loss of appetite and drug therapy. Clients often need to be managed by nutrition support and ultimately may require resection of the diseased portion of the small intestine. The emotional stress of this disease can be debilitating. Despite compliance with medical and nutritional therapies the disease often progresses. The time and effort needed to control the disease is considerable. Repeated hospitalizations and drug therapy cause a financial drain as well.

3. Label reading is an integral part of managing gluten intolerance. However, labels are not always specific enough to alert the client with celiac disease. Clients with celiac disease need to avoid the obvious wheat, oats, rye and barley. But many labels list "protein extenders", malt flavoring (which is made from malted barley) or emulsifier/stabilizers (which could be a wheat based product). Clients who are extremely sensitive to gluten may also have problems with grain based alcohol flavorings used in, for example, ice cream or distilled grains, as in beer. Initially after diagnosis, clients with celiac disease may also have a secondary lactose intolerance and need to avoid milk based products. Listed below are three products "labels" with an analysis of product for use in a client with celiac disease.

Grape Frozen Fruit Bar
Ingredients: water, sugar, grape juice concentrate, corn syrup, citric acid, natural flavor, stabilizer (locust bean and guae gum), and ascorbic acid.

Based on the information listed on this product, clients with celiac disease could consume it safely. A stabilizer is added, but it is specified as locust bean and guar gum.

Chocolate Mint Ice Cream
Ingredients: milk, cream, sugar, vegetable shortening (partially hydrogenated soybean and peanut oil), corn flour, cocoa, invert sugar, syrup, dextrose, corn starch, salt, whey, high fructose corn syrup, and peppermint oil flavor.

When a client with celiac disease is newly diagnosed or has a flare up when an incompletely labeled food is consumed, a secondary lactose intolerance develops. During this time, ice cream would be restricted. The use of this product otherwise, may be complicated by the process by which the peppermint oil is made. Alcohol based oils may be distilled from grains, such as barley and add trace amounts of gluten. Clients with an extreme sensitivity may become symptomatic.

An acceptable substitute for chocolate mint ice cream would be plain chocolate ice cream. For a client who cannot have ice cream, applesauce would be one example of a substitute.

Chicken Terriyaki
Ingredients: chicken, rice, broccoli, pea pods, water chestnuts, red pepper, soy sauce (water, soybeans, alcohol), sugar, sake (rice wine), modified corn starch, spice, garlic, xantham gum, and salt.

The use of soy sauce makes this product questionable in the diet of a client with celiac disease. Malted barley syrup may have been used for coloring and the alcohol may be grain based. An alternative may be to omit the soysauce or contact the manufacturer to inquire about the coloring and alcohol. The Celiac Sprue Association/United States of America (CSA/USA) is also a valuable source of information regarding the gluten content of foods and additives. As you can see, the gluten restricted diet is more involved than just restricting wheat, oats, rye and barley. It requires, not only label reading, but often contacting the food manufactures to pinpoint any possible source of gluten contamination.

CASE STUDY - PANCREATITIS

In describing pancreatitis, a review of the etiology is important. Pancreatitis is caused by alcohol, hypertriglyceridemia, biliary tract disease, and surgery. In Mrs. Corey's case, alcohol appears to be the primary culprit. Alcohol, therefore, is strictly prohibited. Mrs. Corey may need professional help to abstain from alcohol and support groups such as Alcoholics Anonymous can be a valuable adjunct. Damage to the pancreas is caused by the leakage of fluid and protein into the pancreatic cells. This fluid and protein causes swelling or edema of the cell. The damaged cell can not release its' enzymes and begins to self digest. Analogies are helpful in explaining this disorder. A leaky roof allows rainwater and other substances into a house causing damage to the contents. Serum amylase is elevated because the blood picks up this enzyme as it accumulates in the cell. Serum amylase is one of the indicators used to determine the severity of the disease. The major factor in Mrs. Corey's medical history that puts her at risk for malnutrition is alcohol abuse. Alcohol alters nutritional status in a variety of ways.

In acute pancreatitis the primary goal is to reduce pancreatic secretions. Oral intake is withheld and some clinicians prefer to begin parenteral nutrition support (PPN), usually by a peripheral route. Upon admission Mrs. Corey may be a candidate for PPN due to her risk of preexisting nutrient deficiencies. If parenteral support is not indicated serum amylase levels are used as an indicator of readiness for oral feeding. When serum amylase levels decline, pain diminishes, bowel sounds return and oral feeding may begin. Clear liquids are started and Mrs. Corey should be advanced as soon as possible to a low fat diet. If oral support can not be initiated within a week's time or calorie goals are not met, enteral or parenteral support is indicated. Enteral support is the preferred method of nutrition support. Elemental or hydrolyzed formulas are indicated as most of these products are very low in fat. Jejunal feedings may be better tolerated as feeding further down into the intestinal tract decreases pancreatic stimulation. If pain is persistent or the pancreatitis is severe, total parenteral nutrition (TPN) is warranted.

For the management of chronic pancreatitis, Mrs. Corey must eliminate alcohol from her diet. Small meals are better tolerated with fat restricted to 50 grams per day. Vitamin B_{12} may need to be given by injection. Assessment of fat soluble vitamin intake is also indicated. Other measures used to assess nutrient digestion and absorption would be monitoring weight, assessing for steatorrhea, and correction of the folate deficiency as indicated by mean corpuscular volume. Albumin levels are slow to correct but could also be used to assess absorption of nutrients.

CASE STUDY - CYSTIC FIBROSIS

Cystic fibrosis is a genetic disorder with three hallmark symptoms: chronic lung disease, malabsorption due to exocrine pancreatic insufficiency and loss of electrolytes in the sweat. Growth failure is a consequence of this disorder because the enzymes needed for food digestion are decreased. Furthermore, as mucous builds up in the lungs, extra calories are needed just to breathe. Extra calories are also needed for the elevated BMR and to replace those lost in malabsorption. As the client with CF becomes malnourished the ability to clear secretions from the lungs become increasingly more difficult. Respiratory infections are common. The accumulated secretions are a medium for bacteria to grow and multiply. Ryan's growth failure is evidenced by this weight below the 5th% tile and his height below the 5th.

Diet therapy focuses on high calorie (20-50% above the RDA for sex and age) and high protein foods. Salted foods are encouraged. If malabsorption becomes a significant problem, increasing the enzyme replacements is the advisable choice. Historically, clients with CF had been advised to decrease dietary fat intake. This modification, however, makes it very difficult to meet calorie goals and reduces the palatability of the food. In order to assess the adequacy of Ryan's diet, regular nutrition assessments should be conducted.

CASE STUDY - CROHN'S DISEASE

Kanisha's ideal body weight is 135 lbs. However, her normal weight is 130 lbs., so her weight loss should be charted as %UBI. Given her current weight, Kanisha is at 92% UBI, which according to Table 15-5 classifies her, based on this parameter alone, as mildly undernourished. Measures that could have prevented this weight loss include modification of foods she does like to increase the calories and protein content, as well as investigation as to why Kanisha would choose not to eat. How is her appetite? Does she have diarrhea or steatorrhea. In essence, a comprehensive diet history would be the first step in the prevention of weight loss associated with a chronic disease. A hydrolyzed diet may be helpful for Kanisha as enteral stimulation provides a growth stimulating effect for the healthy small intestine and prevent bacterial translocation. As Kanisha is suffering from severe PEM, preventing bacterial translocation lessens the likelihood of infection. Hydrolyzed diets also provide nutrients in a predigested form which may be advantageous when absorption is compromised. However, the predigestion of nutrients, particularly amino acids, often makes this form of nutrition less palatable. Adding flavorings, and serving ice cold or in a "slush" form enhances the flavor. Covering the glass with plastic wrap and serving with a straw minimizes the smell and also increases acceptance. The use of a nasogastric feeding route however insures a more reliable delivery of nutrients and minimizes the need for Kanisha to meet prescribed calorie and protein goals. She still should be encouraged to take the supplement by mouth. Hydrolyzed diets tend to be hyperosmolar and feeding into the stomach allows for normal emptying and minimizes the "dumping syndrome" seen in clients fed nasoenterically. Long-term dietary management includes the integration of Kanisha's preferences into plan derived from the general guidelines for the management of inflammatory bowel disease. These includes low lactose, low fat, high calorie and high protein. Fiber and residue are modified as needed.

Drug therapy for Crohn's disease usually includes sulfasalazine which can cause blood loss and malabsorption. Therefore, additional supplementation with folate, iron and B_{12}. Steatorrhea can be controlled with a low fat diet. However, if steatorrhea persists Kanisha can lose valuable calcium, magnesium and zinc. Excessive oxalate absorption is also known to occur and the avoidance of high oxalate foods may be indicated. Weight goals for Kanisha should be targeted at ½ - 1 lb. per week. Due to the complexity of this disorder Kanisha's progress should be evaluated and re-assessed at regular intervals.

CASE STUDY - INTESTINAL SURGERY

Tim's resection has allowed for the preservation of the ileocecal valve. This allows for nutrient absorption and reduction of watery diarrhea. However, after resections diarrhea can be caused by limited contact with mucosal surfaces resulting from inadequate mixing of chyme as well as limited exposure of chyme to intestinal epithelium.

As Tim is started on enteral nutrition, there is no consensus as to the optimum form of nutrition support type. Total parenteral nutrition is a valuable adjunct to care as it can correct nutrient deficiencies and restore body weight during the post-operative period. As the gut heals and tolerance to enteral nutrition is established, Tim can be weaned off the TPN. Non-elemental diets are thought to be absorbed as well as elemental. Therefore, if Tim finds the elemental diet unpalatable, experimentation with polymeric formulas, that are lactose free and modified in fat (MCT oil) may be indicated. Glutamine enriched formulas are also known to have a trophic effect on the small bowel. Short chain fatty acids produced by anaerobic bacterial metabolism, are trophic primarily for the colon and have a more limited effect potentiating intestinal mucosal growth and adaptation. None the less, enteral feeding would be of benefit to him. As oral intake progresses, Tim should be started on a high calorie, high protein, lactose free, reduced fat diet given in smaller frequent feedings. A minimal residue modification may be helpful initially, but long term is not needed or useful. However, if the intestinal lumen is narrowed, the fiber type and content should be individualized. Additionally, Tim may have concerns about gas forming foods. An individual approach would include a diet history focusing on foods historically causing flatulence for Tim. Other helpful tips for reducing gas include eating slowly, chewing with the mouth closed and avoidance of using a straw. These tips decrease the amount of air swallowed (aerophagia) and may reduce the formation of gas. Odor can be minimize by the use of odor proof pouches and adequate stomal hygiene. The usual ileostomy stool is weakly acidic in nature and generally not unpleasant. Sexuality is a concern as Tim may fear rejection due to his altered body image. An enterostomal therapist may be able to address these issues with Tim and discuss sexual issues with him.

CASE STUDY - DIVERTICULAR DISEASE

Diverticular disease is a general term for the development of pockets or balloonings of the intestinal mucosa. Research indicates that a low fiber diet is implicated in the development of diverticula. Diverticulitis is an acute inflammatory process which causes pain and often fevers and chills. The management of this acute form of the disease includes bed rest, pain relief, and control of infection. Dietary modification progresses from NPO to a soft diet in the acute phase. Diverticulosis is the chronic, asymptomatic form of the disorder. Diverticula are present but not inflamed. The dietary management includes gradually increasing the fiber from the typical 10-13 grams per day to approximately 40 grams. Fluid intake is also encouraged to prevent constipation. Mr. Akimoto should also be instructed to allow an uninterrupted time to have a bowel movement. Mr. Akimoto's symptoms are typical of an episode of diverticulitis, but less than 25% of clients with diverticula will develop diverticulitis (Burrell, 1992). As Mr. Akimoto is being prepared for discharge, simple diagrams can best illustrate diverticular disease. Furthermore, as he adds fiber to his diet he should be cautioned to make changes slowly so that he can adapt to this change uneventfully and avoid or minimize gastrointestinal discomfort.

Burrell, L. O. (ed.). (1992). <u>Adult nursing</u> (p. 1446). East Norwalk, CT: Appleton Lange.

TEACHING STRATEGIES

Have the students visit a stress reduction clinic.

Have everyone bring a gluten free dish to a pot-luck meal.

Throughout the United States there are several organizations that offer information and recipes for clients with celiac disease. Contact one of the organizations and share with the class the information.

The Gluten Intolerance Group of North America
P.O. Box 23053
Seattle, WA 98102-0353
206-325-6980

Celiac Sprue Association/United Stated of America (CSA/USA)
P. O. Box 31700
Omaha, NE 68131-0700
402-558-0600

Celiac Disease Foundation
P. O. Box 1265
Studio City, CA 91614-0265
213-654-4085

USA Rice Council
P. O. Box 740121
Houston, TX 77274

Crohn's & Colitis Foundation of America, Inc.
386 Park Ave. South
New York, NY 10016
1-800-932-2423

CHAPTER 25
NUTRITION AND DISORDERS OF THE LIVER

Scope

This chapter details the metabolic derangement, physiological consequences, and nutritional requirements of clients suffering from liver disorders. Alcohol, drugs, and toxins play a central role in the development of this disorder. Alterations in protein metabolism are of paramount importance in liver disease. As liver disease progresses the ability to metabolize and tolerate protein diminishes and the provision of dietary protein declines. However, although the tolerance to protein declines, the need for protein does not. The clinician therefore walks a fine line between protein tolerance and PEM. Calorie requirements remain high, partly due to the protein sparing nature of carbohydrates. Indeed, many clients with liver disease do develop malnutrition secondary to dietary restrictions as well as anorexia. Esophageal varices, ascites and elevated ammonia levels add additional dietary modification and complexity to the regimen. The nutritional assessment process is complicated by the role of the liver in the synthesis of serum proteins and the invalidity of weight as an indicator of body tissue gains or losses. Diet histories become more focused in nature in order to pinpoint protein needs and tolerances.

Objectives

1. Describe the metabolic alterations associated with hepatitis and the appropriate nutritional therapy.
2. Discuss the physiological and metabolic consequences of cirrhosis and the necessary dietary alterations.
3. Calculate the kcal and protein requirements of clients with liver disease.
4. Plan diets/meals for clients needing sodium restriction in liver disease.
5. Describe the alterations in the nutritional assessment process for clients with disorders of the liver.

Chapter 25 Nutrition and Disorders of the Liver

OUTLINE

TA
14 The Liver
122 The Liver's Circulatory System

I. Normal liver function

    A. Process and synthesize nutrients
    B. Storage of vitamins
    C. Serum protein synthesis
    D. Bile synthesis
    E. Metabolism of drugs

II. Disorders of the liver

    A. Fatty liver
    B. Hepatitis
        1. Consequences
        2. Diet therapy
    C. Cirrhosis

123 The Consequences of Cirrhosis

        1. Etiology
        2. Consequences
            a. Portal hypertension
            b. Esophageal varices
            c. Ascites
            d. Elevated ammonia levels

124 Ammonia Production in the Body

        3. Diet therapy

125 Examples of Aromatic and Branched Chain Amino Acids

            a. Calories
            b. Protein
            c. Fat
            d. Vitamins and minerals
            e. Fluid and sodium

III. Liver transplantation

    A. Nutritional status prior to transplant
    B. Nutrition following transplant

IV. Nutrition assessment

    A. Diet history
        1. Protein
        2. Alcohol
    B. Weight/Anthropometries
        1. Fluid gains
        2. Invalid measure
    C. Laboratory values
        1. Albumin
        2. Ammonia
        3. Blood urea nitrogen

KEY TO CLINICAL APPLICATION QUESTIONS

Exchange lists containing protein
  milk
  bread
  vegetables
  meat
  fat (nuts/seeds)

Exchange lists without protein
  fruit
  fat (oils, margarine, butter)

On a 40 gram protein diet, the groups adequately covered according to the Daily Food Guide or Food Guide Pyramid would be the fruit group and the miscellaneous group, assuming the client chooses pure oils and sugars from that group rather than combination foods such as doughnuts and chips. A client on a 40 gram protein diet most likely would be lacking adequate servings from the meat, dairy, bread and vegetable groups. The list of nutrient deficiencies is comprehensive. Potential deficiencies include, iron, zinc, calcium, riboflavin, folic acid, niacin, thiamin, B_{12}, pyridoxine. Careful meal planning may decrease the possibility of deficiencies, but often vitamin/mineral supplements are prescribed. Fats and sugars can add valuable calories needed for protein sparing. Oils, butter and margarine enhance flavor and palatability. Sugars, such as syrups, hard candy and jelly beans also may enhance acceptance.

Fluid and sodium restrictions added to a 40 gram protein diet further decrease choices and contribute to the likelihood of nutrient deficiencies. Meat choices now eliminate cured meats, regular canned tuna and prepared meat or protein salads such as chicken salad and egg salad. Condiments are limited, but the diet does not have to be bland. Creative use of herbs and spices may compensate some for the flavor lost with the elimination of salt. Fluid restrictions often limit the client's ability to drink plain water as the emphasis is placed on caloric fluids.

CASE STUDY - CIRRHOSIS

Mr. Sloan's laboratory data are consistent with those commonly found in cirrhotic liver disease. In explaining cirrhosis to Mr. Sloan, it is important to underscore the pivotal role that alcohol plays in the etiology and the progression of cirrhosis. This discussion should be designed to be informative not judgmental or condemning. To explain complex physiology to clients, analogies are often helpful. Cirrhosis results in scarring, similar to scars on the outside of the body, but with the difference being this scar is located in a dynamic metabolic factory through which 1½ qts of blood travel through each minute. The build up of scar tissue diminishes the

The body attempts to bypass the diseased liver by creating new vessels called collaterals, but as the fluid and pressure build varicosities develop. The varicosed veins can occur throughout the GI tract, particularly in the esophagus. These varicosed veins are prone to rupture.

From the information provided, Mr. Sloan is likely to be malnourished. He has lost 30 lbs., and ascites complicates obtaining an accurate "dry weight". Loss of weight via diuresis is a method by which clinical improvement can be noted. Measurement of abdominal girth can also be used.

Mr. Sloan should receive a high calorie, adequate protein diet (higher than the RDA, but often lower than usual consumption). Fat should not be restricted unless steatorrhea develops. As the condition deteriorates, with rising ammonia levels, protein is restricted to 40-60 grams per day. Additionally, neomycin and lactulose are given to minimize ammonia absorption from the gut. If necessary, protein may be restricted further, but if protein is kept at very low levels for prolonged periods, lean body mass may be catabolized and itself become a source of ammonia.

Mr. Sloan is likely to develop ascites as rising pressure in the portal vein forces plasma into the abdominal cavity. This leakage of fluid contributes to hypovolemia. Hypovolemia triggers the synthesis of aldosterone which causes retention of sodium and water. Sodium restriction reduces the edema.

Mr. Sloan's ammonia level is high as he is unable to synthesize urea adequately. As collateral circulation develops, some ammonia bypasses the liver and accumulates in the blood. Because he is showing signs of impending hepatic coma, an "advanced form" of cirrhosis, ammonia levels are elevated.

Portal hypertension develops when the diseased liver can not handle the large volume of blood normally flowing through the liver. Blood "backs up" causing an increase of pressure in the portal vein. Collaterals develop to compensate increase in pressure and often bulge into the esophagus. A soft diet is indicated for clients with esophageal varices. Clients with esophageal varices requiring nutrition support are often given parenteral solutions to decrease the risk of bleeding when a nasoenteric tube feeding is placed.

TEACHING STRATEGIES

Have the students plan a 40 gram protein diet using vegetarian foods.

Have the student plan a 2000 calorie diet with a 50 gram fat restriction. Discuss the problems and possible solutions associated with these restrictions.

CHAPTER 26
NUTRITION, DIABETES, AND HYPOGLYCEMIA

Scope

The purpose of this chapter is to describe the pathophysiology of diabetes mellitus (DM) and the role that the proper balance of diet, drug therapy, and exercise plays in controlling this disease process. Insulin-dependent and noninsulin-dependent diabetes are differentiated and the treatment of each is described. Insulin-dependent diabetes mellitus (IDDM) occurs when the pancreas loses the ability to synthesize insulin. The treatment of IDDM consists of a careful balance of diet, exercise, and insulin therapy. Initial insulin doses are calculated based on body weight and then adjusted according to blood glucose levels, food intake and exercise patterns. The use of regular and intermediate acting insulin, with multiple daily injections, helps simulate a normally functioning pancreas. Blood glucose monitoring during the day, is used to measure an individual's response to insluin. Fasting blood sugars and glycosylated hemoglobins are used to assess compliance with the diabetes regimen. Meal planning is based on the exchange system with carefully controlled amounts of protein, fats and carbohydrates to be eaten at specific times that coincide with insulin onset and peak.

Noninsulin-dependent and diabetes mellitus (NIDDM) occurs when insulin cell receptors become less sensitive to or resistant to insulin. The majority of people with NIDDM are overweight, which contributes to insulin cell receptors resistance to insulin. The goal of treatment for NIDDM is weight loss and a carefully controlled diet based on the exchange system. Dietary fats are restricted to prevent high lipid levels that are associated with NIDDM and contribute to the high incidence of cardiac disease in these clients. Oral hypoglycemic agents are used to stimulate insulin production and increase sensitivity of insulin receptors. Insulin therapy is initated for clients who continue to run high blood glucose levels despite traditional treatment.

Chapter 26 Nutrition, Diabetes, and Hypoglycemia

The detection and treatment of acute and chronic complications of DM are also addressed. Acute complications of diabetes include hyperglycemia, dehydration, and ketosis. Chronic complications include vascular disease, microangiopathies and neuropathies. Consistent control of glucose levels within the normal range helps prevent and/or retard the complications of diabetes. The unique needs of special populations of diabetics such as the elderly, children and pregnant women are explained.

Objectives

1. Differentiate between the pathophysiology of insulin-dependent and noninsulin-dependent diabetes mellitus.
2. List the physiological tests that measure glucose control.
3. Plan a diet for a client with IDDM.
4. Describe the desired balance between activity, insulin, and food intake in IDDM.
5. Develop a plan for detecting and treating hyperglycemia and hypoglycemia in a diabetic client.
6. Describe the special needs of children and the elderly with IDDM.
7. Plan a diet for a client with NIDDM.
8. Describe the desired balance between activity, drug therapy, and food intake in NIDDM.
9. Describe the prenatal care for women with existing diabetes and gestational diabetes.
10. Describe the nutritional assessment for a diabetic client.

OUTLINE

TA

I. Diabetes Mellitus

    A. Insulin-dependent
    B. Noninsulin-dependent   126 Obesity Diagram
    C. Acute complications
        1. Hyperglycemia and glycosuria
        2. Dehydration
        3. Ketosis in IDDM   127 Metabolic Consequences of Untreated IDDM & NIDDM
        4. Weight gain in NIDDM
    D. Chronic complications
        1. Vascular diseases
        2. Microangiopathies
        3. Neuropathy

II. Treatment of IDDM

    A. Goals of therapy
    B. Glucose measurements
    C. Insulin
    D. Diet
    E. Physical activity
    F. Treating hyperglycemia
    G. Treating hypoglycemia
    H. Children with IDDM
    I. Elderly with IDDM

III. Treatment of NIDDM

    A. Goals of therapy
    B. Diet
    C. Physical activity
    D. Pharmacological agents

IV. Treatment of diabetes during pregnancy

    A. IDDM and NIDDM
    B. Gestational diabetes

V. Hypoglycemia

    A. Reactive
    B. Fasting

VI. Treatment of hypoglycemia

    A. Reactive
    B. Fasting

VII. Nutritional assessment

KEY TO CLINICAL APPLICATION QUESTIONS

1. Her IBW at 5'9" is 145 lbs. Therefore, weight reduction is indicated. Calories for weight reduction can be estimated using IBW x10. An appropriate calorie level would be 1450 rounded to 1500 calories. Based on the distribution of 55% from carbohydrate, 20% from protein and 25% from fat the calorie division would be:

    1500 x .55 = 825 ÷ 4 kcal/gm = 206 gm

    1500 x .20 = 300 ÷ 4 kcal/gm = 75 gm

    1500 x .25 = 375 ÷ 4 kcal/gm = 42 gm

Chapter 26 Nutrition, Diabetes, and Hypoglycemia

Day's Exchanges

Exchange Group	Number of Exchanges	CHO g	Protein g	Fat g
Milk	2	24	16	--
Fruit	2	30	--	--
Vegetables	4	20	8	--
Bread	9	135	27	--
Meat	3	--	21	15
Fat	5			25
		209	72	40

Total Calories 1484   836   288   360

The division of these exchanges depends on the onset, peak and duration of the insulin given. Another variable to consider, in an effort to individualize, is the client's blood sugar pattern.

2. Treatment of hypoglycemia consists of having the client ingest 10-15 grams of carbohydrate such as 4 oz. orange juice, 3 oz. apple juice, 4 oz. of a regular soft drink, 5-6 lifesavers or glucose tablets or gel. Some clinicians prefer 8 oz. of milk, because in addition to the 12 grams of carbohydrate, milk contains protein which can serve as a source of glucose (via gluconeogenesis), if needed. In this respect, protein can be considered "time released" glucose. The causes of hypoglycemia include taking drugs such as propranolol, skipping all or a portion of meals, taking too much insulin and exercise. Exercise can continue to be a threat for 24-36 hours after the activity as the body rebuilds glycogen stores used during exercise from the glucose in the bloodstream. If a client has a regular exercise schedule, such as Monday, Wednesday, Friday, it may be desirable to decrease the insulin that is peaking at the time of exercise. This is particularly desirable for the client who is overweight. In this way, extra food to treat hypoglycemia becomes unnecessary.

Hyperglycemia is caused by eating too much, other medications such as furosemide and corticosteriods, taking too little insulin, altering/decreasing exercise, or by physiological stress such as an illness.

If the cause is eating too much, the preferred solution is to decrease the food intake, as increasing the insulin to chronically cover increased food intake will result in weight gain. Taking too little insulin will result in hyperglycemia and may be done accidently or purposely. Clients may have difficulty drawing up insulin and be underdosing. Some clients use hyperglycemia and its resultant caloric loss as a method of weight loss. This form of eating disorder has life-threatening implications. Hyperglycemia can occur if regular exercise is omitted or decreased and a sliding scale may be the most appropriate method of correcting this problem. Hyperglycemia can also be caused by exercising when blood sugars are too high. When blood glucose values are greater than a 300 mg/dl, the cells are actually starving and the increase in physiological demand from exercise, causes an *increase* in blood glucose rather than the expected decrease. As a general rule of thumb, if blood sugars are greater than 300 mg/dl or urinary ketones are present, exercise should be postponed until blood glucose control has improved. Physiological stress, such as infection, is a significant cause of hyperglycemia. In this case, increasing insulin is the treatment of choice. Decreasing food intake does little to reduce the hyperglycemia of stress.

CASE STUDY - CHILD WITH IDDM

Kathy's physical symptoms were consistent of those of diabetic ketoacidosis. The metabolic events that lead to a diagnosis of IDDM include a gradual loss of pancreatic beta cell function due to a combination of genetics and a disordered immune system. As insulin production declines, the body loses a major anabolic hormone that is involved in the transport and synthesis of carbohydrate, protein, fat, and electrolytes. Without insulin, the cells starve. This cellular starvation, leads to an increase in glucagon, therefore gluconeogenesis occurs (from protein and fat), in an attempt to provide increased sources of cellular fuel. None of this increased fuel reaches the cell; it is lost in the urine. Extra fluid is needed to clear the glucose and fluid needs are increased. The client experiences polyphagia, polyuria, and polydipsia. If this chain of events is not reversed with insulin, fluid and electrolytes replacement, fat is catabolized at a faster rate than can be metabolized and fatty acids are condensed into ketones. Ketones or ketoacids cause the metabolic acidosis and decease in serum pH. This acidosis is often corrected by the administration of bicarbonate ion (base).

Diabetic ketoacidosis can be distinguished from insulin shock by the following:

DKA	hypoglycemia
3 P's	hunger
nausea	restlessness
headache	numbness around mouth
dry itchy skin	rapid onset
Kussmaul respiration	diaphoretic pale
positive ketones	blood glucose < 60 mg/dl
gradual onset	negative ketones
blood glucose > 240 mg/dl	

If in doubt and blood glucose can not be checked, the health care professional should treat as hypoglycemia. Four ounces of orange juice will not significantly alter the clinical outcome of diabetic ketoacidosis, but the administration of insulin mistakenly to someone in insulin shock can be a fatal error.

To prevent further incidences of DKA, the health care professional needs to investigate the current cause. In general, frequent blood sugar monitoring, especially during illness can determine early warnings. If blood sugars are greater than 240 mg/dl, the urine should be checked for ketones.

If Kathy had never received dietary instructions a comprehensive nutrition assessment is indicated. Her readiness to learn, stress level, acuity, and family/social support are critical elements to determine how much instruction Kathy receives at this time. Basic instruction should include the purpose and goals of the diabetic diet, specifically to keep blood glucose within normal range, thereby preventing chronic complications. The diet has controlled levels of carbohydrate, protein and fat. This diet is tailored to her personal preferences, lifestyle and medical management. The type of insulin with its onset, peak and duration determine the times of her meals. Kathy's age provides different challenges to the health care team. Entering adolescence, teens strive to separate from their family of origin and exert their independence. Diabetes, especially newly diagnosed diabetes, promotes dependence and invites conflict regarding drawing up and administering insulin as well as monitoring diabetes. Every effort to promote independence and self-responsibility may help her to deal with this struggle. Dietary goals may need to be modified. Camps for children with diabetes exist nationwide and share the goals of self-management and responsibility.

The current research from the Diabetes Control and Complications Trial (DCCT) demonstrates the importance of glycemic control in the prevention of chronic diabetes complications. Diet contributes to this control by attempting to match carbohydrate content to the insulin. Diet, by decreasing the saturated fat content and sodium content, also aids in the prevention of macrovascular disease. The diabetic diet being high in water soluble fiber helps to lower cholesterol levels. All of these dietary modifications may help in preventing diabetic complications.

CASE STUDY - ADULT WITH NIDDM

Mr. Kozak fits the typical pattern associated with NIDDM. Clients with NIDDM are usually overweight (60-90%) or have a history of obesity. Non-insulin dependent diabetes has a strong genetic component and is likely to "run in families". It generally occurs in adulthood. The primary difference between IDDM and NIDDM is the ability of the body to make insulin. In IDDM, the ability to produce insulin is lost, therefore, the person with IDDM is absolutely dependent on exogenous insulin for life. The client with NIDDM can produce insulin but is resistant to using this insulin. This explanation may motivate Mr. Kozak to continue to lose and monitor his weight after the fast. Caloric restriction and weight loss are the most importance elements in the control of NIDDM and often the only intervention needed. Caloric restriction is often successful in lowering blood glucose levels even before significant weight loss occurs. Caloric restriction and weight loss improve insulin resistance.

Factors in Mr. Kozak's history, predisposing him to diabetes, are his age and weight. Also, his family history may be a key determinant. Therefore, the primary objective of diet therapy for Mr. Kozak is weight loss. Mr. Kozak's IBW is 172 lbs., therefore a weight caloric level of IBW x10 (1700 calories) is appropriate. An appropriate diet for Mr. Kozak would include:

1700 kcal x .55 = 935 ÷ 4 kcal/gm = 234 grams carbohydrates

1700 kcal x .20 = 340 ÷ 4 kcal/gm = 85 grams protein

1700 kcal x .25 = 425 ÷ 9 kcal/gm = 47 grams fat

Day's Exchange

Exchange Group	Number of Exchanges	CHO g	Protein g	Fat g
Milk	2	24	16	--
Fruit	4	60	--	--
Vegetables	2	10	4	
Bread	9	135	27	
Meat	5		35	25
Fat	4			20
		229	82	45
Total Calories	1649	916	328	405

Controversy exists as to the optimal distribution of carbohydrate, protein and fat for clients with NIDDM. Therefore, adjustments in the distribution may need to be made depending on Mr. Kozak's blood sugar and lipid values.

The rationale for the fast is to achieve rapid glycemic control as well as a rapid initial weight loss. This is helpful physiologically and may also be of important psychological and motivational benefit. Non-insulin dependent diabetes can usually be controlled by diet. If diet is ineffective, exercise may be of benefit as would an oral hypoglycemic agent.

The health care team can be of tremendous support for Mr. Kozak. Acceptance of a chronic disease is a difficult process. However, with diabetes the client has a significant amount of control over his disease process. Although weight loss is difficult, it can provide the key to the prevention of complications and control of the disease. Continued support via clinic visits and telephone calls is critical.

TEACHING STRATEGIES

Compare the label of sugar-free candies and candy bars to comparable market brands. Notice the fat content of the sugar-free brands.

Prepare a sugar-free cake from a commercial mix (found in the dietetic/low calorie section in the grocery store). Discuss the changes in color and texture in this cake.

Plan a project to assess the glycemic index of foods preferred by the students. Obtain a baseline blood sugar and three subsequent blood sugars at 15 minutes intervals. Determine which food caused the greatest mg/dl rise in blood glucose and discuss the reasons why.

Chapter 26 Nutrition, Diabetes, and Hypoglycemia

ADDITIONAL RESOURCES*

American Dietetic Association
216 Jackson Blvd.
Chicago, IL 60606-6995
1-800-877-1600

> Publications:
> Exchange List for Meal Planning
> Health Food Choices
> Professional Guide: Diabetes Nutrition Education and Counseling

American Association of Diabetes Educators (AADE)
500 North Michigan Ave., Suite 1400
Chicago, IL 60611
312-661-1700

> Publications:
> Position Statements
> National Community Resource Guidelines for Diabetes Education
> National Standards for Diabetes Patient Education Programs

Centers for Disease Control
Division of Diabetes Control
Freeway Park, Building 1600B
Atlanta, GA

> Publications:
> Developing Patient and Professional Education Programs
> The Prevention and Treatment of Five Complications of Diabetes

Juvenile Diabetes Foundation (JDF)
60 Madison Ave.
New York, NY 10010
1-800-223-1138

> Publications:
> Parent to Parent: Your Child Has Diabetes
> Parent to Parent: Your Baby Has Diabetes
> Your Student Has Diabetes

National Diabetes Information Clearinghouse
Box NDIC
Bethesda, MD 20892
301-468-2162

    Publications:
    Bibliographies of patient education materials on a variety of topics including:
        Cookbooks
        Sports & Exercise
        Spanish language materials

HCF Diabetes Foundation
P. O. Box 22124
Lexington, KY 40522

    Publications:
    High Fiber Diabetes Resources
    Plant Fiber in Foods

*NOTE: Not all of the above resources are free but are generally low cost items.

CHAPTER 27
NUTRITION AND DISORDERS OF THE HEART AND BLOOD VESSELS

Scope

This chapter begins by explaining the development of atherosclerosis and its widespread effects on the rest of the body. When arterial plaques form they narrow the lumen of arteries so that oxygenated blood cannot flow to the tissues without extra work by the heart. The kidneys, needing fluid to perform their usual filtering function respond by raising the blood pressure. This sudden rush of blood through the body injures the arteries further, causing clots and more plaques to form. Then when clogged injured arteries can no longer take this abuse they burst or become completely obstructed, causing death to the tissues that they supply. Also, prolonged strain on an overworked heart can cause it to fail. Thus health professionals encounter clients with congestive heart failure, strokes, and heart attacks.

Chapter 27 discusses factors which make individuals prone to develop atherosclerosis. Some risk factors are fairly well established while findings of ongoing research suggest that others may not pose a risk unless some additional factor is present. Thus, preventive measures such as diet, behavior change or medication may act directly to reduce a risk or may do so by their effect on a co-factor.

Atherosclerosis is not the only condition that damages the cardiovascular system. Hypertension and heart failure can occur for other reasons; for example, heredity, salt sensitivity or the presence of chronic lung disease. Preventive and interventive measures, including diet will be based on these differences in etiology.

The broad spectrum of topics in Chapter 27 reflects the complicated relationships among body systems. The authors have presented a nutrition assessment tool that takes into account the fact that each client will be at risk for or will have already experienced a different configuration and degree of system damage. Dietary planning ranges from the preventive to crisis management to long-term maintenance.

Chapter 27 Nutrition and Disorders of the Heart and Blood Vessels

Nurses and dietitians frequently encounter clients whose damaged pulmonary and cardiovascular systems have had severely disabling consequences. Such clients may no longer be able to exercise, chew, swallow or feed themselves and are now at risk for obesity or malnutrition. Children's developmental needs are at risk of being unmet, since feeding behaviors pave the way for normal speech. Thus Chapter 27 concludes with recommended methods for helping disabled clients of all ages to feed at their highest level of function.

Objectives

1. Identify modifiable and non-modifiable risk factors for coronary heart disease.
2. Describe recommendations for detecting and improving blood lipids using the following strategies:
   screening
   diet
   physical activity
3. Discuss the nutritional problems and their appropriate interventions for a client with a cardiovascular or pulmonary disease.
4. Plan a diet for a client with a cardiovascular or pulmonary disease.

OUTLINE

TA

I. Atherosclerosis: A self accelerating process

   A. From fatty streaks to plaques   128 The Formation of Plaques on Arteries
   B. How plaques affect blood pressure
   C. Effects of blood pressure on arterial walls
   D. Response of the kidneys
   E. How clots form
   F. Coronary and cerebral thrombosis

II. Risk factors for atherosclerosis

   A. Direct (independent)
   B. Indirect (interactive)

III. The role of dyslipidemia in heart disease

   A. Low density lipids (LDL)   130 HDL and LDL compared
   B. High density lipids (HDL)
   C. Triglycerides
   D. How co-factors interact with dyslipidemia   102 Diet/Lifestyle Risk Factors and Degenerative Diseases
      1. Sex
      2. Age
      3. Diabetes
      4. Obesity
      5. Inactivity
      6. Oxidation

Chapter 27 Nutrition and Disorders of the Heart and Blood Vessels

IV. Implications of research findings for modification of risk factors

    A. How physical activity helps
    B. The role of antioxidant nutrients
    C. The pros and cons of alcohol
    D. Diet vs medication
    E. Treatment of co-existing diseases

V. Screening for dyslipidemia

    A. Factors affecting reliability of lab data
    B. Validity of lipid measurement in children

VI. The preventive role of diet

    A. Weight control
    B. Restrictions on fat intake
    C. Nutritional adequacy

    25 Comparison of Dietary Fats
    26 Hydrogenation
    27 Structural Formulas for Omega 3 and Omega 6 Fatty Acids
    29 Cholesterol
    129 How Normal Blood Pressure Supports Fluid Exchange

VII. Long range effects of atherosclerosis

    A. How hypertension develops
    B. Relationships between hypertension and obesity
    C. How heart failure occurs
    D. How aneurysms develop
    E. How strokes occur
    F. How the kidneys fail

VIII. Established risk factors for hypertension

    A. Age
    B. Heredity
    C. Obesity and fat distribution
    D. Physical inactivity
    E. Salt sensitivity

IX. Research findings on factors that may prevent hypertension

    A. Potassium intake
    B. Calcium intake
    C. Fat restriction
    D. Alcohol restriction
    E. Magnesium intake
    F. Diabetes control
    G. Vitamin C intake

Chapter 27   Nutrition and Disorders of the Heart and Blood Vessels

X.   Treatment of hypertension

    A.   Weight reduction
    B.   Types of exercise and how they help
    C.   How to control salt intake
    D.   Sources of potassium
    E.   Desired and adverse effects of diuretics

XI.   Myocardial infarctions (MI)

    A.   The pathological process
    B.   Nutritional interventions during the crisis
    C.   Meeting individual long-term dietary needs

XII.   Strokes

    A.   How strokes occur
    B.   How strokes affect long-term nutrition
    C.   Dietary interventions

XIII.   Congestive heart failure (CHF)

    A.   How CHF occurs
    B.   How CHF affects nutrition
    C.   How dietary interventions reduce the cardiac workload

XIV.   Chronic obstructive pulmonary disease (COPD)

    A.   Risk factors
    B.   Types of COPD
    C.   Effects on nutrition status
    D.   Risks of overfeeding
    E.   How respiratory failure occurs
    F.   Goals of dietary intervention
    G.   Roles of glucose, fat and protein

XV.   Assessment of individual nutritional needs

KEY TO CLINICAL APPLICATION QUESTIONS

1.   The possible interrelationships among risk factors are endless. Clients presenting with cardiovascular disease require comprehensive and ongoing assessment and evaluation. For example, a post-menopausal woman with NIDDM and hypertension is 5'4" and weighs 152 lbs. At the present time, her cholesterol is 210 mg/dl, LDL is 159, HDL is 35 mg/dl, and triglycerides are 400 mg/dl. Goals for her would include weight reduction, exercise, and possibly a sodium restriction. On the surface, her care may seem straight forward. However, drug therapy requires closer scrutiny. Many drugs used to treat cardiovascular disease may adversely affect diabetes control, such as beta blockers and thiazide diuretics. Post-menopausal estrogen replacement is followed by a decrease in

HDL cholesterol; therefore her risk of coronary heart disease increases. Elevations in triglycerides can be caused by obesity, poorly controlled diabetes, a high fat diet, alcohol and a diet high in simple sugars. Therefore, an analysis of the risk factors and their interrelationships provides a basis for sophistocated management of her care. It serves to focus the assessment process and dictates the needed interventions and patient education.

2. Many factors influence the determination of the calorie needs for a client with a severe stress and respiratory failure. The Harris Benedict equation can be used to determine resting energy expenditure but controversy exists as to the most appropriate stress factor to use for respiratory failure. It is strongly recommended, therefore to determine calorie requirements using indirect calorimetry. The use of indirect calorimetry avoids overfeeding which is undesirable for clients in respiratory failure. The factors influencing nutrient needs include nutritional status pre-injury, severity of the injury, sepsis, fever, and respiratory failure. Clients requiring significant calories have difficulty meeting these requirements via tube feeding. For example, if this client required 4000 calories, he would need approximately four liters of a standard polymeric tube feeding. Seriously ill clients often exhibit hypoperistalsis and high gastric residuals and delivering this large volume of fluid is not possible. The benefits of enteral feeding, even partial, include preservation of gut mass, immunologic function, decrease in bacterial translocation, and the consistent provision of glutamine. Glutamine is not only needed by the gut mucosa but also by the pulmonary artery endothelial cells (Austgen and Souba, 1991). Additionally, enteral support is less expensive. The possible disadvantages of tube feeding include the inability to meet full calorie needed, the increased likelihood of diarrhea and the increased risk of aspiration. Parenteral nutrition's primary advantages are the ease of modification of the solution and full calorie/protein delivery. The disadvantages of parenteral nutrition include gut atrophy, increased risk of bacterial translocation, infection and cost. The special problems associated with respiratory failure and nutrition support include the absolute need to avoid overfeeding. Overfeeding increases the respiratory quotient. The respiratory quotient is the ratio of carbon dioxide produced to oxygen consumption during macronutrient or substrate utilization. The higher the respiratory quotient, the more CO_2 produced. The respiratory quotient for protein is 0.8, carbohydrate 1.0 and fat 0.7. This indicates that a high fat diet produces less CO_2 and may be of benefit to clients in respiratory failure. However, overfeeding and subsequent lipogenesis has a RQ of 8.0. Therefore, overfeeding produces the most CO_2 and should be avoided. However, based on respiratory quotient alone, many clinicians advocate the use of low carbohydrate/high fat regimens. Protein energy malnutrition can also reduce respiratory muscle strength and ventilatory drive. Ongoing nutritional assessments are needed to monitor nutritional status and intervene as indicated.

Austgen, T. R., & Souba, W. W. (1991). The effects of endotoxin on lung glutamine metabolism in vivo. <u>Journal of Trauma, 31</u>, 742-751.

CASE STUDY - CORONARY HEART DISEASE

Mr. Garrett's risk factors for coronary heart disease include his age, gender, genetics, elevated LDL and triglycerides, obesity, diet, cigarette smoking and physical inactivity. His modifiable risk factors include his blood lipids, obesity, diet, smoking, physical inactivity, and hypertension. By altering his diet, he can reduce his weight and blood lipids. Additionally, diet is a valuable adjunct to control his blood pressure. Complications expected would be an advancement of his

CHD with a likelihood of a myocardial infarction or stroke. Initially, Mr. Garrett would be placed on a Step 1 diet. Calorie level appropriate for weight reduction would be IBW x 10 (148 x 10) = 1480 or 1500. The calorie reduction will facilitate weight reduction useful in decreasing LDL, triglycerides and blood pressure. Mr. Garrett needs a reduction in his total fat to less than 30% with saturated fat to less than 10% of calories. These reductions will aid in controlling blood lipids and possibly blood pressure. A sample 24 hour menu to illustrate these recommendations would include:

	Kcal	Fat
toasted oat cereal	110	.5
skim milk	90	.5
½ grapefruit with sugar	75	.0
4 oz. orange juice	60	.0
roast beef sandwich (2 oz.) with grilled	150	10.0
onions, lettuce, tomato, mustard	25	.0
French bread	160	.0
apple	60	.0
non-fat frozen yogurt	150	.5
tea		.0
4 oz. baked salmon with dill	300	20.0
rice pilaf	125	5.0
steamed broccoli with lemon	25	.0
skim milk	90	.5
angel food cake	150	.0
with fresh strawberries	60	.0
	1630	36.5

This is within the calorie level needed for weight reduction and the % of calories from fat. This diet is modified to meet the dietary goals for blood pressure in that no salt is used in cooking or at the table and minimally processed foods are used. By avoiding highly processed foods, Mr. Garrett may retain potassium and magnesium and his sodium can be controlled. Non-fat and low-fat dairy products add needed calcium. Regular monitoring of weight, blood pressure, total cholesterol, LDL and HDL could provide valuable feedback, reinforcement and guidance for Mr. Garrett as his weight loss decreases. Physical activity is a valuable adjunct to weight control and improvement of blood pressure, HDL cholesterol, and possibly LDL cholesterol. However, the exercise should provide an aerobic cardiovascular workout. Weight lifting or straining is contraindicated. Additional nutritional interventions would be needed if Mr. Garrett suffered a heart attack. Immediately after the event, Mr. Garrett would be NPO. Once stable, he would receive a low-calorie liquid diet. The diet eliminates gas forming foods and avoids foods at temperature extremes. Caffeine may be restricted depending on practitioner and institutional preferences. Sodium is restricted to approximately 2 grams. To prepare Mr. Garrett for discharge, an assessment of understanding of his previous restrictions and compliance is needed. If adherence to his Step I did not lower his lipids, he may be a candidate for a Step II diet and lipid lowering medications. If he was not compliant, exploring the barriers to compliance is indicated. Reinforcement of the Step I diet (with a sodium restriction) would be appropriate. If Mr. Garrett were to suffer a stroke, assessment for dysphagia is critical. Dysphagia, as described in Chapter 23, can contribute to malnutrition as well as increase the likelihood of aspiration. Mr. Garrett may also need an occupational therapy consultation to evaluate the mechanical aspects of eating. Long-term diet therapy would be the same as above. Congestive heart failure provides a distinct set of challenges. Edema is a problem that complicates the use of weight as a marker of malnutrition. Weight loss is indicated for Mr. Garrett as are small frequent meals. If the congestive heart failure becomes severe, cardiac cachexia is a possibility and Mr. Garrett should be evaluated frequently. Elevated blood lipids and hypertension are part of the etiology of these disorders as occlusion of the vessels increases peripheral resistance and aggravates high blood pressure. Decreasing blood flow to the kidney increases fluid retention and the workload on the heart. Mr. Garrett should be empowered to prevent these complications by changing his lifestyle.

TEACHING STRATEGIES

Have each student record a 24 hour diet history and evaluate it for total fat, saturated fat, cholesterol, and sodium. Each student should then identify in this diet the three main dietary sources of these items and suggest possible alternatives.

ADDITIONAL RESOURCES

American Heart Association
7320 Greenville Ave.
Dallas, TX 75231
Check phone book for local affiliate

McDonald's Nutrition Information
McDonald's Corporation
Oak Brook, IL 60521
708-575-FOOD

Fleischman's Margarine
Standard Brands, Inc.
625 Madison Ave.
New York City, NY 10022

Have the student visit the grocery store to evaluate how processing a food adds to its sodium content. For example, the more "instant" a food becomes, generally the more sodium it contains. Do a "sodium evaluation" of one or more foods beginning with fresh to frozen to canned.

Have small groups of students plan a Step I diet for a client to include one meal each from a different restaurant including fast food. Provide time for each group to present its work to the class. Encourage comparisons of menu items with respect to ease of modification. Predict likelihood of taste and texture appeal in the meals.

CHAPTER 28
NUTRITION AND DISORDERS OF THE KIDNEYS

Scope

This chapter deals with the nutritional challenges of caring for clients with acute or chronic renal disease. The pathophysiology behind renal failure and nephrotic syndrome is covered along with the special dietary considerations for each disorder. The kidneys' primary responsibilities are eliminating waste products and maintaining fluid and electrolyte balance.

Renal failure occurs when the nephrons are no longer able to maintain these functions. There are two types of renal failure, acute and chronic. Acute renal failure has a sudden onset and is usually precipitated by physiological stress that decreases renal blood flow. Congestive heart failure, stroke, infection or an urinary tract obstruction can be the causative factors. Symptoms that hallmark the onset of acute renal failure are a sudden drop in urine output and glomerular filtration rate. The client becomes hypercatabolic and hyperkalemic. Associated signs of nausea, vomiting, and anorexia make nutritional support a primary concern. Total parenteral or enteral feedings are prescribed that provide the appropriate amounts of protein, electrolytes and fluid while the underlying disorder is being treated.

Chronic renal failure has a gradual onset with extensive damage to nephrons before symptoms appear. Fluid overload, metabolic acidosis, hyperkalemia and hyperphosphoremia are hallmarks of this condition. Clients have an altered nutritional status due to loss of nutrients from nausea, vomiting, diarrhea and altered absorption ability. In addition, dietary restrictions to correct the physiological processes of renal failure are often unpalatable. A renal diet is high in energy with individualized restrictions on protein, phosphorus, sodium, potassium and fluids. Vitamins and minerals are often supplemented. Since renal diets are restrictive, special emphasis is placed on working with the client to gain acceptance of the food plan.

Chapter 28 Nutrition and Disorders of the Kidneys

Clients in severe renal failurerequire dialysis to take over the function of the kidneys. An alternative to dialysis is a kidney transplant which brings about a new set of dietary challenges. Because kidney recipients are immunosupressed, they experience fluid retention, carbohydrate intolerance and muscle wasting from a negative nitrogen balance. Diets are aimed at restricting sodium and providing enough protein to counteract the catatonic state.

Nephrotic syndrome is characterized by low albumin levels, fluid retention and elevated lipids. It occurs most frequently in children who have experienced glomerulonephritis, renal thrombosis, and diabetes. Dietary interventions are aimed at providing enough energy to prevent further protein loss and restricting sodium and fat.

Urinary tract infections (UTIs) are treated with antimicrobials and increased fluids. Low urinary pH can be beneficial in the treatment of UTIs. The controversy of the use of cranberry juice to alter urinary pH is addressed. The chapter concludes with a section on the nutritional assessment of clients with renal disorders.

Objectives

1. Differentiate between the symptoms and treatment of acute and chronic renal failure.
2. Explain the therapeutic options in acute renal failure and their impact on nutritional support.
3. Describe the long-term nutritional problems associated with chronic renal failure and appropriate interventions.
4. Plan a diet for a client in chronic renal failure.
5. Explain dietary guidelines following a kidney transplant.
6. Explain the dietary guidelines for nephrotic syndrome.
7. Describe the assessment of a client with a disorder of the kidney.

OUTLINE

TA

I. Functions of the kidney

    A. Blood filtration
    B. Blood pressure regulation
    C. Red blood cell production
    D. Calcium and bone metabolism

131 Events Leading to Osteodystrophy

II. Renal failure

    A. Acute renal failure
        1. Physiological responses
        2. Treatment
            a. Nutrient needs
            b. Fluids and electrolytes

B. Chronic renal failure
   1. Physiological responses
   2. Treatment
      a. Nutrient needs
      b. Dietary planning
C. Kidney transplants
   1. Immunosuppressants
   2. Diet therapy

III. Nephrotic syndrome

132 Consequences of Nephrotic Syndrome

   A. Physiological responses
   B. Diet therapy

IV. Urinary tract infections

   A. Fluids
   B. Cranberry juice

V. Nutrition assessment

KEY TO CLINICAL APPLICATION QUESTIONS

1.

	Severe Stress	Resp. Failure	Liver Disease	Renal Failure
kcal	35-40 kcal/kg	35-40 kcal/kg	35-45 kcal/kg	35-50 kcal/kg
protein	1.5-2.0 gm/kg	1.5-2.0 gm/kg	.6-.8 gm/kg (40-60 gm)	.5-.6 gm/kg (30-40 gm)
fat	25-30% of total energy intake	50%	25-30% unless steatorrhea develops	25-30%
fluid	retained	retained	retained	retained
other	increased need for B vitamins. Glutamine may be helpful. Omega 3 fatty acids may be helpful.		Malabsorption of fat soluble vitamins. Increased needs for B vitamin.	Fluid and sodium severely restricted. Potassium restricted.

The nutrient modifications that are common to all of the above conditions are the need for increased kcalorie and protein. Additionally, each of the disorders may need a fluid and sodium restriction. However, as organs begin to fail, tolerance rather than physiological requirement dictates the amount of nutrient delivered. For example, a client in renal failure is hypercatabolic and needs increased protein but due to poor urine output can only tolerate 30-40 grams per day. The delivery of protein therefore is determined by tolerance rather than need. The final decision on how to feed an individual in multi-system organ failure is determined on a case by case basis. Indirect calorimetry is extremely helpful in the calculation of the appropriate calorie level. Laboratory values, specific to each disease, are analyzed to determine nutrient distribution and the form of the nutrient needed. For example, a high fecal fat level may signal the need to modify the form of fat delivered i.e., a change from a polyunsaturated fat to MCT oil. Continued surveillance of lab data and serial nutrition assessments are indicated.

2. Suggestions to improve the renal diet are summarized in Table 28-5. Other suggestions would be to try flavored vinegars as marinades for meats or vegetables. Refrigerated mouthwashes are helpful, but avoid those with a high alcohol content as they dry out the mouth. Lemon drop candy may increase saliva flow and help prevent dry mouth. The modification of favorite recipes by a registered dietitian is helpful and proves invaluable during the holiday season.

CASE STUDY - ACUTE RENAL FAILURE

The most probable cause of Mrs. Calley's acute renal failure is hypovolemia due to the large amount of blood she lost. Other causes of acute renal failure include but are not limited to heart failure, drug overdose, sepsis, toxins and environmental pollutants. In the initial phase of acute renal failure little or no urine is produced and protein, sodium, potassium and fluids are restricted. As the client enters the diuretic phase, the potassium, sodium and fluid restrictions are liberalized. Mrs. Calley's calorie and protein needs are high. Calorie needs range between 1989 and 2809. However, because of this wide range, indirect calorimetry could pinpoint the need and avoid under or overfeeding. Protein needs are also high but if urine output is low and dialysis is not initiated, tolerance is low. Monitoring of BUN and creatinine clearance is important as findings are often used to institute dialysis. Monitoring serum potassium is of paramount importance. Hyperkalemia can cause fatal arrhythmias. Her fractured leg and broken ribs also increase her calorie and protein requirements. If she becomes febrile or develops an infection, her calorie and protein requirements will increase further. If dialysis is instituted, more protein, sodium and potassium will be allowed. As diuresis commences, large volumes of fluid are lost; blood urea nitrogen and creatinine will slowly decrease. The client may even become hypokalemic and develop metabolic alkalosis.

CASE STUDY - CHRONIC RENAL FAILURE

Chronic renal failure is defined as a significant decrease in the glomerular filtration that occurs over a period of years or even decades. Up to 80% of renal function ceases before signs and symptoms appear. As the glomerular filtration falls the body is unable to excrete waste products and blood urea nitrogen climbs. Uremic syndrome is characterized by increased susceptibility to infection, pruritus, anorexia and vomiting, skeletal manifestations secondary to a decreased production of vitamin D, and iron deficiency anemia. In comparison to children, Yusuf's height is at the $\approx$ 45% tile and weight at 25% tile. Growth can be compromised in children with renal failure for many reasons. Anorexia and nausea contribute to poor intake. Calorie intake less than 80 kcal/kg does not support reasonable growth. His energy intake should be minimally 2000 kcal. Currently his intake is 44 kcal/kg. Growth may also be compromised secondary to decreased production of vitamin D and the development of metabolic bone disease. Anemia also contributes to fatigue and often a poor appetite. Prior to dialysis, Yusuf received a diet that restricted sodium, potassium, fluid, and controlled the amount of protein he consumes. Fluid and electrolytes are restricted because the kidney is no longer able to clear the waste products effectively. Research suggests that controlling the amount of protein, to avoid excesses, may delay the progression of chronic renal failure. As Yusuf begins hemodialysis, his blood level of blood urea nitrogen will fall and to a certain degree, his appetite will improve. Protein allowances will increase to levels somewhat above the RDA to meet growth and development needs and to compensate for amino acid loss in the dialysate. If Yusuf is given a transplant most restrictions are lifted, but many practitioners continue sodium restrictions, advocate adequate protein and monitor calories to prevent excessive weight gain. As with all chronic disease, the stress on the family is enormous. The increase of financial burdens, repeated hospitalizations, and dietary restrictions make routine family life very complex. If there are siblings in the family, they may feel anger and resentment toward their brother and family. Continual support from the health care team is vital and may come in a variety of forms. Honest open communication may alleviate the fear of the unknown. Allowing Yusuf's family to ventilate their concerns and fears without passing judgement is also helpful. Support groups may also fill that need. Referrals to mental health professionals, including psychologists, psychiatric social workers, nurse practitioners, or psychiatrists may also be indicated.

TEACHING STRATEGIES

Have the students divide into groups. Have each group collect dietary information on at least two clients being seen by two different physicians. Have the students report their findings to the class. Compare and contrast the clients and their prescribed nutritional therapy. Point out how protein restrictions vary depending on client and health care practitioner.

Collect a cycle of lab data on a dialysis client. Have the students evaluate the effectiveness of the dialysis.

Assign a research project on the use of cranberry juice to prevent urinary tract infections. Have the students collect data from a health food store employee, a lay person, and a health care professional. Require documentation from both lay and professional journals.

Give students a set of lab values from a renal client. Have them plan an appropriate diet. Ask the students to follow that diet for a two day period. Have a group discussion about the appeal and palatability of the diet.

Modify a favorite holiday food recipe to lower the sodium, potassium content, and then calculate the sodium potassium and phosphorus content of the original and modified version.

Analyze the protein, sodium and potassium content of a 60 gram protein vegetarian diet. Discuss the problems encountered and possible solutions when the renal diet must accomodate vegetarian restrictions.

CHAPTER 29
NUTRITION AND WASTING DISORDERS: CANCER AND AIDS

Scope

Chapter 29 addresses the challenging task of providing nutritional support for clients who have cancer and AIDS. Both conditions affect multiple systems which can interfere with nutrient absorption and delivery. Also with both conditions, clients may have nutritional deficiencies that can be directly attributed to their treatment therapy.

The introductory material to the cancer section discusses current theory on the development of cancer. Decreasing exposure to substances that may play a role in the development of cancer such as environmental hazards and food sources is advocated. The American Cancer Society's recommendations of a high-fiber, low-fat diet that includes a variety of fruits and vegetables to decrease the risk of cancer is reviewed.

Cancer treatment can include radiation therapy, drug therapy including chemotherapy, surgery and bone marrow transplants. Each modality is effective in the war against cancer yet each has an impact on the client's nutritional status. Types of alternative therapies and the rationale for their use is discussed.

Anorexia and inadequate nutrient intake in cancer patients has multiple causes. Clients are often fatigued, in pain, or under increased stress. Additionally, surgery, chemotherapy, and radiation therapy can further decrease nutrient intake by causing anorexia, nausea, vomiting, stomatitis, taste blindness, and food aversions. When a cancer client does eat, nutrients are often lost due to malabsorption or problems with digestion. Inactivation of digestive enzymes as in Zollinger-Ellisen syndrome, radiation enteritis, nausea and vomiting, and diarrhea all effect digestion and absorption of nutrients.

Chapter 29 Nutrition and Wasting Disorders: Cancer and AIDS

Altered metabolism, despite adequate nutritional support, accounts for the muscle wasting that is seen in people with cancer. Clients are often hypermetabolic, or even if they are not, their tumors use energy inefficiently to support growth. After glycogen stores are depleted the body uses protein as energy which explains the negative nitrogen balance seen in cancer patients. Hyperlipidemia along with vitamin and mineral deficiencies are also frequently seen.

Nutrition support for clients with cancer can improve their quality of life but it cannot cure cancer nor is it a primary treatment. Actual protein and energy needs are individualized. The Harris-Benedict equation can be used to calculate energy needs, and protein requirements are usually between 1.5 to 2.0 grams/kg/ideal body weight. Cancer patients are supported by oral diets, enteral, and parenteral feedings. Antiemetics play a major role in increasing food intake. Tables are used to display suggestions for improving food intake and special dietary considerations that account for the location of the cancer and the resulting disability. At the end of this section, ethical considerations of feeding a terminally ill client is addressed.

Recipients of bone marrow transplants are often given TPN with glutamine added to prevent translocation of bacteria. When the client is able, a lactose-free, low-residue, low-fat liquid diet is introduced and the diet is then progressed as tolerated. Since the client is immunosuppressed, a high protein and calcium diet is recommended.

The second part of this chapter deals with HIV/AIDS related infections. The progression of HIV infection into AIDS, associated symptoms, and treatments are discussed. Two goals for dietary intervention are to delay the PEM and wasting seen in AIDS clients.

Anorexia and inadequate nutrient intake are common in clients with HIV. Severe psychological stress, thrush, oral and esophageal lesions, use of oxygen devices, side-effects of drugs, lethargy, and dementia all contribute to the problem. Nutrients taken in are not completely absorbed or are lost due to diarrhea and a high gastric pH. Hypermetabolism associated with frequent, recurring infections also affects the client's nutrient status. Additionally, clients with HIV and cancer will have altered metabolism as discussed previously.

Dietary interventions are centered around providing enough protein, energy, vitamins, and minerals for HIV infected clients. Oral diets are used as long as possible. Dietary modifications are given for managing diarrhea and malabsorption. Nutritional support is begun early to help prevent catabolism. With HIV infected individuals, aggressive nutrition support has been found to be effective for regaining lean body mass. Enteral and parental products are used to provide nutrition. The risks and benefits of using TPN in an immunocompromised client are discussed.

The chapter concludes with nutritional assessment pointers specific for clients with cancer and AIDS. PEM is a frequent problem to assess for. Also the use of alternative therapies and possible nutrient interactions is another key area in assessment.

Objectives

1. Describe dietary factors associated with cancer.
2. Describe the use of foods as cancer antipromoters.
3. Explain the nutritional consequences of cancer and cancer treatments.
4. Describe the goal of nutrition support for a client with cancer.

Chapter 29 Nutrition and Wasting Disorders: Cancer and AIDS

5. Describe interventions to improve nutrient intake and prevent nutrient loss in a cancer client.
6. Explain the dietary considerations for a bone marrow recipient.
7. Explain the nutritional consequences of HIV/AIDS.
8. Describe the goals of nutrition support for a client with HIV/AIDS.
9. Relate the nutritional assessment factors that are the key to detecting nutrient deficiencies in clients with cancer or HIV/AIDS.

OUTLINE

TA

I. Cancer

   A. How cancer develops
   B. Cachexia
      1. Mechanisms of cachexia
      2. Effects of cachexia   133 Consequences of the Cancer Cachexia Syndrome
   C. Cancer prevention
      1. Risk factors
      2. Carcinogens
      3. Cancer promoters
      4. Antipromoters
      5. Diet
   D. Treatment of cancer
      1. Radiation
      2. Chemotherapy   105 Two Antivitamins used as Drugs
      3. Other drug therapy
      4. Surgery
      5. Bone marrow transplants
      6. Unproven treatment

II. Nutritional consequences of cancer

   A. Anorexia and inadequate nutrient intake
      1. Early satiety
      2. Fatigue   103 Interrelationships between Illness and Malnutrition
      3. Pain
      4. Psychologic stress
      5. Obstructions
      6. Altered taste perception
      7. Stomatitis
      8. Mouth blindness
      9. Esophagitis
      10. Fistula
      11. Food aversions
      12. Mechanical problems
      13. Combined effects

B. Nutrient losses
  1. Maldisgestion and malabsorption
  2. Vomiting and diarrhea
  3. Radiation enteritis
C. Metabolic alterations
  1. Altered energy metabolism
  2. Protein
  3. Carbohydrate
  4. Lipid
  5. Other metabolic effects
     a. Vitamin deficiencies
     b. Anemias

III. Nutrition support

  A. Role of nutrition in cancer treatment
  B. Dietary interventions
    1. Nutrient needs
    2. Oral diets
    3. Enteral and parenteral feedings
    4. Drug therapy
    5. Ethical issues

IV. Bone marrow transplants

  A. Parenteral nutrition
  B. Oral diets

V. HIV and AIDS

  A. Consequences of HIV infection
  B. Treatment
  C. HIV wasting syndrome
  D. Anorexia and inadequate nutrient intake
    1. Psychological stress
    2. Thrush
    3. Herpes virus and Kaposi's sarcoma
    4. Respiratory infections
    5. Drug therapy
    6. Lethargy and dementia
  E. Nutrient losses
    1. HIV infection
    2. Other infections
    3. Malnutrition
    4. Cancer and cancer therapy
    5. Other
  F. Metabolic alterations

VI. Nutrition support for HIV

  A. Early nutrition support
  B. Dietary interventions
     1. Oral diets
     2. Treatment of diarrhea
     3. Aggressive nutrition support
     4. Enteral nutrition
     5. Parenteral nutrition

VII. Nutrition assessment
  A. PEM
  B. Drug - nutrient interactions
  C. Laboratory values

KEY TO CLINICAL APPLICATION QUESTIONS

1. Nutrition plays a primary role when diet is an integral part of the treatment. Diabetes and coronary artery disease are examples where diet therapy can alter the course of the disease as well as control symptoms. In oncology and HIV disease, diet plays a supportive role and may provide symptom relief, support the immune system, aid in the prevention of PEM, and possibly help the individual better tolerate the medical therapies which are the cornerstone of treatment. However, nutrition is not curative. Quality of life may be improved by helping clients keep their "strength up" and take care of personal issues of importance to them.

2. The prevention of PEM is crucial in clients with cancer and HIV disease. Clients with cancer and HIV disease often present with some degree of weight loss. Cachexia and malnutrition have been found to be the actual cause of death in approximately 22% of clients with advanced cancer. Significant weight loss is present in two-thirds of clients with advanced disease (DeWys et al., 1980 and Warren, 1932). Protein energy malnutrition causes anergy, a negative nitrogen balance, and decrease in serum proteins and the increased susceptibility to infection. Research suggests that an albumin level of less than 2.2 gm/dl is predictive of anergy (Harvey, et al., 1981) and there is 12 fold increase in mortality in clients with hypoalbuminemia over those with a normal albumin (Doweiko et al., 1991). Therefore, PEM contributes to the incidence of infection and mortality.

DeWys, W. D., Begg, C., & Lavin P. T. (1980). Prognostic effect of weight loss prior to chemotherapy in cancer patients. American Journal of Medicine, 68, 683-690.

Warren, S. (1932). The immediate cause of death in cancer. American Journal of Medical Science, 184, 610-615.

Harvey, K. B., Moldaiver, L. L., & Bistrian, B. R. (1981). Biologic measures for the formulation of a hospital prognostic index. American Journal of Clinical Nutrition, 34, 2013-2022.

Doweiko, J. P., & Nompleggi, M. D. (1991). The role of albumin in human physiology and pathophysiology. Part III: Albumin and disease states. <u>Journal of Parenteral and Enteral Nutrition.</u> <u>15</u>, 476-483.

CASE STUDY - CANCER

Mr. Weisman's ideal body weight is 166 lbs. At his current weight he is at 75% IBW. Given he has kwashiorkor-marasmus mix, he would have a depressed albumin and lymphocyte count. Triceps skinfold thickness and midarm muscle mass would also be below normal. Mr. Weisman's history of chronic nicotine and alcohol abuse places him at risk for B vitamin deficiencies. A detailed dietary history would be useful to determine how his alcohol consumption affected his dietary habits. His cancer can affect his nutrition status in many ways. Cancer can cause anorexia, increased nutrient losses and metabolic alterations specifically by increasing metabolic rate and decreased energy efficiency. Hyperglycemia and lactic acid accumulation can further depress appetite. Radiation therapy can alter Mr. Weisman's ability to consume adequate nutrition orally. Damage to teeth and bones, esophagitis and strictures, nausea and vomiting, taste alterations, such as loss of taste and thick salivary secretions all pose difficult challenges. Radical head and neck surgery may increase the likelihood of dysphagia, cause disfigurement and loss of speech. Pain and depression are important causes of anorexia. Mr. Weisman may need a gastrostomy to facilitate the delivery of long-term nutrition. Cancer cachexia is multifactorial. Possible causes include reduced food intake secondary to anorexia, excessive losses of nutrients secondary to drug therapy and malabsorption and altered energy metabolism. The benefits of preventing or correcting cachexia include possible increase in weight and strength, better tolerance to therapies and improvement in the immune system. If Mr. Weisman were able to consume foods by mouth, small frequent meals of nutrient dense foods are indicated. The foods should have a high-moisture content, be easy to swallow, and non-acidic. An example would be a cheese omelet and a biscuit with jelly and pear nectar. Mr. Weisman must capitalize on periods when he is feeling good or not fatigued to increase his calorie and protein intake. Again, if this is not possible, a gastrostomy is indicated.

CASE STUDY - HIV INFECTION

Nutrition status is compromised by HIV infection. Reduced food intake is caused by depression, fever, pain, dysphagia, mouth ulcers, obstructions and lesions, drug therapy and dementia. Nutrient loses can be caused by AIDS enteropathy and opportunistic infections causing diarrhea. Drug therapy, megadoses of vitamins, home remedies such as colonics (enemas) reduce gastric acid secretions and bacteria also contribute to nutrient losses. Depression, however, should not be overlooked as a potential cause. Nutritional strategies for dealing with thrush include choosing soft moist non-acidic easily swallowed foods. Milkshakes are often well accepted. The dietary management of diarrhea generally includes the reduction of dietary fat, lactose and residue. However, clients with HIV/AIDS often have secretory type of diarrhea that does not decrease when food intake is limited. If the dietary interventions do not decrease the diarrhea, the health care team should be notified. Kevin's weight loss should be evaluated by using his usual body weight. He has lost 10 lbs., with a current weight of 158 lbs. His percent usual body weight is 94%. Using his ideal body weight of 178 lbs., his percent of ideal body weight is 88%. He has lost 10 lbs. or 6% over the last four months. He certainly is at risk of malnutrition but aggressive nutrition support is not indicated at this time. To prevent further weight loss, kevin needs a comprehensive nutrition assessment as well as education to provide him with accurate nutrition information. Kevin needs education on safe food handling and food preparation to prevent food borne illnesses.

TEACHING STRATEGIES

Visit a health food store and identify a supplement or herbal preparation marketed to boost the immune system. Discuss the pros and cons of the supplement.

Have the students develop a teaching plan for a client who was receiving chemotherapy. The plan should include an appropriate diet along with methods for increasing food intake and controlling nausea and vomiting.

Have the students research common alternative therapies for cancer and HIV. Their papers/reports should include the therapies' impact on the client's nutritional status and whether or not the alternative therapies are thought to be safe.

ADDITIONAL RESOURCES

Tyler, V. E., Brady, L., & Robbers, J. E. (1985). Pharmacognosy. Philadelphia: Lea & Febiger. This book provides insight into the pharmocological action of herbs.

American Cancer Society
90 Park Avenue
New York City, NY 10016

FDA Consumer
U.S. Food & Drug Administration
DHHS-PHS
Order from : Superintendent of Documents
Washington, D.C. 20402-9371

Videotape (available through Ross Products)
    Taking Charge, Nutrition for Cancer Patients

Running Time
22 min.

HANDOUTS

Prepared by:

Lori Waite Turner, M.S., R.D.
Tallahassee Community College

| List Food and Amount | Indicate Number of Servings from Each Food Group ||||||
	Bread/Cereal	Fruit	Vegetable	Meat	Milk	Miscellaneous
Breakfast:						
Snack:						
Lunch:						
Snack:						
Dinner:						
Snack:						
Total:						

HANDOUT 2-1

Compare Your Food Intake to the Daily Food Guide

©1994 West Publishing Company

ORGAN OR GLAND	Secretion	TARGET	PRIMARY ACTION
SALIVARY GLANDS	*saliva*	MOUTH	starch —*amylase*→ maltose
GASTRIC GLANDS	*gastric juice*	STOMACH	protein —*pepsin/HCl*→ smaller polypeptides
INTESTINAL GLANDS	*intestinal juice*	SMALL INTESTINE	carbohydrate —*carbohydrase*→ monosaccharides
LIVER	*bile*		
GALL BLADDER	*bile*	SMALL INTESTINE	fats —*bile*→ (emulsified fat)
PANCREAS	*pancreatic juice*	SMALL INTESTINE	protein —*protease*→ dipeptides, tripeptides, amino acids lipase: monoglycerides, glycerol & fatty acids

HANDOUT 3-1
Digestive Secretions and Their Actions
©1994 West Publishing Company

Transport of Nutrients into Blood

Water-soluble nutrients
  Carbohydrates
    Monosaccharides   Directly into blood
  Lipids
    Glycerol   Directly into blood
    Short-chain fatty acids   Directly into blood
    Medium-chain fatty acids   Directly into blood
  Proteins
    Amino acids   Directly into blood
  Vitamins
    Vitamins B and C   Directly into blood
  Minerals   Directly into blood
Fat-soluble nutrients
  Lipids
    Long-chain fatty acids   Made into triglycerides
    Monoglycerides   Made into triglycerides
    Triglycerides   To lymph, then blood
    Cholesterol   To lymph, then blood
    Phospholipids   To lymph, then blood
  Vitamins
    Vitamins A, D, E, K   To lymph, then blood

HANDOUT 3-2
Transport of Nutrients into Blood
©1994 West Publishing Company

Sugar	Relative Sweetness[a]
Fructose	170[b]
Sucrose	100
Glucose (dextrose)	70
Maltose	46
Lactose	35
Galactose	32

[a] Sucrose is the standard by which the approximate sweetness of other sugars is compared.

[b] The sweetness of fructose depends on the temperature and acidity of the foods in which it occurs.

Source: Adapted from H. L. Sipple and K. W. McNutt, *Sugars in Nutrition* (New York: Academic Press, 1974), pp. 44–46, as cited in *Sugars and Your Health—A Report by the American Council on Science and Health* (Summit, N.J.: American Council on Science and Health, May 1986), p. 7.

HANDOUT 4-1
Sweetness of Sugars
©1994 West Publishing Company

Fruits: about 3 g of fiber per portion

Apple, 1 small	Grapes, 30
Apricots, 5	Orange, 1 small
Banana, 1 1/2	Peach, 1 1/2 small
Blackberries, 1/3 c	Pear, 1/2 small
Blueberries, 3/4 c	Pineapple, 1 1/2 c
Cantaloupe, 1/2	Plums, 3 small
Cherries, 1 c	Prunes, 4
Dates, 5	Raisins, 1 1/2 oz
Figs, 1 1/2	Raspberries, 1/3 c
Grapefruit, 3/4	Strawberries, 3/4 c

Grains and Cereals: about 3 g of fiber per portion

All-bran, 1/3 oz	Raisin bran, 1/2 c
Barley, 3/4	Rice, 1 c
Bulgur, 1/4 c	Rye bread, 1 1/2 slices
Cracked wheat bread, 3 slices	Shredded wheat, 1/2 c
Granola, 1/4 c	Wheat bran, 1/4 c
Grape-nuts, 1/3 c	Whole-wheat bread, 1 1/2 slices
Oatmeal, 3/4 c	

Vegetables: about 3 g of fiber per portion

Artichoke, 1/3	Corn on the cob, 5-inch piece
Asparagus, 12 spears	Green beans, 1 c
Beets, 3/4 c	Lettuce, 1/3 head
Broccoli, 1/2 spear	Potato, 1/2 (with skin)
Brussels sprouts, 1/2 c	Spinach, 1 1/2 c raw
Cabbage, 1 1/2 c raw	Squash, 1 c
Carrots, 1 1/2	Tomato, 1 1/2 medium
Collards, 3/4 c cooked	

Legumes: about 8 g of fiber per portion

Baked beans, 1/2 c	Lentils, 1 c
Black beans, 1/2 c	Lima beans, 1 c
Black-eyed peas, 1 c	Navy beans, 1/2 c
Garbanzo beans, 1 c	Pinto beans, 1/2 c
Kidney beans, 1/2 c	

Miscellaneous: about 1 g of fiber per portion

Nuts, 1/2 oz	Peanut butter, 1 tbs
Olives, 5	Pickle, 1 large

HANDOUT 4-2

Foods to Include on a High-Fiber Diet

©1994 West Publishing Company

	Calories per Serving	% Calories from Fat	Grams Fat per Serving	Proportion of Saturated Fat
DAIRY				
Whole milk, 8 oz. (1 glass)	159	47	8	High
Ice cream, ¾ cup	143	48	11	High
Eggs, 2 large	164	64	12	Moderate
Cheddar cheese, 2 oz.	228	73	19	High
Swiss cheese, 2 oz.	214	73	16	High
Cream cheese, 2 Tbsp	99	88	10	High

The following cheeses also contain a minimum of 60% calories from fat and 8 to 9 grams fat per ounce: Bleu, Brick, Brie, Caraway, Edam, Gouda, Gruyere, Limburger, Monterrey, Muenster, Port du Salut, Provolone, Romano, Roquefort; also pasteurized processed American, Pimento or Swiss.

	Calories per Serving	% Calories from Fat	Grams Fat per Serving	Proportion of Saturated Fat
FISH				
Sockeye (red) salmon, 4 oz.	194	49	11	Low
Herring (Pacific), 4 oz.	235	59	16	Low
Mackerel (Pacific), 4 oz.	204	50	11	Low
Sardines (Atlantic) in oil, drained, 4 oz.	230	49	12	Low
RED MEAT *				
Beef, rib roast (well-trimmed), 4 oz.	278	52	16	High
Beef, club steak (well-trimmed), 4 oz.	234	42	11	High
Pork, loin roast (well-trimmed), 4 oz.	271	53	16	High
Pork, Boston butt (well-trimmed), 4 oz.	290	59	19	High
Lamb chops (well-trimmed), 4 oz.	239	45	12	High
Liverwurst, 2 oz.	186	78	16	High
Hot dog, 2 oz. (one), Beef & Pork	183	82	17	High
NUTS & SEEDS				
Peanut butter, 2 Tbsp.	188	73	16	Low
Sunflower seeds, ⅛ cup	100	71	9	Low
Almonds, ⅛ cup	123	77	11	Low
Walnuts, black, ⅛ cup	98	79	9	Low
BAKED GOODS				
Croissant, 1, about 1 oz.	109	50	6	Usually high
Apple pie, ⅛ of pie	302	38	13	Usually high
Danish pastry, ⅛ ring	179	49	10	Usually high
OTHER				
Avocado, ½ fruit	188	82	19	Low
Coconut, 1 piece, 2" x 2" x ½"	156	85	16	High
Milk chocolate, 1 oz.	147	53	9	High
Cream of mushroom soup, 10 oz. (prepared with water)	150	66	11	Variable

*All values for fresh meat represent cooked portions of choice grade. The information is based on *averages* of samples analyzed by the U.S. Department of Agriculture. These figures represent the "lean" of the meat only; every possible bit of outside fat has been removed.

Almost all of the information in this chart is based on USDA food tables. However, in a few cases, information supplied by food companies was used.

HANDOUT 5-1

Exposing Hidden Fat

©1994 West Publishing Company

How to Modify A Recipe (Lasagne)

Original	Modified
⅓ c olive oil (to sauté vegetables)	[omit oil]
1½ c diced onions	1½ c onion, 1 green pepper, ½ lb mushrooms
2 cloves garlic	2 cloves garlic
1½ lb ground chuck	¾ lb ground round
2 t salt	[omit salt]
2 lb tomato sauce	use no-added-salt type
28 oz canned tomatoes	use no-added-salt type
6 oz canned tomato paste	use no-added-salt type
1 tbsp oregano	2 t oregano, 2 t basil, ¼ c fresh parsley
2 tsp onion salt	[omit salt]
1 lb lasagne noodles	1 lb whole wheat lasagne noodles
2 tbsp olive oil (to cook noodles)	[omit oil]
16 oz ricotta	16 oz low-fat cottage cheese, pureed
8 oz mozzarella	8 oz part skim mozzarella
10 oz parmesan	4 oz parmesan
oil to grease pan	spray to grease pan

Yield 16 servings (2 9" × 12" pans)

Analysis	Original	Modified
Energy (cal)	513	281
Protein (g)	35	21
Fat (g)	29 (6 t)	7 (1.4 t)
Sodium (mg)	1121	380
Cholesterol (mg)	73	32
Fat as % of calories	51	24

Source: Culinary Hearts Kitchen Course, Tallahassee, Fla., as taught by Sandi Woodruff, M.S., R.D., with permission.

HANDOUT 5-2

How to Modify a Recipe

©1994 West Publishing Company

Food	Amount	Protein (g)	Energy (kcal)
THESE ARE THE FOODS PEOPLE USUALLY THINK OF WHEN THEY THINK OF PROTEIN:			
Cheese:			
Cheddar[a]	1 oz	7	115
Cottage	1/2 c	12 to 15	85 to 130
Egg	1 large	7	80
Fish, light and dark, cooked	3 oz	20 to 25	125 to 175
Meat, cooked:			
Ground beef	3 oz	20 to 23	185 to 235
Heart, kidney, liver[a]	3 oz	23 to 28	160 to 215
Pork	3 oz	23 to 28	310
Poultry (without skin), light and dark, cooked	3 oz	25	145 to 175
Milk:			
Nonfat	1 c	9	90
Whole[a]	1 c	9	160
THESE ARE OTHER GOOD SOURCES OF PROTEIN THAT YOU COULD USE INSTEAD:			
Vegetables, cooked:			
Broccoli	1 medium stalk	6	45
Brussels sprouts	1 c	7	55
Cauliflower	1 c	3	30
Greens	1 c	3 to 7	30 to 65
Legumes:			
Dried, cooked	1/2 c	7 to 8	90 to 115
Mung sprouts, raw	1/2 c	2	20
Tofu (soybean curd)	4 oz	9	85
YOU CAN ALSO GET SIGNIFICANT QUALITIES OF PROTEIN FROM THESE FOODS (IF YOU CAN AFFORD THE KCALORIES):			
Ceareal grain products:			
Barley, whole grain, cooked	1/2 c	4	135
Bran, unprocessed	1/2 c	4	55
Bran cereal (100% bran), uncooked	1/2 c	5	90
Breads	1 slice	2 to 3	60 to 80
Cornmeal, unrefined ground, uncooked	1/2 c	5	215
Millet, whole grain, cooked	1/2 c	3	95
Oatmeal, cooked	1 c	5	155 to 200
Pasta, enriched, cooked	1 c	5 to 7	225 to 230
Rice, cooked	1 c	4 to 5	225
Wheat, bulgur, cooked	1/2 c	7	110
Wheat, cracked, cooked	1/2 c	4	110
Wheat berries, cooked	1/2 c	5	
Starchy vegetables			70
Corn	1 medium ear or 1/2 c	3	115
Peas, fresh	1 c	9	145
Potato, baked	1 large	4	130
Winter squash, baked	1 c	4	
Miscellaneous:			95
Nut butters[a]	1 tbs	4	80 to 115
Nuts[a]	2 tbs	2 to 5	95 to 100
Seeds[a]	2 tbs	3 to 5	40 to 45
Yeast, brewer's	2 tbs	6	

[a]These items are high in fat and should be used in moderation.

Source: Adapted from Society for Nutrition Education materials.

HANDOUT 6-1

Protein Sources

©1994 West Publishing Company

Glycolysis

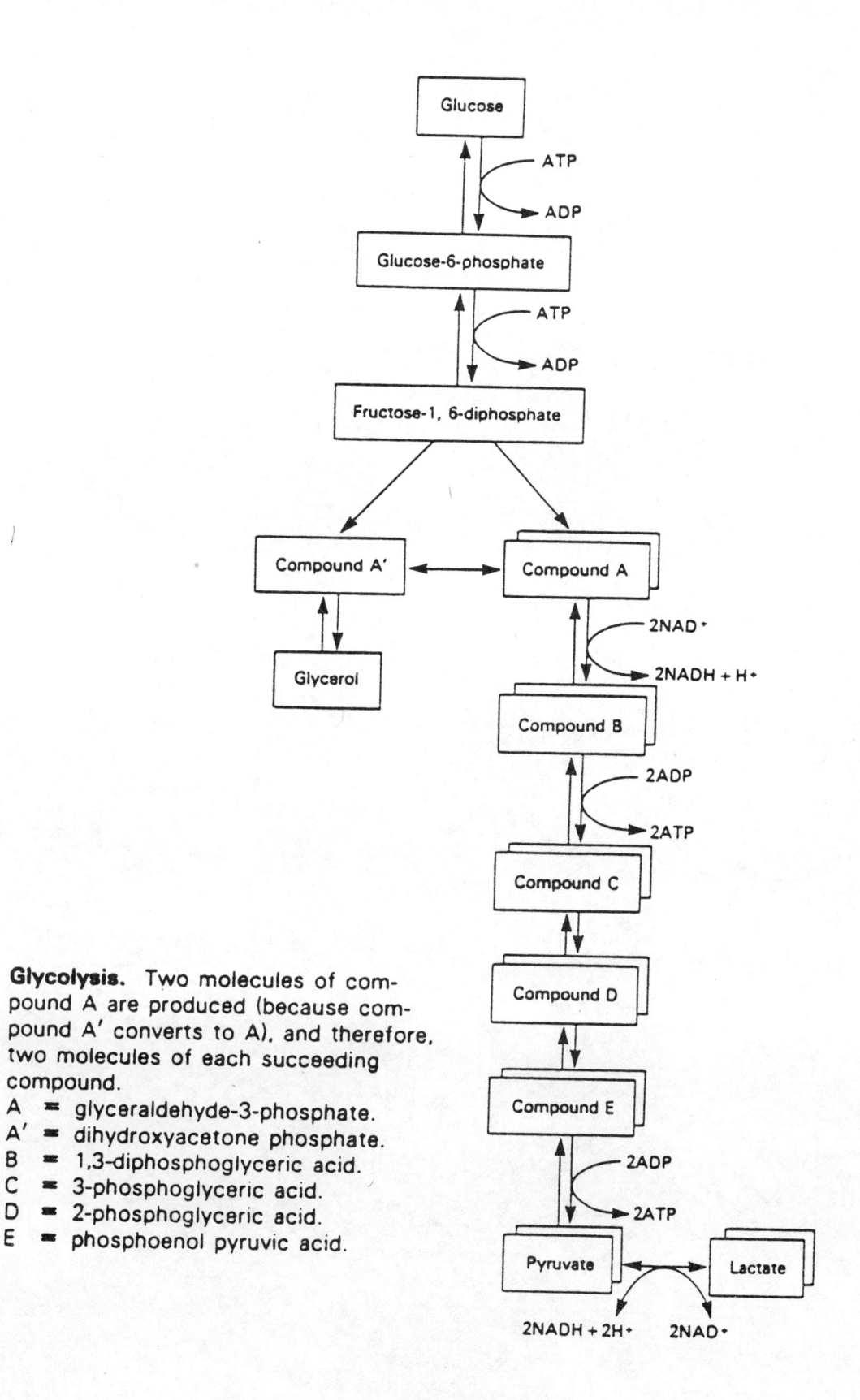

```
                    Glucose
                      ↑↓  ⟶ ATP
                          ⟶ ADP
              Glucose-6-phosphate
                      ↑↓  ⟶ ATP
                          ⟶ ADP
            Fructose-1, 6-diphosphate
                    ↙        ↘
          Compound A' ⟷ Compound A
               ↑↓              ↑↓  ⟶ 2NAD⁺
            Glycerol               ⟶ 2NADH + H⁺
                            Compound B
                              ↑↓  ⟶ 2ADP
                                  ⟶ 2ATP
                            Compound C
                              ↑↓
                            Compound D
                              ↑↓
                            Compound E
                              ↑↓  ⟶ 2ADP
                                  ⟶ 2ATP
                           Pyruvate ⟷ Lactate
                              2NADH + 2H⁺  2NAD⁺
```

Glycolysis. Two molecules of compound A are produced (because compound A' converts to A), and therefore, two molecules of each succeeding compound.

- A = glyceraldehyde-3-phosphate.
- A' = dihydroxyacetone phosphate.
- B = 1,3-diphosphoglyceric acid.
- C = 3-phosphoglyceric acid.
- D = 2-phosphoglyceric acid.
- E = phosphoenol pyruvic acid.

HANDOUT 7-1

Glycolysis

©1994 West Publishing Company

SELF-ASSESSMENT TEST FOR ALCOHOLISM

Give yourself one point for each "yes" answer.

1. Do you feel you are not a normal drinker? (By *normal* we mean you drink less than or only as much as most other people.)
2. Do friends or relatives think you are not a normal drinker?
3. Are you unable to stop drinking when you want to?
4. Does your wife, husband, a parent, or other near relative ever worry or complain about your drinking?
5. Have you ever attended a meeting of Alcoholics Anonymous?
6. Has drinking ever created problems between you and your wife, husband, a parent, or other near relative?
7. Have you ever gotten into trouble at work because of drinking?
8. Have you ever neglected your obligations, your family, or your work for two or more days in a row because you were drinking?
9. Have you ever gone to anyone for help about your drinking?
10. Have you ever been in a hospital because of drinking?
11. Do you ever feel guilty about your drinking?
12. Have you ever been arrested for drunken driving, driving while intoxicated, or driving under the influence of alcoholic beverages?
13. Have you ever been arrested, even for a few hours, because of other drunken behavior?

A score of 0 or 1 indicates no alcohol problem. A score of 2 indicates possible alcoholism, and a score of 3 or more indicates alcoholism. This test is highly accurate but is for screening purposes only. Final diagnosis should be made by an alcoholism expert.

Source: Michigan Alcoholism Screening Test (MAST), developed by Dr. Melvin L. Selzer of the University of Michigan, as cited in Test shows alcoholism, *Tallahassee Democrat,* 29 October 1975, p. 10. There are longer tests, but this short one is valid, detecting from 94 to 99% of people with alcoholism.

HANDOUT 7-2

Self-Assessment for Alcoholism

©1994 West Publishing Company

Medical Problems Associated With Obesity

- Hypertension
- Renal Disease
- Gallbladder Disease
- Diabetes Mellitus
- Pulmonary Disease
- Problems With Anesthesia During Surgery
- Osteoarthritis and Gout
- Breast and Endometrial Cancer
- Abnormal Plasma Lipid and Lipoprotein Concentrations
- Impairment of Cardiac Function
- Menstrual Irregularities and Toxemia of Pregnancy
- Psychological Trauma
- Flat Feet and Infection in Fatfolds
- Organ Compression by Adipose Tissue
- Impaired Heat Tolerance

Source: Art Gilbert, Director, Wellness Fitness Institute, University of California, Santa Barbara, with permission.

HANDOUT 8-1

Medical Problems Associated With Obesity

©1994 West Publishing Company

Eating Attitudes Test

Name _____ Date _____ Age _____
Present Weight _____ Height _____ Gender _____
Highest Past Weight _____ How long ago? _____
Lowest Past Weight _____ How long ago? _____

Answer these questions using the following responses:
A = Always   U = Usually   O = Often
S = Sometimes R = Rarely   N = Never

_____ 1. I am terrified about being overweight.
_____ 2. I avoid eating when I am hungry.
_____ 3. I find myself preoccupied with food.
_____ 4. I have gone on eating binges where I feel that I may not be able to stop.
_____ 5. I cut my food into very small pieces.
_____ 6. I am aware of the calorie content of the foods I eat.
_____ 7. I particularly avoid foods with a high carbohydrate content.
_____ 8. I feel that others would prefer if I ate more.
_____ 9. I vomit after I have eaten.
_____ 10. I feel extremely guilty after eating.
_____ 11. I am preoccupied with a desire to be thinner.
_____ 12. I think about burning up calories when I exercise.
_____ 13. Other people think I am too thin.
_____ 14. I am preoccupied with the thought of having fat on my body.
_____ 15. I take longer than other people to eat my meals.
_____ 16. I avoid foods with sugar in them.
_____ 17. I eat diet foods.
_____ 18. I feel that food controls my life.
_____ 19. I display self-control around food.
_____ 20. I feel that others pressure me to eat.
_____ 21. I give too much time and thought to food.
_____ 22. I feel uncomfortable after eating sweets.
_____ 23. I engage in dieting behavior.
_____ 24. I like my stomach to be empty.
_____ 25. I enjoy trying new rich foods.
_____ 26. I have the impulse to vomit after meals.

Scoring: 3 for never, 2 for rarely, 1 for sometimes, 0 for always, usually and often. Total scores under 20 points indicates abnormal eating behavior.

Source: J. A. McSherry, Progress in the diagnosis of anorexia nervosa, Journal of the Royal Society of Health 106 (1986): 8-9. (Eating Attitudes Test developed by Dr. Paul Garfinkel.)

HANDOUT 8-2
Eating Attitudes Test
©1994 West Publishing Company

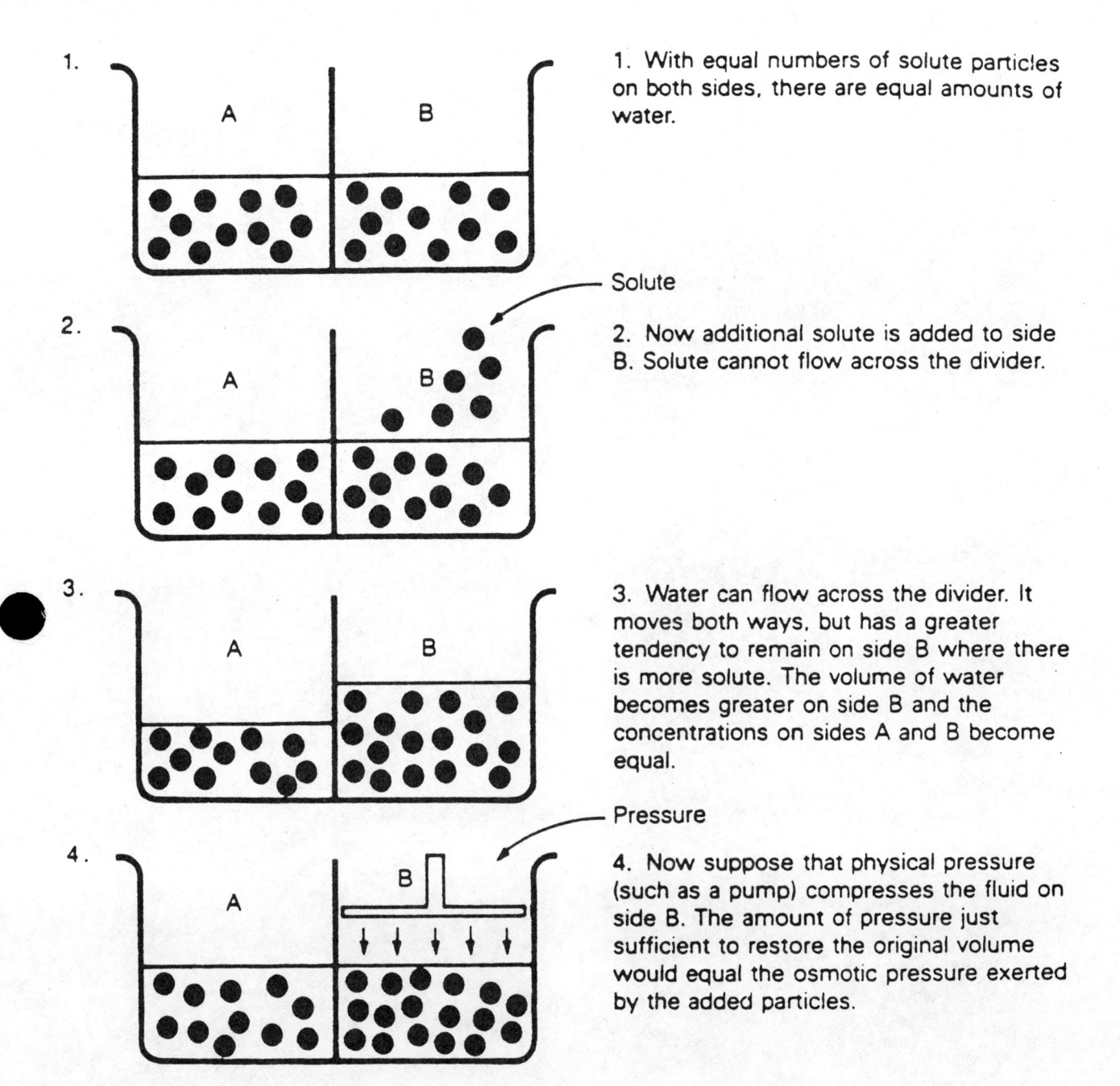

1.

1. With equal numbers of solute particles on both sides, there are equal amounts of water.

— Solute

2.

2. Now additional solute is added to side B. Solute cannot flow across the divider.

3.

3. Water can flow across the divider. It moves both ways, but has a greater tendency to remain on side B where there is more solute. The volume of water becomes greater on side B and the concentrations on sides A and B become equal.

— Pressure

4.

4. Now suppose that physical pressure (such as a pump) compresses the fluid on side B. The amount of pressure just sufficient to restore the original volume would equal the osmotic pressure exerted by the added particles.

HANDOUT 11-1
Osmotic Pressure
©1994 West Publishing Company

```
                    ┌─────────────────┐
                    │ Person can't or │
                    │ won't drink milk│
                    └─────────────────┘
         ┌──────────────────┼──────────────────┐
         ▼                  ▼                  ▼
   ( If allergic to )  ( If lactose    )  ( If unexplained )
   ( cow's milk,    )  ( intolerant,   )  ( intolerance    )
   ( select options )  ( select options)  ( or dislike,    )
   ( with altered   )  ( with altered  )  ( select these   )
   ( protein        )  ( carbohydrate  )
         │                  │                  │
         ▼                  ▼                  ▼
   ┌───────────┐      ┌───────────┐      ┌───────────────┐
   │Boiled milk│      │  Enzyme   │      │Calcium-fortified│
   │or goat's  │      │treated    │      │soy milk       │
   │milk       │      │milk       │      │               │
   └───────────┘      └───────────┘      └───────────────┘
         │                  │                  │
      (and/or)           (and/or)           (and/or)
         │                  │                  │
         ▼                  ▼                  ▼
   ┌───────────┐      ┌──────────────┐   ┌────────────────┐
   │Milk cooked│      │Smaller       │   │Emphasis on foods│
   │into foods │      │portions of   │   │containing the  │
   │           │      │milk more often│  │calcium of milk │
   └───────────┘      └──────────────┘   └────────────────┘
         │                  │                  │
      (and/or)           (and/or)         (Last resort)
         │                  │                  │
         ▼                  ▼                  ▼
   ┌────────────────┐ ┌──────────────┐   ┌───────────┐
   │Emphasis on foods│ │Yogurt and    │   │Nutrient   │
   │containing the  │ │other fermented│   │supplements│
   │calcium of milk │ │dairy products │   └───────────┘
   └────────────────┘ └──────────────┘
         │                  │
    (Last resort)         (and/or)
         │                  │
         ▼                  ▼
   ┌───────────┐      ┌────────────────┐
   │Nutrient   │      │Emphasis on foods│
   │supplements│      │containing the  │
   └───────────┘      │calcium of milk │
                      └────────────────┘
                             │
                        (Last resort)
                             │
                             ▼
                      ┌───────────┐
                      │Nutrient   │
                      │supplements│
                      └───────────┘
```

HANDOUT 11-2

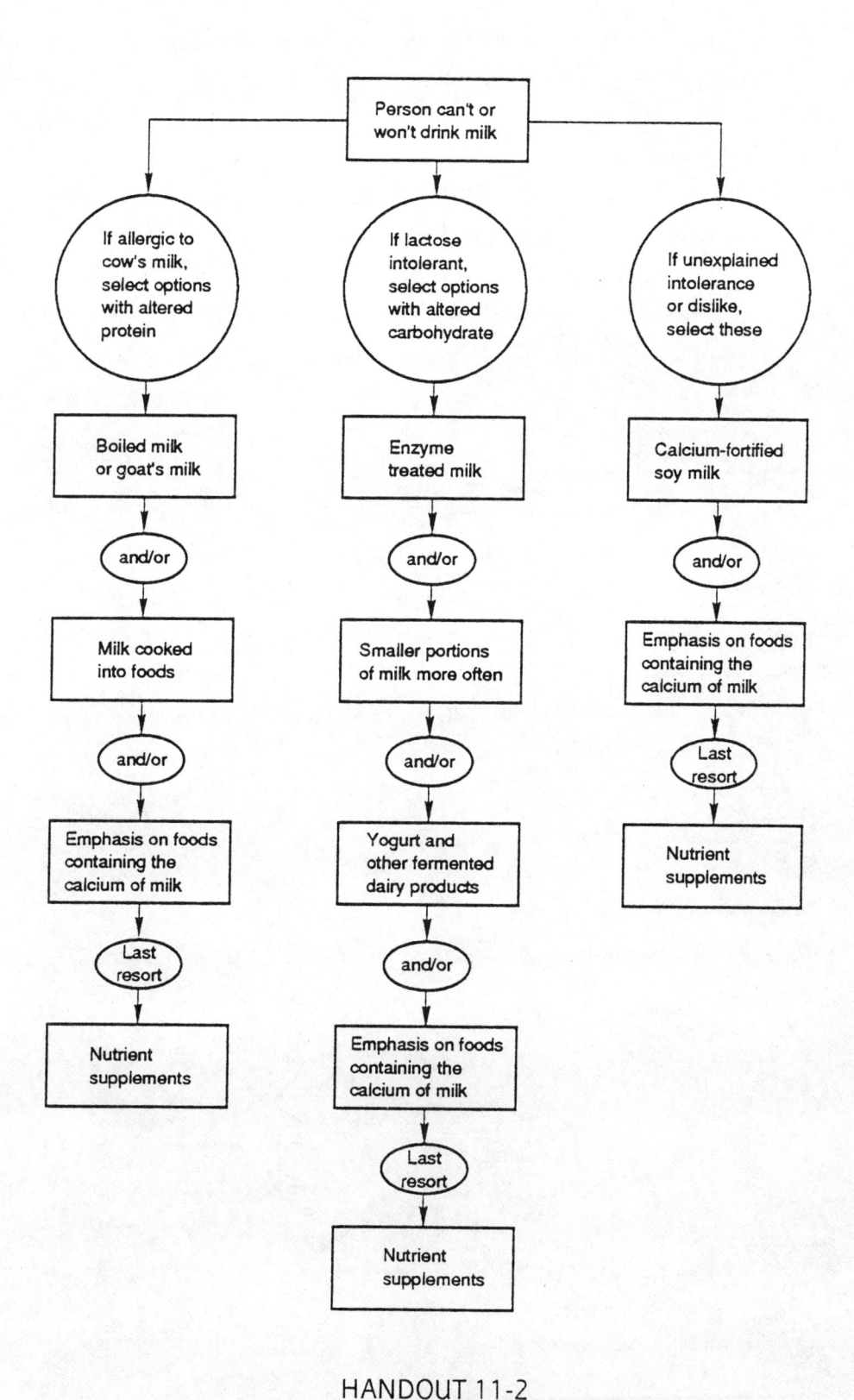

Choosing a Milk Substitute

©1994 West Publishing Company

Ways to Include Exercise in a Day

Join a corporate fitness program; use half of your lunch hour to exercise.

Join a social fitness club.

Develop friendships with people who help one another stay fit.

Play sports in schools; play with children; coach a sport.

Get credit hours for dance, sports, or physical-conditioning courses.

Improve your swim stroke.

Join a nature, hiking, or biking club; join a YMCA program.

Walk to nearby stores.

Park a few blocks from your destination and walk the rest of the way.

Take stairs instead of elevators.

Stretch many times during the day.

Lift small weights, pedal an exercise bike, or row a rowing machine while watching television or talking on the phone.

Garden; mow the lawn with a push mower, do your own vigorous yard work or household chores.

Wash your car with extra vigor.

Bend and stretch to wash your toes in the bath.

HANDOUT 13-1

Ways to Include Exercise in a Day
©1994 West Publishing Company

How to Evaluate a Fitness Program

You can evaluate fitness programs objectively by using your knowledge of what fitness is and how it is gained and maintained. The following are some questions that can help in your evaluation. Start with 100 points and subtract the points indicated for shortcomings.

1. Does the program include sufficient aerobic exercise for cardiovascular fitness (about 20 minutes, three days a week)? If not, *minus 10*.

2. Does the program include exercises that promote muscle strength, such as sit-ups, push-ups, or weight training? If not, minus 5. Are strengthening exercises given for all large muscle groups? If some parts are left out, *minus 5*.

3. Does the program include exercises for flexibility, such as gentle stretches? If not, *minus 10*.

4. Does the program allow for varying initial fitness levels; that is, can you start out slowly and work your way up? If not, *minus 10*.

5. Does the program give adequate exercises within a reasonable time each day--say at least 20 minutes, but less than an hour--at least three days per week? If not, *minus 10*.

6. Does the program include a warm-up period? If no, *minus 10*.

7. Can the program be performed with only basic equipment, such as shoes, small weights, or a jump rope? Must you join an expensive club to participate? If specific or unusual products must be used, or if a large membership fee is required, *minus 10*.

8. Is the program safe? If it suggests bouncy stretches or straight-leg sit-ups, give it a *minus 10*. If it advocates clearly hazardous practices, such as running in heavy or rubber clothing, don't even consider using it, its total score is zero.

9. Does the promoter make only claims backed up by legitimate research? If unorthodox claims are made, such as "no-work fitness," *minus 10*.

10. Does the program promote a lifetime fitness plan based on a variety of enjoyable activities? If the program is monotonous, it will soon become boring and hard to stay with, so give it a *minus 10*.

HANDOUT 13-2

How to Evaluate a Fitness Program

©1994 West Publishing Company

MEAT	Celsius	Fahrenheit
FRESH BEEF		
Rare	60	140*
Medium	71	160
Well Done	77	170
Ground Beef	77	170
FRESH VEAL	77	170
FRESH LAMB		
Medium	77	170
Well Done	82	180
FRESH PORK	77	170
POULTRY		
Chicken	82-85	180-185
Turkey	82-85	180-185
Boneless		
Turkey Roasts	77-80	170-175
Stufing (inside or outside)	74	165
CURED PORK		
Ham, raw		
(cook before eating)	77	170
Ham, fully cooked		
(heat before serving)	60	140
Shoulder		
(cook before eating)	77	170
GAME		
Deer	71-77	160-170
Rabbit	82-85	180-185
Duck	82-85	180-185
Goose	82-85	180-185

*Rare beef is popular, but you should know that cooking it to only 140°F means some food poisoning organisms may survive.

Source: M. A. Parmley, The Safe Food Book, United States Department of Agriculture, Home and Garden Bulletin Number 241, 1984.

HANDOUT 14-1

Safe Internal Temperatures for Meat and Poultry

©1994 West Publishing Company

Nutrient	Deficiency Effect
Energy	Low infant birthweight
Protein	Reduced infant head circumference
Folate	Miscarriage and neural tube defect
Vitamin D	Low infant birthweight
Calcium	Decreased infant bone density
Iron	Low infant birthweight and premature birth
Iodide	Cretinism (varying degrees of mental and physical retardation in the infant)
Zinc	Congenital malformations

Source: Adapted from L. K. DeBruyne and S. R. Rolfes. *Life Cycle Nutrition: Conception through Adolescence*, ed. E. N. Whitney (St. Paul, Minn.: West, 1989), p. 68.

HANDOUT 17-1

Effects of Nutrient Deficiencies During Pregnancy

©1994 West Publishing Company

Supervised Food Activities for Preschoolers

Children's muscle development determines their abilities to perform activities involving foods. The ages listed here are average ages; individual children develop on their own schedules.

A two-year-old can use large muscles of the arms to:

- ☐ scrub vegetables
- ☐ tear lettuce
- ☐ snap beans

A three-year-old can use hand muscles to:

- ☐ wrap foods in foil; wrap cheese slices around bread sticks
- ☐ pour beverages from a small pitcher into a cup
- ☐ mix cereal snacks in a large bowl with clean hands
- ☐ mix bread or muffin batters with a wooden spoon
- ☐ shake juices together in a small, sealed container or make a drink
- ☐ spread peanut butter, cream cheese, or jelly on bread with a dull butter knife or small spatula

A four-year-old can use the small muscles in the fingers to:

- ☐ peel the shells from hard-boiled eggs or the skins from oranges
- ☐ roll out a ball of ground meat or dough with clean hands
- ☐ juice citrus fruit by pushing down and turning the fruit on a hand juicer
- ☐ crack raw eggs by tapping the center of the egg against the side of a bowl
- ☐ mash a bowl of bananas or cooked beans for dip

A five-year-old can use eye-hand coordination to:

- ☐ measure ingredients with measuring spoons and cups
- ☐ cut semisoft foods such as soft cheese or bananas with a dull butter knife and practice keeping fingers away from the blade
- ☐ grind chunky peanut butter or cooked meats in a hand-turned food grinder, or turn a hand-cranked ice cream maker
- ☐ grate carrots or cheese on an upright grater with fingers far from the grater to avoid cuts

Source: Adapted from A.A. Hertzler, Preschoolers' food handling skills--motor development, *Journal of Nutrition Education* 21 (1989): 100B-100C.

HANDOUT 17-2

Supervised Food Activities For Preschoolers

©1994 West Publishing Company

	You probably cannot change these:	You probably can slow or prevent these changes by exercising, maintaining other good health habits, and planning ahead.
Appearance		
Greying of hair	X	
Balding	X	
Drying and wrinkling of skin		X
Nervous System		
Impairment of near vision	X	
Some loss of hearing	X	
Reduced taste and smell	X	
Reduced touch sensitivity	X	
Slowed reaction (reflexes)	X	
Slowed mental function	X	
Mental confusion		X
Cardiovascular System		
Increased blood pressure		X
Increased resting heart rate		X
Decreased oxygen consumption		X
Body Composition/Metabolism		
Increased body fatness		X
Raised blood cholesterol		X
Slowed energy metabolism		X
Other Physical Characteristics		
Menopause (women)	X	
Loss of fertility (men)	X	
Joints: loss of flexibility		X
Loss of teeth; gum disease		X
Bone loss		X
Accident/Disease Proneness		
Accidents		X
Inherited diseases	X	
Lifestyle diseases		X
Psychological/Other		
Reduced self-esteem		X
Loss of sex drive		X
Loss of interest in work		X
Depression, loneliness		X
Reduced financial status		X

HANDOUT 18-1

Changes With Age: Preventable Versus Unavoidable

©1994 West Publishing Company

CANADIAN NUTRITION INFORMATION

Prepared by
MARGARET HEDLEY, M.Sc., R.D.
University of Guelph

CANADIAN NUTRITION INFORMATION

CONTENTS

INTRODUCTION	1
CANADIAN GOVERNMENT DEPARTMENTS AND LEGISLATION	3
SI METRIC UNITS	5
TEACHING CANADIAN INFORMATION: *CHAPTER 1: AN OVERVIEW OF NUTRITION	7
Adjusting for SI Metric Units	7
Nutrition Recommendations in Canada	7
Surveys of Populations	8
HIGHLIGHT 1: WHO SPEAKS ON NUTRITION? THE QUALIFIED VERSUS THE QUACKS	10
Dietitians' Credentials in Canada	10
CHAPTER 2: FOOD CHOICES AND DIET-PLANNING GUIDES	11
Canada's Food Guide to Healthy Eating	11
Good Health Eating Guide	12
Nutrient Enrichment in Canada	12
The Guidelines Applied to Ethnic Diets	16
Self-Study - Calculate Your Nutrient Intakes	16
HIGHLIGHT 2: FOOD LABELS	19
Food Labelling in Canada	19
Nutrition Labelling in Canada	21
CHAPTER 4: THE CARBOHYDRATES: SUGAR, STARCH AND FIBRES	23
Carbohydrate and Dietary Fibre Recommendations	23
Estimating Carbohydrate using Food Groups of Good Health Eating Guide	23
HIGHLIGHT 4: ALTERNATIVES TO SUGAR	26
CHAPTER 5: THE LIPIDS: TRIGLYCERIDES, PHOSPHOLIPIDS, AND STEROLS	27
Recommendations about Fats	27
Estimating Fat using Food Groups of Good Health Eating Guide	28
HIGHLIGHT 5: ALTERNATIVES TO FATS	29

* All subsequent chapters refer to **Teaching Canadian Information**

CHAPTER 6: PROTEIN: AMINO ACIDS	31
Protein and Health	31
Estimating Protein using Food Groups of Good Health Eating Guide	31
Amino Acid Supplements	33
HIGHLIGHT 6: HEALTH ASPECTS OF A MEATLESS DIET	34
HIGHLIGHT 7: ALCOHOL AND NUTRITION	35
CHAPTER 8: ENERGY BALANCE AND WEIGHT CONTROL	37
SI Energy Units	37
Healthy Weights	37
Eating Plans with the Good Health Eating Guide	38
HIGHLIGHT 8: EATING DISORDERS - ANOREXIA AND BULIMIA	40
CHAPTER 9: THE WATER-SOLUBLE VITAMINS: B VITAMINS AND VITAMIN C	41
Vitamins in Canadian Foods	41
Vitamin Recommendations	41
CHAPTER 10: THE FAT-SOLUBLE VITAMINS: A, D, E, AND K	43
Fat-Soluble Vitamins in Canadian Foods	43
HIGHLIGHT 10: VITAMIN AND MINERAL SUPPLEMENTS	44
CHAPTER 11: THE BODY FLUIDS AND THE MAJOR MINERALS	45
Sodium and Potassium Recommendations	45
Sodium Content of Packaged Food	45
Calcium	45
Phosphorus	46
CHAPTER 12: THE TRACE MINERALS	47
Trace Mineral Recommendations	47
Iron Enrichment	47
HIGHLIGHT 12: OUR CHILDREN'S DAILY LEAD	49
CHAPTER 13: FITNESS: PHYSICAL ACTIVITY, NUTRIENTS AND BODY ADAPTATIONS	51
Canadian Programs and Studies	51
HIGHLIGHT 13: SUPPLEMENTS AND ERGOGENIC AIDS ATHLETES USE	53
CHAPTER 14: CONSUMER CONCERNS ABOUT FOODS	55
Food-Borne Illnesses	55
Environmental Contaminants, Natural Toxicants and Pesticides	56
Food Additives and Allergens	56
Food Irradiation	57
Consumer Concerns about Food Safety and Nutrition	58

HIGHLIGHT 14: ENVIRONMENTALLY CONSCIOUS FOODWAYS   58
    Agricultural Methods in Canada   58

CHAPTER 15: NUTRITION ASSESSMENT   59
    SI Units in Nutrition Assessment   59

HIGHLIGHT 15 - U.S. AND WORLD HUNGER   60
    Hunger in Canada   60

CHAPTER 16: NUTRITION CARE STRATEGIES   61
    Diet Manuals in Canada   61

CHAPTER 17: LIFE CYCLE NUTRITION: PREGNANCY, LACTATION AND INFANCY   63
    Canadian Guidelines and Programs   63

HIGHLIGHT 17: FETAL ALCOHOL SYNDROME   65

CHAPTER 18: LIFE CYCLE NUTRITION: CHILDHOOD, ADOLESCENCE, AND THE LATER YEARS   67
    Dietary Fat and Children   67
    School Food Policy   67
    Child Hunger   67
    Programs for the Elderly   68

HIGHLIGHT 18: CAFFEINE: THE BREWING CONTROVERSY   69

HIGHLIGHT 19: DIET AND HEALTH   71
    Nutrition Recommendations   71
    Canadian Consensus Conference on Cholesterol   71
    Health Promotion   71

CHAPTER 26: NUTRITION, DIABETES, AND HYPOGLYCEMIA   73
    Canadian Food Choice System   73

CHAPTER 29: NUTRITION AND WASTING DISORDERS: CANCER AND AIDS   75

HIGHLIGHT 29: HEALTH CARE REFORM, COST CONTAINMENT, AND NUTRITION SERVICES   76

RESOURCE GROUPS   77

REFERENCES   82

CANADIAN INFORMATION

INTRODUCTION

Nutrition education in Canada uses many of the same concepts and principles used in the United States. Different social and political approaches to health and cultural issues have led to differences in government regulations which affect the food supply, nutritional standards and policies which influence the management of nutrition education programs in Canada. Free trade agreements between Canada and the United States will result in more similarities, for example food labels. This section highlights Canadian regulations, standards, programs and resources which affect nutrition, by chapter or topic. Examples of the food group system of the Canadian Diabetes Association Good Health Eating Guide are included. Readings are suggested to support the Canadian perspective for teaching nutrition courses in Canada.

CANADIAN GOVERNMENT DEPARTMENTS AND LEGISLATION

This overview of national government departments identifies general responsibilities. Specific applications of legislation, e.g. nutrition labelling will be described according to the chapters in *Understanding Normal and Clinical Nutrition, Fourth Edition*. The following national departments are involved with the development and administration of food and nutrition regulations. With many issues, several departments work together to develop and administer regulations.

HEALTH CANADA

Health Protection Branch

The Health Protection Branch is responsible for administering the health and safety aspects of the *Food and Drugs Act and Regulations*[1]. This legislation deals with food safety and quality, and economic fraud, and affects nutrient enrichment/composition, food additives, chemical contaminants, microbiological contaminants, nutrition labelling and health claims. The act and regulations are described in the publication, *Health Protection and Food Laws*[2]. The Food Directorate is responsible for program policies and standards related to food safety and nutritional value for the legislation and recommends standards for nutrient intake. It also provides advice on nutrition and food safety for other departments, such as with agricultural chemicals for Agriculture Canada. The Field Operations Directorate promotes compliance with the legislation.

Health Services and Promotion Branch

The **Nutrition Programs Unit, Health Promotion Directorate** promotes sound nutritional practices through implementing the *Nutrition Recommendations* and *Canada's Guidelines for Healthy Eating*, revising *Canada's Food Guide to Healthy Eating* and promoting an integrated approach to healthy weights, of enjoyable healthy eating, enjoyable physical activity, and a positive body image. The unit recommends strategies; analyzes and documents nutrition components of health promotion programs; gives technical and professional advice on nutrition; plans, implements and evaluates projects that involve building professional and institutional support for nutrition programs; and consults and maintains a network of contacts with professional groups, voluntary associations, academic institutions, and health agencies.

Medical Services Branch

The Indian and Northern Health Services Directorate provides health services to the registered Indian and Inuit population of Canada. The nutritionist is with Epidemiology and Community Health Specialties. Nutritionists in the Regional Offices provide public health and health promotion programs to meet the regional needs. Nutrition treatment services are also provided in areas which do not have access to other sources of service, such as provincial or territorial health services.

AGRICULTURE AND AGRI-FOOD CANADA

Food Production and Inspection Branch

Food Production and Inspection Branch, Agriculture and Agri-food Canada administers the *Meat Inspection Act and Regulations, Pest Control Products Act, and Canada Agricultural Products Act and Regulations*. The latter includes regulations for veal and beef grading, dairy products, eggs, fresh fruits and vegetables, honey, maple products, processed poultry and other processed products. This department is also administers the labelling, packaging, and advertising aspects of the *Food and Drugs Act and Regulations* and *Consumer Packaging and Labelling Act*, which had previously been the mandate of Consumer and Corporate Affairs Canada. There is now a single contact in Agriculture and Agri-food Canada which is responsible for food labels and advertisements. Consumer and Corporate Affairs Canada published an interpretation of the legislation and regulations for labelling and advertising foods, *Guide for Food Manufacturers and Advertisers*[3]. This includes the guidelines for nutrition labelling and claims to comply with the *Guidelines in Nutrition Labelling* in the *Food and Drugs Act and Regulations*[1].

Policy Branch

The Policy Branch publishes information on trends in food consumption and food prices, including costs for Nutritious Food Baskets in cities across Canada[4,5]. Since food intakes in Canada are not monitored regularly, this food consumption information is a major source of information on Canadian food intake trends. The Food Industry Development Division of the **Agri-food Development Branch** assists the Canadian agri-food industry to promote development, marketing and consumption of Canadian food products. It publishes research on consumer attitudes to food and food packaging and consumer food trends[6].

FISHERIES AND OCEANS CANADA

Fisheries and Oceans Canada ensures the safety and quality of fish and shellfish products through the administration of the *Fish Inspection Act and Regulations*.

PROVINCIAL, TERRITORIAL AND MUNICIPAL GOVERNMENTS

Health services are the responsibility of the provincial and territorial governments and are implemented at the municipal level. Each of the ten provinces and two territories has specific legislation for the provision of health services and programs. Public health nutrition issues across Canada are identified and discussed by the Network of the Federal/Provincial/Territorial Group on Nutrition. This group is comprised of the chief nutritionists from the provinces and territories and representatives from three branches of Health Canada. Addresses of the group members are listed at the end of this section. The network has supported the development of national guidelines for stages in the lifecycle, such as pregnancy and preschool years.

Public health departments provide health promotion programs, including nutrition education. Local offices provide educational materials, or information on how to get nutrition education resources, to support teaching nutrition in your locality.

SI METRIC UNITS

The Metric Commission of Canada adopted the units of le Système international d'unités (SI) for use by all Canadians. Metric units for volume, length, and weight are the standard measures. The changeover from the Imperial system of quarts, feet, pounds, etc. is a continuing process with units from both systems being used for many labels, signs and publications. Today SI measures of weights or volumes are required on labels and in advertisements, with the Imperial units optional. Health professionals use SI units in their practice, including molar concentrations for laboratory tests. The conversion factors for units which are commonly used by consumers are listed in Appendix D of the textbook.

The joule is the SI unit used for all forms of energy and thus the kilojoule was adopted to replace the kilocalorie as the food energy unit.

1 joule is the energy expended when 1 kg is moved 1 metre by 1 newton.

1 newton is the force which accelerates 1 kg by 1 m per sec^7.

Since consumers have a better understanding of the concept of calories than joules, food labelling and nutrition information for the public uses both units. The following energy units are used by Health Canada.

For all:
  joules (J), kilojoules (kJ), megajoules (MJ)

For the general public:
  kilocalories which are expressed as Calories or Cal.

For scientific/technical purposes:
  kilocalories, kcalories, or kcal

  1 calorie = 4.184 joules

  1 kilocalorie = 4184 J = 4.184 kJ = .004184 MJ

The Mole

In SI Metric, the mole (mol) is the unit for quantifying the amount of substances, replacing milliequivalent or mg/dL.

One mole (mol) of material is its grams divided by its relative atomic or molecular mass.

TEACHING CANADIAN INFORMATION: CHAPTER 1
AN OVERVIEW OF NUTRITION

1.1 ADJUSTING FOR SI METRIC UNITS

a) Convert the weight of human body materials to kilograms. Students could start by converting their own weight from pounds to kilograms using the example in Appendix D as a guide.

Body weight	150 lb =	68 kg
Water	90 lb =	41 kg
Fat	30 lb =	14 kg
Other components	30 lb =	14 kg

b) Define joule and convert energy values from kcalories to kJ. You might provide the preceding information, *SI Metric Units*, in handout form for your students.

1.2 NUTRITION RECOMMENDATIONS IN CANADA

The 1990 Nutrition Recommendations, developed by the Scientific Review Committee for Health and Welfare Canada[8], present the revised Recommended Nutrient Intakes for Canadians (RNI) with the revised Nutrition Recommendations. Advice for preventing individual nutrient deficiencies has been combined with advice on dietary patterns to reduce chronic diseases[9]. This approach was used to produce a single set of recommendations which could be used by all health professionals and health organizations, thus reducing the confusion resulting from several different recommendations. The Nutrition Recommendations for Canadians are printed in Appendix I. You will note that there is no reference to cholesterol in the Nutrition Recommendations. The Scientific Review Committee chose to emphasize decreasing total fat intake and saturated fat as the most important measure for lowering blood cholesterol[8]. It also assumed that dietary cholesterol intake will decrease with the lower fat intake. For the first time, there is a quantitative recommendation for limiting alcohol intake.

Table 1 on pages 28-30 of the Report of the Communications/Implementation Committee summarizes the recommendations which have been directed to the Canadian public from 1977 to 1989[10]. This list demonstrates the potential for confusing the public. To reduce confusion the Nutrition Recommendations have been adopted by health organizations and are included in nutrition education material for health professionals. The report, *Nutrition Recommendations*[8] includes the rationale for the recommendations and a summary of the research related to each of the nutrients, as well as alcohol, aspartame, and caffeine.

The philosophy for establishing the RNI is similar to that for the Recommended Dietary Allowances (RDA). It should be noted that some of the RNI values in Appendix I differ from those published in the summary tables of the first printing of the Nutrition Recommendations[8]. The Appendix I values include the corrections made by Health and Welfare Canada. Most of these corrections were published in the *Journal of The Canadian Dietetic Association*[9].

While the Scientific Review Committee developed the Nutrition Recommendations to be used by the scientific and professional community, the Communications/Implementation Committee (CIC) was translating the scientific statements into Canada's Guidelines for Healthy Eating[10] to communicate the message to consumers. These guidelines are found in Appendix I. The wording of the guidelines focuses on foods and eating suggestions rather than amounts of nutrients. The Committee also completed a thorough review of Canada's Food Guide and recommended a revision to the guide with a new food guidance system to reflect a total diet approach and support the Guidelines for Healthy Eating[11]. *Action Towards Healthy Eating... Technical Report*[12] provides more detailed information about food and nutrition trends in Canada and issues related to developing a food guidance system. The new Canada's Food Guide for Healthy Eating was published in November 1992 and is included in the textbook.

The CIC developed 106 recommendations for a comprehensive and coordinated implementation of Canada's Guidelines for Healthy Eating by all levels of government, nutrition and health professionals and organizations, the food industry, the food services sector, non-governmental organizations, and the public[10]. The strategies for accomplishing the implementation include development of comprehensive food and nutrition policies, multi-sectorial and community-based nutrition intervention programs, nutrition education in schools, worksites, restaurants and supermarkets and nutrition research and surveillance. The key to effective implementation is the adoption of a single set of guidelines plus cooperation and coordination among the stakeholders.

Reading

NIN Rapport, Vol. 5, NO.4 October 1990 includes several articles on the Nutrition Recommendations and comparison between RDA and RNI.

1.3 SURVEYS OF POPULATIONS

Canada does not have data available on food consumption such as HANES and NFCS. The most recent national survey of food intake was Nutrition Canada completed from 1970 to 72. Under the Canadian Heart Health Initiatives, several provincial surveys have been completed.

Since methods of data collection vary with the surveys, the results of these studies cannot be compiled nationally or used for comparisons between regions. Check with your provincial or territorial health department to see if the results for your area are available. The nutrition community is lobbying the federal government for a national nutrition monitoring system.

Some food disappearance data is available from the Policy Branch, Agriculture and Agri-food Canada. This can estimate average food intake at the household level but cannot be used for estimating the intake of individuals.

Reading

Summaries of survey results in Nova Scotia, Quebec and Ontario have been published in *NIN Rapport* Vol. 8, No. 4, 1993.

HIGHLIGHT 1 - WHO SPEAKS ON NUTRITION? THE QUALIFIED VERSUS THE QUACKS

Dietitians' Credentials in Canada

The qualifications for admission to The Canadian Dietetic Association are similar to those for the American Dietetic Association. Although the dietetic associations in Canada are working on the issue, there is no single designation of title, or initials for Canadian dietitians. Provincial government legislation determines the professional designation for health professionals who practise in the province. All provinces include the word "dietitian" or "diététiste" in the title. The following lists the designation for dietitians in each of the provinces:

Alberta	- R.D. (Registered Dietitian)
British Columbia	- R.D.N. (Registered Dietitian Nutritionist)
Manitoba	- R.D. (Registered Dietitian)
New Brunswick	- P.Dt. (Professional Dietitian)
Newfoundland	- R.Dt. (Registered Dietitian)
Nova Scotia	- P.Dt. (Professional Dietitian)
Ontario	- R.D. (Registered Dietitian)
Prince Edward Island	- P.Dt. (Professional Dietitian)
Quebec	- dt.p. (diététiste professionnelle)
Saskatchewan	- P.Dt. (Professional Dietitian)

Addresses for The Canadian Dietetic Association and the provincial associations are listed with the Resources at the end of this Section.

Reading

Benedetti, P. Donsbach's Canadian connection. *Nutrition Forum* 8(1991):30-31. This article describes the dubious credentials and groups involved with promoting nutrition in Canada, including the Nutritional Consultants Organization of Canada and the Canadian Nutrition Institute The latter should not to be confused with the National Institute of Nutrition which is often cited in this Section as a reliable nutrition resource.

TEACHING CANADIAN INFORMATION: CHAPTER 2
FOOD CHOICES AND DIET-PLANNING GUIDES

2.1 CANADA'S FOOD GUIDE TO HEALTHY EATING

Canada's Food Guide to Healthy Eating was introduced in 1992. The new guide is based on Canada's Guidelines for Healthy Eating and includes many of the recommendations of the Health and Welfare Communication Implementation Committee[10]. It uses a total diet approach with a broader range of servings to accommodate individuals with higher nutritional needs. The new guide recognizes the use of foods which don't fit into the four food groups with the "Other foods" category. Canada's Food Guide to Healthy Eating is presented on a two-sided tear sheet, as in Appendix G of the text. You will find the rainbow design handy for emphasizing the grain products and vegetables and fruit food groups. This is particularly useful for athletes with higher energy needs who should include good sources of complex carbohydrate. If you have plastic food models available, use them to teach the concept of serving size. The number of servings recommended from the food groups often appear very high until students realize that their portion size may be equal to two or three "Canada's Food Guide Servings".

The consumer booklet, *Using the Food Guide*, describes the rationale for the Food Guide and how to use the range of servings to meet individual needs. This is an important handout for most nutrition courses since the Food Guide is such an important educational tool. Order copies for your students from your local or provincial public health department.

Food Guide Facts: Background for Educators and Communicators includes fact sheets to help you interpret the information in the guide to your students. The information will help to teach the concepts of the guide and explain reasons for the recommendations. If you expect that your students may teach the Food Guide when they complete their program, you should consider

12   Canadian Information: Chapter 2

ordering copies to give to the students.

An interesting activity is for students to compare Canada's Food Guide to Healthy Eating to the Food Guide Pyramid in the textbook. You will note that the Canadian Guide has a single group for vegetables and fruit, while the Pyramid has separate groups. Students can also compare their food intake for one day to the recommendations of Canada's Food Guide to Healthy Eating.

2.2 GOOD HEALTH EATING GUIDE

The Canadian Diabetes Association Good Health Eating Guide involves a Food Group System using the exchange concept[13]. The food groups and their nutrient content differ from the United States exchange system. Table 2.1 summarizes the energy nutrient content of the food groups. The complete exchange lists for the Good Health Eating Guide are in Appendix G.

If you refer to the exchange lists when teaching about carbohydrates, lipids and proteins, please remind students about the differences for the Good Health Eating Guide. This is especially important for the carbohydrate content for milk, which uses a 1/2 cup (125 mL) serving instead of 1 cup (250 mL) and fruits and vegetables, which is a single group instead of separate groups.

At the time of this printing, the Good Health Eating Guide is in the process of being revised. Check with your local branch of the Canadian Diabetes Association about the status of the revision.

Table 2.1 Energy Nutrient Content of Food Groups in the Good Health Eating Guide[13]

Food Group Choice	Protein (g)	Fat (g)	Carbohydrate (g)	Energy kJ (kcal)
Protein Foods Choice	7	3	-	230 (55)
Starchy Foods	2	-	15	290 (68)
Milk: whole	4	4	6	320 (76)
2%	4	2	6	240 (58)
skim	4	-	6	170 (40)
Fruits and Vegetables	1	-	10	190 (44)
Extra Vegetables	-	-	< 3.5	< 60 (14)
Fats and Oils	-	5	-	190 (44)
Extras	-	-	< 2.6	< 61 (15)

2.3 NUTRIENT ENRICHMENT IN CANADA

The addition of nutrients to foods is mentioned in The Guidelines Applied. Canadian policies on the addition of nutrients are identified here so that you may alert students to the differences early in the course, before they calculate their food intakes. You may want to refer to this information when teaching individual vitamins and minerals in Chapters 10, 11, 12 and 13 or with Chapter 14, Consumer Concerns about Foods.

Canadian Information: Chapter 2   13

The *Food and Drug Regulations*[1] in Canada specify the foods to which nutrients may or must be added and the amounts which may be added. These differ from the amounts of nutrients which are added to foods in the United States. The policy requires or permits the addition of a nutrient to a food when there is need to:[2]

- correct a demonstrated nutrient deficiency in the population using an appropriate food (See Table 2.2);

- replace nutrients which are lost when the food is processed (See Table 1.1); and

- ensure the nutritional quality of products sold as substitutes for traditional foods, e.g. egg substitutes, or as sole sources of nourishment. Nutrient composition of the substitute should be comparable to the food being replaced. Sole sources of nourishment, e.g. meal replacements, infant formulas, or formulated liquid diets must contain essential nutrients, including energy, in amounts related to the purpose of the food (See Table 2.3).

The difference in the enrichment legislation means that the nutrient composition of some foods sold in Canada are significantly different from those sold in the United States. Thus nutrient values from food composition tables and computerized nutrient analysis programs based on United States data do not accurately reflect Canadian foods and nutrient intakes. Breakfast cereals are the most common examples of this variation, especially for vitamins A and D and iron.

Tables 2.2 and 2.3 summarize the foods to which nutrients must or may be added in Canada. These two pages could be used as a student handout.

Table 2.2 Foods to Which Nutrients May Be Added[a]

Foods	Nutrients that <u>must</u> be added	Nutrients that <u>may</u> be added
Alimentary pastes (pasta)	-	Thiamine, riboflavin, niacin or niacinamide, iron.
Apple juice, reconstituted apple juice, grape juice, reconstituted grape juice, pineapple juice, concentrated fruit juice, apple juice and any other fruit juice	-	Vitamin C
Breakfast Cereals	-	Thiamine, niacin, vitamin B_6, folic acid, pantothenic acid, magnesium and iron.
Dehydrated Potatoes	-	Vitamin C
Enriched vitamin B white flour	Thiamine, riboflavin, niacin or niacinamide, iron.	
Flavoured beverage mixes and bases for adding to milk	-	Vitamin A, thiamine, niacin or niacinamide, vitamin C, iron.
Flour, white flour, enriched flour or enriched white flour	Thiamine, riboflavin, niacin, iron.	Vitamin B_6, folic acid, d-pantothenic acid, calcium, magnesium.
Fruit nectars, vegetable drinks and bases and mixes for them, mixture of vegetable juices	-	Vitamin C
Fruit drinks and bases, concentrates and mixes for them, sold as substitutes for fruit juices	Vitamin C	Folic acid, thiamine, iron, potassium
Infant cereal products	-	Thiamine, niacin or niacinamide, riboflavin, iron, calcium, phosphorus, iodine.

[a] Adapted from Health and Welfare Canada. *Departmental Consolidation of the Food and Drugs Act and the Food and Drug Regulations with Amendments to December 30, 1988*, pp 132-133.

Table 2.2 Foods to Which Nutrients May Be Added (Continued)

Foods	Nutrients that <u>must</u> be added	Nutrients that <u>may</u> be added
Goats milk, all forms	-	Vitamin D.
In addition: Skimmed or partly skimmed (fresh, canned or powdered) form	-	Vitamins A and D.
Evaporated - skimmed or partly skimmed	-	Vitamins C, folic acid.
Margarine and other butter substitutes	Vitamins A and D	Alpha-tocopherol.
Milk, all forms including flavoured milks	Vitamin D	-
In addition: Skimmed and partly skimmed (fresh, canned, powdered, flavoured)	Vitamin A	
Canned evaporated	Vitamin C	
Mineral water, spring water, water in sealed containers, prepackaged ice	-	Fluorine
Precooked rice	-	Thiamine, niacin, vitamin B_6, folic acid, pantothenic acid, iron.
Table salt, table salt substitutes	Iodine	

Table 2.3 Substitute and Formulated Foods with Nutrition Standards[b]

Formulated liquid diets
Infant formulas
Meal replacements, whether or not for use in a weight reduction diet
Products simulating whole egg
Ready breakfast, instant breakfast, similar breakfast replacement foods
Simulated meat and poultry products, meat and poultry product extenders

[b] Standards described in Health and Welfare Canada. *Departmental Consolidation of the Food and Drugs Act and the Food and Drug Regulations with Amendments to December 30, 1990.*

2.4 THE GUIDELINES APPLIED TO ETHNIC DIETS

Canada, like the United States, is comprised of people from many nations. Native Indians and the Inuit have been in the country for many centuries. Others nationalities have immigrated more recently, starting with the French and English in the 1700s and followed by other European, Asiatic and African cultures. Each group has brought their food preferences and adapted them to their new homeland, providing a variety of food specialties across the country.

The French Canadians in Quebec enjoy pea soup, tourtière, sugar pie and poutine. The latter is french fried potatoes served with cheese curds and gravy. Newfoundlanders eat cod tongues and brewse. Most provinces have some traditional products for which they are known. Surveys of food consumption trends identify differences in amounts and types of foods consumed in different regions of Canada.

Recent immigration patterns have increased the number of Canadians from different cultural backgrounds. Eating patterns of the immigrants are similar to those described in the textbook. Many Canadians are in various stages of adapting their ethnic food habits to the foods and eating styles of this country. Nutrition classes are often comprised of students from a variety of ethnic backgrounds. Group projects on different cultural food patterns can help students gain a better understanding about different eating habits and their nutritional implications.

Health promotion for native people focuses on encouraging healthy selection of common native foods, including sea and land animals, supporting their cultural heritage. These programs use specially designed educational materials with pictures and food models using country foods and available store foods. Videos, audiotapes, and written materials are produced in the various native languages. In the North West Territories materials are requested in their 8 official languages. The Department of Health for the Northwest Territories and the Regional Offices for the Medical Services Branch are sources of information about nutrition education projects which support the cultural eating patterns of native people.

Readings

National Institute of Nutrition *Rapport* Vol. 9, No. 1, Winter 1994. Nutritional Health of Canada's Aboriginal Peoples.

Organization for Nutrition Education BULLETIN, Vol. 9, No. 3, Spring, 1990 is based on the theme, Nutrition Education in the Multicultural Community.

2.5 SELF-STUDY - CALCULATE YOUR NUTRIENT INTAKES

Because this self-study or a similar exercise is important for applying and reinforcing nutrition knowledge, it is important that nutrient intake values are as accurate as possible. Several adaptations can increase the accuracy for Canadian students.

Variations in nutrient composition of foods

a) Use Canadian nutrient composition data. *Nutrient Value of Some Common Foods*[14] provides data for many of the foods regularly consumed in Canada and can be purchased from the Canadian Government Publishing Centre. The publication is based on the Canadian Nutrient

Canadian Information: Chapter 2   17

Data File which is described in two articles in the *Journal of The Canadian Dietetic Association*[15,16]. A number of computer nutrient analysis programs based on the Canadian Nutrient Data File are also available.

b) Use the United States nutrient composition data, substituting nutrient values from nutrition labelling for breakfast cereals, and carefully selecting the appropriate foods, e.g. fortified milk, without added solids. Students should refer to the RDI on Table H2.1 on the Nutrition Labelling handout for estimating amounts of vitamins and minerals listed on the label. This method lets students use either Appendix H in the textbook or *West Diet Analysis '91* to complete this exercise. It also teaches students how to use Canadian nutrition labelling, which is described in Highlight 2 of this section. The resulting analysis may not be quite as accurate as the method using Canadian nutrient data because it does not consider other differences in food composition, e.g. fat content of meats.

Analysis of Energy Intake

It is important for Canadian students to be familiar with kilojoules as a unit of food energy. If Canadian nutrient data is used in the self-study exercise, energy values will be available in both calories and kilojoules. The Self-Study Form could be adapted by adding an additional energy column for kilojoules or substituting kilojoules for calories. If United States nutrient data is used, kilojoules could be calculated for each food or for the total energy intake, using the formula 1 kcal. = 4.184 kJ (or 4.2 kJ). The Self-Study Form could be adapted accordingly.

Analysis of Niacin Intake

Since the Recommended Nutrient Intake for niacin is stated in **niacin equivalents**, the analysis of the niacin intake should use this unit, especially if niacin intake appears low. The Canadian Nutrient Data File uses niacin equivalents for describing niacin content of foods[14] Niacin content of foods in Appendix H and in the *West Diet Analysis '91* nutrient data is expressed as mg niacin. As suggested in Chapter 9, point 3 of Evaluate your Water-soluble Vitamin Intake, niacin equivalents from protein can be estimated from the protein intake in excess of the protein RNI.

The following example shows the calculations to estimate the additional niacin equivalents from protein.

Total protein intake	80 g
Protein RNI	55 g
	===
Estimated "leftover" protein	25 g
Potential tryptophan available (25 g/100)	.25 g or 250 mg
Potential niacin from tryptophan (250 mg/60)	4.2 mg or NE

Comparison to Standard

Nutrient intakes for Canadian students should be compared to the 1990 RNI. *West Diet Analysis '91* is available in a Canadian version with the 1990 RNI. If manual calculation of RNI is preferred, the following points should be considered to allow for individual variations.

- For more accurate estimates for individual RNI, students should calculate RNI for energy, based on kcal/kg or MJ/kg from Table 1 in Appendix I, and protein based on 0.86 g/kg body weight.

- The RNI for vitamin B_6 is based on 0.015 mg/g dietary protein intake and requires individual calculation since no example is included the tables of examples in Appendix I.

- The RNI for thiamin, riboflavin, and niacin are based on energy expenditure. For students who have unusually high energy expenditures, as indicated by a high energy intake or activity level, the RNI for these B vitamins can be calculated using the following:

Thiamin	0.40 mg/1000 kcal	0.48 mg/5000 kJ
Riboflavin	0.5 mg/1000 kcal	0.6 mg/5000 kJ
Niacin	7.2 NE/1000 kcal	8.6 NE/5000 kJ

HIGHLIGHT 2 - FOOD LABELS

Food Labelling in Canada

Food labelling in Canada is regulated under the *Food and Drugs Act and Regulations*. Agriculture and Agri-food Canada enforces the food labelling regulations. The *Consumer Packaging and Labelling Act and Regulations*, administered by Agriculture and Agri-food Canada, also applies to food packaging and labels. The Guidelines on Nutrition Labelling are printed in Annex E of the *Guide for Food Manufacturers and Advertisers*[3]. Regulations for making nutrition claims are described in Part C of that publication. All label information required by the regulations must appear in both English and French. The article *Nutrition Labelling of Foods: A Global Perspective*[17] compares the proposed regulations for the United States (1990) with the regulations for Canada, the European Community and Codex Alimentarius.

Ingredient Labelling

Food ingredients are listed, using their common name, in descending order of proportion or percentage of the packaged product. For some foods, such as vegetable oils or spices, the class rather than the common name is permitted. If an ingredient is optional or can be substituted for another one in a product, the label must list all the ingredients that are likely to be used in the product within a one-year period. The label must indicate that all of these specific ingredients may not be present in each package of the food. This is often seen on cracker labels when the source of oil or fat varies with the market.

Biological Role of Nutrients

The *Food and Drugs Act and Regulations* specifies the nutrients for which claims of the biological activity are permitted. The biological role claims may include generally accepted functions of nutrients associated with maintaining normal metabolism and good health, with the precise wording at the discretion of the manufacturer. Drug-like claims or claims pertaining to the prevention, treatment of cure of a disease are not permitted. The nutrient content of a serving of the food must be included under "Nutrition Information" when a biological role claim is made. Regulations for making health claims for foods on labels or in advertising in Canada are more restrictive than those in the United States.

Food Labelling and Advertising

Regulations for food advertising are similar to those for food labelling and more restrictive than those in the United States. Since many Canadians have access to United States radio and television stations, it is often difficult to know the source of the commercial. Students enjoy learning about the Canadian regulations by comparing commercials from each country.

Teaching Canadian Nutrition Labelling

The information on nutrition labelling starts on a new page so that it can be copied as a student handout. An example of a food label which complies with the labelling regulations is included as a Handout at the end of this Section.

Using Food Labels to Choose Foods for Healthy Eating is a useful handout when teaching about food labels. Copies are available from the Regional Offices of the Health Protection Branch, Health Canada. Addresses and phone numbers for these offices are under Resource Groups at the end of this section. Look for the sample Canadian label and nutrition information at the end of this section. Students should be encouraged to collect and/or discuss interesting food labels. Many enjoy finding labels which do not comply with the regulations.

Additional Resources on Nutrition Labelling and Claims

Consumer and Corporate Affairs Canada. *Guide to Nutrition Labelling*. Ottawa: Supply and Services Canada, 1991. A free pamphlet available from the Regional Office of Consumer and Corporate Affairs Canada and suitable as a student handout.

Available from Food Directorate, Health Protection Branch, Health Canada:
Guidelines for Health Information Programs Involving the Sale of Foods and General Principles for Labelling Advertising Claims that Relate to the Nutrition Recommendations.

Reid, D.J. and Hendricks, S. Consumer awareness of nutrition information on food package labels. *J Can Diet Assoc* 54(1993):127-131.

NUTRITION LABELLING IN CANADA

Nutrition labelling in Canada is voluntary for food manufacturers. It is displayed under the heading of "Nutrition Information", followed by the serving size in grams or millilitres. The equivalent household measure, e.g. cup, or common unit, e.g. slice, may also be given. The amount of each of the declared nutrients is then listed for the stated serving size. If the manufacturer chooses to make a nutrition claim on the label of a product, or in an advertisement, the regulations on how to list the claim must be followed. For some nutrition claims a "Nutrition Information" section is not required.

- **Core List** - The minimum information required for nutrition labelling is the core list:
    Energy - in both Calories (Cal) and kilojoules (kJ)
    Protein - in grams (g)
    Fat - in grams (g)
    Carbohydrate - in grams (g)

- **Sodium and Potassium** - If one of these minerals is declared, both sodium and potassium content (mg) are to be listed following the core list.

- **Fatty Acids and Cholesterol** - If any of the following are declared, the content of each of the following must be listed under fat: polyunsaturates (g), monounsaturates (g), saturates (g), cholesterol (mg). Linoleic acid contents (g) is the only single fatty acid which may be declared and then it must be accompanied by the other four fat components. Trans fatty acids are not included in the components or listed separately.

- **Carbohydrate Components** - The declaration of carbohydrates is based on the total carbohydrate, including dietary fibre. The content of one or more of the carbohydrate components (g), e.g. sugars, starch, may be declared following the declaration of total carbohydrates.

- **Vitamins and Minerals** - The content of a vitamin or mineral may be declared if a Recommended Daily Intake (RDI) has been established for that nutrient if it is expressed as percent of the RDI. (See Table H2.1)

Descriptive Claims

Criteria for descriptive claims have been developed so that labels can provide useful information for consumers without being misleading. When these claims are made, the amount of the nutrient must also be presented as "Nutrition Information". The criteria include:

- **fat, fatty acids and cholesterol content**
    "**low fat**" - not more than 3 g fat per serving and not more than 15% fat in dry matter
    "**low saturates**" - not more than 2 g saturated fatty acids per serving and not more than 15% energy from saturated fatty acids
    "**low cholesterol**" - not more than 20 mg cholesterol per serving and per 100 g, and low in saturated fatty acids
    "**cholesterol free**" - not more than 3 mg cholesterol per 100 g and low in saturated fatty acids

- **dietary fibre content**
  "**source**" or "**moderate source**" - at least 2 g per serving
  "**high source**" - at least 4 g serving
  "**very high source**" - at least 6 g per serving

- **vitamin and mineral content** per serving
  "**contains**"of "**source**" - at least 5% RDI
  "**high**" or "**good source**" - at least 15% (vitamin C - 30%) RDI
  "**very high**" or "**excellent source**" - at least 25% (vitamin C - 50%) RDI

Criteria are also specified for the use of the following terms:
  "low", "light in" or "free" for energy, fat, sugar, sodium/salt
  "gluten-free"
  "no sugar added", "unsweetened", "no salt added", "unsalted"
  "lean"
  "light/lite", "Calorie-reduced", "low-Calorie"

Table H2.1 Reference Standard for Nutritional Labelling

Recommended Daily Intakes (RDI)*

Nutrient	RDI for Persons 2 years of age or older	RDI for Infants or Children less that 2 years of age
Vitamin A	1000 RE	400 RE
Vitamin D	5 mcg	10 mcg
Vitamin E	10 mg	3 mg
Vitamin C	60 mg	20 mg
Thiamine	1.3 mg	0.45 mg
Riboflavin	1.6 mg	0.55 mg
Niacin	23 NE	8 NE
Vitamin B_6	1.8 mg	0.7 mg
Folacin	220 mcg	65 mcg
Vitamin B_{12}	2 mcg	0.3 mcg
Pantothenic acid	7 mg	2 mg
Calcium	1100 mg	500 mg
Phosphorus	1100 mg	500 mg
Magnesium	250 mg	55 mg
Iron	14 mg	7 mg
Zinc	9 mg	4 mg
Iodide	160 mcg	55 mcg

* based on the **Recommended Nutrient Intakes for Canadians, 1983.**

Source: Tables to Divisions 1 and 2, Part D, *Food and Drugs Act and Regulations*, Health and Welfare Canada, 1988. Reprinted with permission.

TEACHING CANADIAN INFORMATION: CHAPTER 4
THE CARBOHYDRATES: SUGAR, STARCH AND FIBRES

4.1 CARBOHYDRATE AND DIETARY FIBRE RECOMMENDATIONS

The 1990 Nutrition Recommendations state that "the Canadian diet should provide 55% of energy as carbohydrate (138 g/1000 kcal or 165 g/5000 kJ) from a variety of sources"[8]. They recommend including sources of carbohydrate which provide complex carbohydrates and a variety of dietary fibre. There is no numerical recommendation for dietary fibre. However, the recommendations assume that the increase in carbohydrate intake will lead to the desired increase in dietary fibre intake. It is recommended that any increase in dietary fibre be a gradual one. *Canada's Guidelines for Healthy Eating*[10] encourage an increased dietary fibre intake by promoting the intake of cereals, breads, other grain products, vegetables and fruits. The guidelines for claims on dietary fibre content are based on the Report of the Expert Committee on Dietary Fibre[18].

4.2 ESTIMATING CARBOHYDRATE USING FOOD GROUPS OF GOOD HEALTH EATING GUIDE

The food groups for the Good Health Eating Guide[13] are different from the Exchange lists. Thus there is a difference in carbohydrate content of the food groups and sample day's intake. Table 2.1 of this section shows the carbohydrate content for each of the food groups. Students who are required to learn the Good Health Eating Guide food groups system could estimate the carbohydrate content of the day's intake in Figure 4-13 of the textbook, using the system. Table 4.1 shows the estimates using the Good Health Eating Guide.

Table 4.1 Estimating Carbohydrate Intake Using the Good Health Eating Guide

Food Intake	Food Group Choices[a]	Carbohydrate (g)
Breakfast 2 shredded wheat biscuits 1 c 1% low-fat milk 1/2 banana sliced (6 in.)	2 starchy foods choices 2 milk choices 1 fruits & vegetables choice	30 12 10

Lunch
 1   turkey sandwich:
      2 slices whole-wheat bread
      2 oz turkey (50 g)
      1 tsp mayonnaise
      1 tsp mustard
 1 c   vegetable juice (canned)
	
	 2 starchy foods choices
	 2 protein foods choices
	 1 fats & oils choices
	 Extras
	 1 fruits & vegetables choices
		
		 30
		 -
		 -
		 -
		 10

Afternoon Snack 4 whole-wheat crackers 1 oz cheddar cheese (25 g) 1 apple	1 starchy foods choice 1 protein foods choice 2 fruits & vegetable choices	15 - 20

Dinner
 Salad:
 1 c   raw spinach leaves, shredded
      carrots, and sliced mushrooms
 1/3 c   garbanzo beans
 5 lg   olives
 1 tbsp ranch dressing
 Entrée:
 1 c   spaghetti with meat sauce
      1 c pasta (cooked)
      1 c tomato sauce
      3 oz ground round (75 g)
 1/2 c   green beans
 2 tsp   butter
 Dessert:
 1 1/4 c strawberries (fresh)
	
	 1 extra vegetables choice
	
	 2/3 starchy foods choice
	 1 fats & oils choice
	 1 fats & oils choice
	
	 2 starchy foods choices
	 1 fruit & vegetables choice
	 3 protein foods choices
	 1 extra vegetables choice
	 2 fats & oils choices
	
	 1 1/4 fruits & vegetable choices
		
		 < 3.5
		
		 10
		 -
		 -
		
		 30
		 10
		 -
		 < 3.5
		 -
		
		 12.5

Bedtime Snack 3 graham crackers 1 c 1% low-fat milk	1 starchy food choice 2 milk choices	15 12
Day's Total		223.5

[a] Based on Food Group Choices from Canadian Diabetes Association Good Health Eating Guide[13]

The fibre content of the food groups in Figure 4-16 in the textbook should be adjusted for the serving sizes of the Good Health Eating Guide groups. The major difference will be for the fruits in the fruits in the fruits and vegetables group.

Canadian Reading on Starch

National Institute of Nutrition. *Starch in Human Nutrition*. NIN Review No. 15, October 1990.

Canadian Information

HIGHLIGHT 4 - ALTERNATIVES TO SUGAR

This highlight presents the regulation status of artificial sweeteners in both Canada and the United States. Note in the Glossary of Alternative Sweeteners, the difference in status for acesulfame potassium, cyclamate, saccharin and sucralose. Sucralose is available as SPLENDA Brand Sweetener, as an industrial ingredient, and SPLENDA Low-Calorie Sweetener for the tabletop in granular and packet form. Information on sucralose is available from the SPLENDA Information Centre, P.O. Box 1390, Guelph, Ontario N1H 7L4.

TEACHING CANADIAN INFORMATION: CHAPTER 5
THE LIPIDS: TRIGLYCERIDES, PHOSPHOLIPIDS, AND STEROLS

5.1 RECOMMENDATIONS ABOUT FATS

The 1990 Nutrition Recommendations state that "The Canadian diet should include no more than 30% energy as fat" and "no more than 10% as saturated fat"[8]. They also recommend that n-6 fatty acids be at least 3% of energy and n-3 fatty acids at least 0.5% of energy with a ratio of n-6 to n-3 fatty acids in the range of 4:1 to 10:17.

The Joint Working Group of the Canadian Paediatric Society and Health Canada published their report *Nutrition Recommendations Update... Dietary Fat and Children*[19] in 1993. This addresses the appropriateness of restricting the fat intake of growing children. The Working Group concluded[19]:

1. Providing adequate energy and nutrients to ensure adequate growth and development remains the most important consideration in the nutrition of children. Small frequent feedings play a significant role in providing energy in the diets of children.

2. During the preschool years nutritious food choices should not be eliminated or restricted because of fat content. During early adolescence an energy intake adequate to sustain growth should be emphasized with a gradual lowering of fat intake. Once linear growth has stopped, fat intake as currently recommended is appropriate.

3. Food patterns which emphasize variety, complex carbohydrate and include lower fat choices are appropriate and desirable for children.

28   Canadian Information: Chapter 5

    4. Physical activity and healthy eating are important lifestyle habits for children.

The following recommendations were made[19]:

    From the age of two until the end of linear growth, there should be a transition from the high fat diet of infancy to a diet which includes no more than 30% energy as fat and no more than 10% of energy as saturated fat.

    During this transition, energy intake should be sufficient to achieve normal growth and development. Food patterns should emphasize variety and complex carbohydrate, and include lower fat foods. Physical activity should be stressed.

You may introduce this report during this chapter or with Chapter 18, Lifecycle Nutrition: Childhood, Adolescence, and the Later Years.

5.2 ESTIMATING FAT USING FOOD GROUPS OF GOOD HEALTH EATING GUIDE

It is possible to estimate the fat content, using the Good Health Eating Guide. To estimate the fat content of the Starchy Foods Group, note the list which identifies foods for which a fats and oils choice must be added, e.g. cookies and muffins. For the Protein Foods Groups, one list identifies choices which contain extra fat, but do not estimate the amount. The estimate for fat intake on Figure 5-21 in the textbook would be similar, using the Canadian system.

HIGHLIGHT 5 - ALTERNATIVES TO FATS

Regulation status of alternatives to fat in Canada is similar to the United States. Look on the labels of low-fat and fat-free products to see if a fat alternative has been used. Starch derivatives are often used to improve the texture of the lower fat products.

TEACHING CANADIAN INFORMATION: CHAPTER 6
PROTEIN: AMINO ACIDS

6.1 PROTEIN AND HEALTH

Nutrition Recommendations[8] address the issue of protein recommendations beyond the level of preventing protein deficiency. The recommended safe and adequate level of protein intake is 0.86 g/kg BW. This is the level which minimizes the risk of a deficiency. However, the current average protein intake in Canada is considerably higher. Because there is no evidence that this higher intake has damaging effects on healthy individuals, the committee emphasized maintaining current patterns of protein intake rather than making drastic changes to the lower safe intake. The recommended proportion of protein is 13-15% of energy throughout adulthood, with an increase for female seniors to 15-20% of energy.

6.2 ESTIMATING PROTEIN USING FOOD GROUPS OF GOOD HEALTH EATING GUIDE

Since the protein content of the food groups in the Good Health Eating Guide is different from the United States Exchange Lists, you could have students to complete the estimate using the Canadian groups. One estimate is seen in Table 6.1.

Table 6.1 Estimating Protein Intake Using the Good Health Eating Guide

Food Intake	Food Group Choices[a]	Protein (g)
Breakfast		
2 shredded wheat biscuits	2 starchy foods choices	4
1 c 1% low-fat milk	2 milk choices	8
1/2 banana sliced (6 in.)	1 fruits & vegetables choice	1
Lunch		
1 turkey sandwich:		
2 slices whole-wheat bread	2 starchy foods choices	4
2 oz turkey (50 g)	2 protein foods choices	14
1 tsp mayonnaise	1 fats & oils choices	-
1 tsp mustard	Extras	-
1 c vegetable juice (canned)	1 fruits & vegetables choices	1
Afternoon Snack		
4 whole-wheat crackers	1 starchy foods choice	2
1 oz cheddar cheese (25 g)	1 protein foods choice	7
1 apple	2 fruits & vegetable choices	2
Dinner		
Salad:		
1 c raw spinach leaves, shredded carrots, and sliced mushrooms	1 extra vegetables choice	-
1/3 c garbanzo beans	2/3 starchy foods choice	2
5 lg olives	1 fats & oils choice	-
1 tbsp ranch dressing	1 fats & oils choice	-
Entrée:		
1 c spaghetti with meat sauce		
1 c pasta (cooked)	2 starchy foods choices	4
1 c tomato sauce	1 fruit & vegetables choice	1
3 oz ground round (75 g)	3 protein foods choices	21
1/2 c green beans	1 extra vegetables choice	-
2 tsp butter	2 fats & oils choices	-
Dessert:		
1 1/4 c strawberries (fresh)	1 1/4 fruits & vegetable choices	1
Bedtime Snack		
3 graham crackers	1 starchy food choice	2
1 c 1% low-fat milk	2 milk choices	8
Day's Total		82

[a] Based on Food Group Choices from Canadian Diabetes Association Good Health Eating Guide[13]

With the emphasis on reducing fat intake and nutrition recommendations encouraging a decreased intake of red meat, some health professionals have been recommending cutting out all red meat or all animal products. The National Institute of Nutrition managed a project to review scientific literature concerning the relationships of red meat and health. The summary of the report, written by Dr. J. Henderson Sabry was published in the NIN Review[20]. The report concluded that moderate intake of lean meat is not a major contributor to chronic diseases in Canada, such as heart disease, cancer, and osteoporosis.

6.3 AMINO ACID SUPPLEMENTS

The regulatory status of single amino acids supplements in Canada is addressed in the textbook. Athletes continue to use amino acid supplements. A recent study of amino acid preparations sold in Canada indicated that the single amino acid content was not consistent with package labelling[21]. The following article by Houston helps put the use of amino acid supplements in perspective.

Canadian Reading

Houston, M.E. Single Amino Acids as Supplements. SPORT MED INFO, Sport Medicine Council of Canada, Ottawa, 1990.

Canadian Information

HIGHLIGHT 6 - HEALTH ASPECTS OF A MEATLESS DIET

The following readings provide some Canadian perspectives on the health aspects of vegetarianism and eating meat and fish.

Canadian Readings

National Institute of Nutrition. *Risks and Benefits of Vegetarian Diets.* NIN Review No.12, January 1990.

National Institute of Nutrition. *Nutritional Aspects of Fish Consumption in Canada.* NIN Review No.16, January 1991.

HIGHLIGHT 7 - ALCOHOL AND NUTRITION

The Nutrition Recommendations for Canadians state that "The Canadian diet should include no more than 5% of total energy as alcohol, or two drinks daily, whichever is less."[8] This indicates the need to limit alcohol intake. The rationale for the recommendation is described on pp. 181-2 of *Nutrition Recommendations*[8]. This is especially important to discuss in relation to pregnancy and fetal alcohol syndrome.

TEACHING CANADIAN INFORMATION: CHAPTER 8
ENERGY BALANCE AND WEIGHT CONTROL

8.1 SI ENERGY UNITS

This chapter focuses on energy units involved with energy balance, using kcalories both as a unit and the term for energy. Since both kilocalories and kilojoules are used in Canada, you may choose the most appropriate terms for teaching energy concepts. If the students are likely to be involved in health care, e.g. dietetics, nursing, etc., it may be appropriate to use kilojoules in calculations and the term "energy" to replace kcalories. Refer to the SI Metric Units, earlier in this Canadian Information Section. These students might practise thinking in kilojoules by estimating their BMR and exercise energy output in kilojoules.

8.2 HEALTHY WEIGHTS

The Body Mass Index (BMI) was adopted by Health and Welfare Canada for assessing health risk from body composition to replace the concept of a single ideal weight[22]. This concept is used in many health promotion programs in Canada. The interpretation of the BMI in Canada is different from that described in Chapter 8.

38   Canadian Information: Chapter 8

Table 8.1 Interpretation of BMI for Evaluation of Weight[22,23]

Under 20   A BMI under 20 may be associated with health problems for some individuals. It may be a good idea to consult a dietitian and physician, especially if there has been a sudden decline in BMI.

20 - 25   This zone is associated with lowest risk of illness for most people. This is a "generally acceptable range" of weight for health.

25 - 27   A BMI over 25 may be associated with health problems for some people. Caution is suggested if your BMI is in this zone. This is a "generally acceptable range" of weight for health.

Over 27   A BMI over 27 is associated with increased risk of health problems such as heart disease, high blood pressure and diabetes. It maybe a good idea to consult a dietitian and physician for advice.

The Expert Committee on Weight Standards also recommended that health professionals also use Waist-Hip Ratio as an indicator of fat distribution when assessing health risk with BMI[22]. The committee also noted that the BMI is not appropriate to use for pregnant women, children and trained athletes and may have limitations for adolescents and adults over 65 years. Issues related to body weight and prevention of weight problems are also addressed in *Promoting Healthy Weights: A Discussion Paper*[24]. These publications are valuable resources to support teaching "Healthy Weights" with this chapter. Some provincial health ministries have published pamphlets which can be used as handouts for this topic.

The Health Services and Promotion Branch, Health Canada introduced the *Vitality* in 1991. This program has three components: enjoyable, healthy eating; enjoyable, physical activity; and positive self and body image. This program involves providing information and promoting activities which support the three components. Additional information about *Vitality* is available from the Health Promotion Directorate, (613) 957-8328.

8.3 EATING PLANS WITH THE GOOD HEALTH EATING GUIDE

A sample eating plan using the Good Health Eating Guide[13] will be different from the plan in Table 8-10 of the textbook. Table 8.2 shows a plan which provides approximately 1400 kcal (5880 kJ) using the Canadian system.

Table 8.2 A Sample Weight-Loss Program Using Good Health Eating Guide[13]

Food Choice	Number of Choices	Carbohydrate (g)	Protein (g)	Fat (g)	Energy kJ (kcal)
Starchy Foods	7	105	14	-	2030 (476)
Protein Foods	5	-	35	24	1150 (275)
Fruits & Vegetables	6	60	6	-	1140 (264)
Extra Vegetables	2	7	-	-	120 (28)
Milk (Skim)	4	24	16	-	680 (160)
Fats & Oils	4	-	-	20	760 (180)
Total		196	64	41	5880 (1382)

Canadian Readings

Canadian Dietetic Association. *Healthy Weight in '88: A Resource Manual for Health Professionals*. Toronto: The Canadian Dietetic Association, 1987.

McCargar, L.J. The effects of weight cycling on metabolism and health. *J Can Diet Assoc* 52(1991):101-106.

National Institute of Nutrition. *Metabolic Consequences of Weight-Reduction Diets*. NIN Review No.6, July 1988.

National Institute of Nutrition. *Assessing Obesity: Beyond BMI*. NIN Review No.19, April, 1992.

Obesity: A case for prevention. Official position of The Canadian Dietetic Association. *J Can Diet Assoc* 49(1988):11-16.

HIGHLIGHT 8 - EATING DISORDERS - ANOREXIA AND BULIMIA

Canadian Resources

The National Eating Disorder Information Centre provides information about eating disoreders and treatment in Canada. See the Resource Groups at the end of this section for its adress and phone number.

Video and supporting manual: Desperate Measures: Eating Disorders in Athletes. 1990. Sports Medicine Council of Canada, 1600 James Naismith Drive, Suite 502, Gloucester, ON K1B 5N4.

Canadian Reading

National Institute of Nutrition. *An Overview of the Eating Disorders Anorexia Nervosa and Bulimia Nervosa.* NIN Review No.8, January 1989.

TEACHING CANADIAN INFORMATION: CHAPTER 9
THE WATER-SOLUBLE VITAMINS: B VITAMINS AND VITAMIN C

9.1 VITAMINS IN CANADIAN FOODS

The major differences in the vitamin content of foods sold in Canada are due to the differences in the regulations for nutrient enrichment. These were discussed in 2.3 Nutrient Enrichment in Canada in this section. A review of this topic may be appropriate with this chapter to help students connect the specific vitamins with foods. If the students are completing the self-study for the water-soluble vitamins, provide information or resources to assist them in finding the accurate Canadian values, e.g. *Nutrient Value of Some Common Foods*[14] or Nutrition Information on the food label.

If nutrient enrichment was not covered earlier in the course, this would be an appropriate time to discuss it, with special emphasis on the water-soluble vitamins.

9.2 VITAMIN RECOMMENDATIONS

A review of the RNI with an emphasis on the differences from the RDA for vitamins can help students learn about vitamins. For example each student could calculate their RNI for vitamin B_6 based on 0.015 mg/g dietary protein intake and compare it to the RDA for that vitamin. The RNI for vitamin C should be noted because of the recommended increase for smokers. This is a new approach for the recommendations and many young people smoke cigarettes. The recommendations for thiamin, riboflavin and niacin are based on energy expenditure with the minimum based on 2000 kcal/day.

Thiamin   0.40 mg/1000 kcal 0.48 mg/5000 kJ   Min. 0.80 mg
Riboflavin 0.5 mg/1000 kcal   0.6 mg/5000 kJ   Min. 1.0 mg
Niacin   7.2 NE/1000 kcal   8.6 NE/5000 kJ   Min. 14.4 NE

Students should use the RNI as the basis for evaluating vitamin intakes in the self-study. The 1990 RNI are used in the Canadian Version of West Diet Analysis '91. Remember that if the Canadian Nutrient Data File is used, e.g. *Nutrient Value of Some Common Foods*, niacin values are given in Niacin Equivalents and thus no calculations are required to estimate potential niacin from tryptophan.

TEACHING CANADIAN INFORMATION: CHAPTER 10
THE FAT-SOLUBLE VITAMINS: A, D, E, AND K

10.1 FAT-SOLUBLE VITAMINS IN CANADIAN FOODS

In the Canadian Nutrient Data File, all food values for vitamin A are in Retinol Equivalents. International Units for fat-soluble vitamins are used in the Drug Section, not the Food Section, of the *Food and Drug Act and Regulations*[1]. These units are also seen on vitamin supplements which are sold as drugs.

The Canadian policy on enrichment is different than the United States for vitamins A and D. In Canada, vitamins A and D is not permitted to be added to cereals. Students completing a self-study of vitamin intake should check the values for vitamin A in their cereal. If it is high, the value is probably based on United States data and higher than the actual content. Students should check the cereal label for the actual content of vitamin A.

It is mandatory for vitamin D to be added to all cow's milk which is sold as fluid milk, and vitamin A to be added to cow's milk which has had fat removed. Vitamins A and D must also be added to margarine. For more details on vitamin enrichment, see Table 2.2 of this section.

Canadian Information

HIGHLIGHT 10 - VITAMIN AND MINERAL SUPPLEMENTS

The Canadian Food and Drugs Act and Regulations[1] set minimum and maximum levels for vitamins in supplements. Some such as vitamin K can be sold only on prescription. Advertising of supplements is also controlled, preventing advertising which recommends high doses. This information is very important for Canadians who may buy vitamins when in the United States where regulations differ.

Reading

National Institute of Nutrition *Folic Acid and Neural Tube Defects Prevention*. NIN Review No. 21, Summer 1993.

TEACHING CANADIAN INFORMATION: CHAPTER 11
THE BODY FLUIDS AND THE MAJOR MINERALS

11.1 SODIUM AND POTASSIUM RECOMMENDATIONS

No quantitative recommendations for sodium and potassium are stated in the Nutrition Recommendations[8]. The text of the Nutrition Recommendations advocates that the Canadian population decrease the current intake of sodium. It advises consumers to do this by minimizing the use of salt in cooking, avoiding its use at the table, and selecting commercial foods low in added salt[8]. Advise students to review the Nutrition Recommendations for Canadians and Canada's Guidelines for Healthy Eating to see how the advice on sodium and salt is worded.

The Nutrition Recommendations also note the potential beneficial effects of increasing potassium intake and suggest a potassium-rich diet which emphasizes fruits and vegetables.

11.2 SODIUM CONTENT OF PACKAGED FOOD

According to the *Food and Drugs Act and Regulations*, the sodium content of a food is only required if a claim is made about the sodium content[1]. When a claim is stated, then the amount sodium and potassium content must also be stated in mg/serving of a stated size. For foods without such labelling, consumers should read the list of ingredients, looking for salt or sodium compounds. This will give some indication of the sodium which has been added to the product.

11.3 CALCIUM

Canadian students should note that the RNI for women over 50 increases to 800 mg from 700 mg in the earlier adult years. This recognizes potential problems with absorption of calcium due to aging and the possibility that a higher intake may moderate bone loss[8]. Canadian students should also note that calcium-fortified fruit juices, soy or rice beverages, or calcium-fortified milk can be sold in Canada.

11.4 PHOSPHORUS

Canadian students should note that the phosphorus RNI for adult women is 850 mg/day and for adult men is 1000 mg/day. The level is higher than the United States RDA. The higher level is recommended because the phosphorus requirement is slightly in excess of the calcium requirement and the requirement for phosphorus is increased by the consumption of a high protein diet.

TEACHING CANADIAN INFORMATION: CHAPTER 12
THE TRACE MINERALS

12.1 TRACE MINERAL RECOMMENDATIONS

The RNI for iron, zinc and iodine are identified in Chapter 12. Although there are no specific RNI for the other trace minerals, Table 12.1 lists the comments or suggestions for trace minerals from the Nutrition Recommendations[8]

12.2 IRON ENRICHMENT

If Canadian students are completing the self-study of trace minerals, they should check the iron content of breakfast cereals. The iron content on the package label, as % RDI, may be lower than the value in Appendix H or the computer printout. Refer to Table H2.1 of this section to calculate the iron content, based on the RDI for iron.

Table 12.1 Recommendations for Trace Minerals[8]

Mineral	Recommendation
Copper	2 mg/day seems adequate and safe for adults
Fluoride	Community water supplies should contain 1 mg/L fluoride. Supplements are recommended for infants and children only if the level of fluoride in drinking water is less than 0.7 mg/L. (See Table 17 in *Nutrition Recommendations* for recommended supplementation[8].
Manganese	There is insufficient data to make a firm recommendations. Present intakes of manganese are deemed sufficient in the absence of evidence of deficiency in the population.
Selenium	There is no recommendation. The normal Canadian intake appears to exceed the selenium requirement. Selenium supplement use is discouraged because of risk of toxicity.
Chromium	There is not sufficient data to make a recommendation.

HIGHLIGHT 12 - OUR CHILDREN'S DAILY LEAD

Lead has also been a concern in Canada. The adulteration of food with lead is addressed in B.15.001 of the *Food and Drugs Act and Regulations*[1]. Many of the cans used for food products no longer contain solder. Leaded gasoline is no longer available for use in cars. Some urban areas have reported on studies of lead in children. You may want to consult the local health department about recent studies in the area to discuss current risks in your community.

TEACHING CANADIAN INFORMATION: CHAPTER 13
FITNESS: PHYSICAL ACTIVITY, NUTRIENTS AND BODY ADAPTATIONS

13.1 CANADIAN PROGRAMS AND STUDIES

The 1988 Campbell's Survey on Well-Being in Canada collected information on aspects affecting well-being, including activities related to fitness, nutrition and health[25]. This survey involved the Canadian Fitness and Lifestyle Research Institute, Health and Welfare Canada, Fitness Canada and Campbell's Soup Company Ltd. It provided updated information to compare to the 1981 Canada Fitness Survey. The results of the study would be of interest to students majoring in recreation or human kinetics. The survey results can be purchased from the Canadian Fitness and Lifestyle Research Institute, Ottawa.

The *Vitality* Program which was mentioned in 8.2 of the Canadian Information Section. The three pronged approach of nutrition, activity and self esteem supports the issues in this chapter.

The Sport Nutrition Advisory Committee of the Sport Medicine Council of Canada has developed and distributes information on nutrition for athletes and active people. Resources include laminated cards on sport nutrition issues, SNAC PAC Newsletter on current topics of interest, videos and a manual for athletes and coaches called Sport Nutrition for the Athletes in Canada. The resources are useful for coaches, fitness leaders and nutrition educators.

Canadian Readings

Barr, S.I. Energy and nutrient intake of elite adolescent swimmers. *J Can Diet Assoc* 50(1989):20-24.

Barr, S.I. Nutrition and athletic performance. *NIN Rapport* 3(1):1-2, 1988.

Bouchard, C. Contribution of physical activity to body weight control. *NIN Rapport* 3(1):5-6, 1988.

52   Canadian Information: Chapter 13

Davis, B. Nutrition and fitness in Canada: Current status and future directions. A PARTICIPaction perspective. *NIN Rapport* 3(1):7, 1988.

Houston, M. Why a high carbohydrate diet? *SNAC PAC* Vol. 1, 1992.

National Institute of Nutrition. *Protein and Amino Acid Needs of Athletes*. NIN Review No. 18, January 1992.

HIGHLIGHT 13 - SUPPLEMENTS AND ERGOGENIC AIDS ATHLETES USE

This is a topic of particular interest to students who are athletes or trying to improve their body shape. Many of the supplements and aids are imported into Canada and may not meet the standards government standards for labelling and content. An interesting activity for students is to prepare a critical review of supplements available from local stores, gyms or fitness clubs. Information on any products which are considered to be illegal could then be sent to the closest office of the Health Protection Branch, Health Canada.

Reading

Sarwar G, Ujiie M, Botting HG. Protein and amino acid analyses of some protein/amino acid preparations sold in Canada. *J Can Diet Assoc* 53(2):159-63, 1992.

TEACHING CANADIAN INFORMATION: CHAPTER 14
CONSUMER CONCERNS ABOUT FOODS

14.1 FOOD-BORNE ILLNESSES

The safety of foods is regulated by the *Food and Drugs Act and Regulations*, and monitored by the Field Operations Directorate of the Health Protection Branch, Health Canada[1] and local public health departments. Mishandling of foods during handling, storage and preparation often permit the growth of pathogens leading to food-borne illness. The Regulations define storage requirements and microbial specifications for foods to be offered for sale. Inspectors for the Field Operations Directorate monitor foods for contamination from extraneous matter such as insects, insect fragments, rodent hair, animal droppings, metal or wood fragments, glass, etc. Educational material to promote food safety is available from the Food Operations Directorate, Health Protection Branch. Provincial or municipal inspectors monitor other regulations for food safety.

Safe handling of foods by foodservice is required to ensure the safety of foods served in restaurants and institutions. These are monitored by local health departments. To help meet the needs of educating food handlers, the Canadian Restaurant and Foodservices Association has established an education program for sanitation in foodservice operations. Similar education programs are offered by some community colleges.

Canadian Readings

Caira, R. Getting the dirt on sanitation: A primer to food sanitation principles. *Foodservice and Hospitality* April, 1992:49-62.

Garrett, R. Providing the industry with information about AIDS. *NIN Rapport* 5(1990):4-5.

Herzog, L. Coming clean on sanitation success. *Foodservice and Hospitality* April, 1992:65-68.

14.2 ENVIRONMENTAL CONTAMINANTS, NATURAL TOXICANTS AND PESTICIDES

Chemical contaminants in foods are monitored and regulated by Health Protection Branch and Agriculture Canada. The government agencies and the agri-food industry are responding to consumer concerns about contaminants through pesticide review, producer education and food product testing. The Fresh for Flavour Foundation and other producer organizations provide information on this use and regulation of pesticides in agriculture. The registration and regulation of pesticides in Canada are described in *Fresh Fact Finder*[26].

Regulation of Pesticides in Canada

- AGRICULTURE CANADA - *Pest Control Products Act* - registers pesticides and is responsible for aspects relating to sale and use of pesticides including safety to the producer, consumer, environment, and product safety.

- Health CANADA - *Food and Drugs Act* - determines the safety and quantity of a pesticide permitted in foods. The Food Directorate decides about the safety of a pesticide for the consumer. The Environmental Health Directorate determines the occupational health and safety of the pesticide for the user and bystander.

The following readings provide some perspective on these issues in Canada.

Agriculture Canada. *Annual Review of Chemical and Biological Tests on Agri-food Commodities, 1990-91*.
From Agri-food Safety and Strategies, Food Production and Inspection, Halldon House, 5th Floor, 2255 Carling Ave., Ottawa, Ontario K1A 0Y9.

Health and Welfare Canada. Natural Toxicants in Plants. Ottawa:Supply and Services Canada., 1984.

Wiley, M. Consumers will benefit from federal pesticide registration review process. *AGCare UPDATE*, Winter 1991:1-4.

14.3 FOOD ADDITIVES AND ALLERGENS

Food additives are regulated in Canada under the *Food and Drugs Act and Regulations*. The approach and regulations are similar those of the United States. The policy on the use of food additives in Canada is consistent with the FAO/WHO Joint Expert Committee on Food Additives. The regulations are summarized in Chapter 9 of *Health Protection and Food Laws*[2].

The safety of food additives is a concern for individuals with allergies or hypersensitivities. The requirement that all ingredients and food additives be included on labels of prepackaged foods helps these individuals to select foods which they can tolerate. The Canadian Restaurant and Foodservices Association has developed an Allergy Program[27] to assist restaurants and foodservice operations to develop a listing of potential allergens in their menu items. Information on this program is available from the Canadian Restaurant and Foodservices Association. (See Resource List at the end of this Section.)   Health Protection Branch, Health Canada uses news releases entitled Allergy Alerts to notify the public about potential allergens, e.g. almonds, which have been found to be included in food products but not on the list of ingredients on the label.

14.4 FOOD IRRADIATION

Food irradiation continues to be an issue of concern for many consumers. Sahasrabudhe provided an overview of food irradiation in the *Journal of the Canadian Dietetic Association*[28]. The reference may help instructors respond to students' questions on this topic.

14.5 CONSUMER CONCERNS ABOUT FOOD SAFETY AND NUTRITION

Several studies are monitoring trends and consumers concerns about food safety. The following readings provide Canadian information to present to students.

Canadian Readings

Campbell, I. Consumer attitudes to food safety. *Visions* 2(1991):1-7.

Consumers' Association of Canada. *Food Safety in Canada: A Survey of Consumer Attitudes and Opinions*.
Ottawa: Consumers' Association of Canada, May 1990.

Grocery Products Manufacturers of Canada. *Grocery Attitudes of Canadians 1992*. Don Mills, Ontario: GPMC, 1992.

HIGHLIGHT 14 - ENVIRONMENTALLY CONSCIOUS FOODWAYS

Agricultural Methods in Canada

Concerns about sustainable agriculture and food safety and global economic conditions are leading to changes in some changes in agriculture production methods in Canada. The agri-food industry, researchers and government agencies are responding to many of the issues raised in Highlight 14. The following references provide Canadian information about environmentally conscious foodways. When reviewing material on this topic it is important to look for information from agricultural scientists and professionals to compare with popular literature of environmentalists to get the full perspective of the issues.

Canadian Readings

Hough, K. Concerns about agricultural nitrates and water quality. *AGCare UPDATE* 2(2)(1992):1-2.

Pelletier, M.C. The Canadian hog industry and the environment. *Meat Probe* 9(1)(1991):1-2.

Strankman, P. The beef cattle industry: Part of an environmentally sustainable agriculture system. *Meat Probe* 9(2)(1991):1 - 3.

Surgeoner, G. A scientist's view of organic farming. *Fresh Fact Finder* (Fresh for Flavour Foundation) 1991.

Wiley, M. First environmental farm plans to be completed in 1993. *AGCare UPDATE* 2(2)(1992):3-4.

TEACHING CANADIAN INFORMATION: CHAPTER 15
NUTRITION ASSESSMENT

15.1 SI UNITS IN NUTRITION ASSESSMENT

SI units are used by most Canadian health professionals. Standards used for assessing deficiencies may differ from those in the text. Standards used for different nutrients tend to vary with the laboratory. Check with the laboratories in your area to find the standards which are currently used. If assessment is an important part of your course, it may be a useful learning experience for students to convert mass concentrations to molar concentrations. See the introduction to S.I. units at the beginning of this section.

Resource

McDonald, J.E. *A Pocket Guide to Physical Examination and Nutritional Assessment* Toronto: W.B. Saunders Canada, 1994.

HIGHLIGHT 15 - U.S. AND WORLD HUNGER

Hunger in Canada

Hunger has become an increasing concern in Canada. There has been a huge increase in the number of food banks and emergency feeding programs. Helping at a local food bank, shelter or emergency feeding centre provides students with an opportunity to gain an understanding of the hunger issue. The following readings provide some perspectives on hunger issues in Canada and the role of nutrition professionals.

Canadian Readings

Campbell, C., Katamay, S., Connolly, C. The role of nutrition professional in the hunger debate. *J Can Diet Assoc* 49(1988):230-235.

Davis, B and CDA Ad Hoc Committee on Hunger and Nutrition. Nutrition and food security in Canada: A role for The Canadian Dietetic Association. *J Can Diet Assoc* 52(1991):141-145.

Dyer, S. How do the poor afford to eat? *NIN Rapport* 4(3)(1989):6-7.

Hunger and food security in Canada: Official Position of The Canadian Dietetic Association. *J Can Diet Assoc* 52(1991):139.

Riches, G. Responding to hunger in a wealthy society: issues and options. *J Can Diet Assoc* 50(1989):150-154.

Riches, G. Food banks, hunger and economic growth: charity of collective security in the 1990s? *NIN Rapport* 4(3)(1989):5-6.

Tarasuk, V. and Woolcott, L. Food acquisition practices of homeless adults: Insights from a health promotion project. *J Can Diet Assoc* 55(1994): 15-19.

TEACHING CANADIAN INFORMATION: CHAPTER 16
NUTRITION CARE STRATEGIES

16.1 DIET MANUALS IN CANADA

There is no single diet manual which is used across Canada. Several provincial dietetic associations publish diet manuals. These are often used by hospitals and nursing homes as the basis for diet therapy. Some institutions adopt specific diet manuals, approved by their institution's medical committee. Before teaching this section, check with the institutions in your area to see which diet manuals are used most often. These can then be used in teaching and case studies.

TEACHING CANADIAN INFORMATION: CHAPTER 17
LIFE CYCLE NUTRITION: PREGNANCY, LACTATION AND INFANCY

17.1 CANADIAN GUIDELINES AND PROGRAMS

Pregnancy and Lactation

The RNI for pregnancy and lactation are different from the RDA and can be found in Appendix I. These are supported by the National Guidelines for Nutrition in Pregnancy[29]. These guidelines assist health professionals in providing advice for women throughout pregnancy. The guidelines are in the form of responses to questions which often arise during pregnancy, including weight gain, salt intake, etc. The guidelines recommend that for the majority of healthy women weight gain should be 10 to 14 kg.

There is no national program to support the nutrition of pregnant women in Canada. Many municipalities provide programs of education and health support to promote healthier mothers and babies. One of the first programs was established at the Montreal Diet Dispensary by Agnes Higgins[30]. Mendelson et al. describe the results of the evaluation of the Healthiest Babies Possible program in Toronto[31]. To find out about programs for pregnant women at nutritional risk in your locality, contact your local public health department. Many public health departments offer prenatal and postnatal education programs to interested members of the community. A new initiative is Brighter Futures, a program of Health Canada. It supports local programs for pregnant women, and parents and caregivers of young children through the Community Action Program for Children. Check to see if there are any of these programs in your community.

64   Canadian Information: Chapter 17

Readings and Resources

National Institute of Nutrition *Folic Acid and Neural Tube Defects Prevention.* NIN Review No. 21, Summer 1993.

Canadian Task Force on the Periodic Health Examination. Periodic health examination, 1992 update: 1. Screening for gestational diabetes mellitus. *Can Med Assoc J* 147(1992):435-443.

Federal-Provincial Subcommittee on Nutrition. *Nutrition in Pregnancy - National Guidelines.* Ottawa: Minister of Supply and Services, 1987.

Promoting breastfeeding: A role for the dietitian/nutritionist. Official position of The Canadian Dietetic Association. *J Can Diet Assoc* 50(1989):211-214.

Sauve, R.S. The WHO Code and its effect on breast-feeding promotion in hospitals.

Infant Feeding

Iron status of infants has been identified as a concern in Canada. Greene-Finestone et al. reported on a study on iron depletion and iron deficiency anemia among infants in Ottawa-Carlton[32]. New guidelines for meeting iron needs have been published by the Canadian Paediatric Society[33]. These recommend that supplemental iron is not needed by term infants who are exclusively breast-fed until they are 6 months old. After they reach 6 months, they should receive extra iron in the form of iron-fortified infant cereals and other iron-rich foods. If solid foods are introduced to these infants before 6 months, they should contain an adequate amount of iron. For term infants who are not breast-fed, iron-fortified infant formula should be given from birth. After 4 to 6 months iron-fortified cereals are a good additional source of iron. Additional iron is recommended for premature infants. Whole cow's milk should not be introduced until 9 to 12 months of age.

At the time of publication, the Canadian Paediatric Society is reviewing the infant feeding guidelines. Check the journals or consult with the local health department for the new guidelines.

Readings and Resources

Health and Welfare Canada. *Feeding Babies. A Counselling Guide on Practical Solution to Common Infant Feeding Questions.* Ottawa: Minister of Supply and Services, 1986.

Infant Nutrition Institute. *In-Touch Newsletter.* This is a quarterly publication established by HJ Heinz of Canada Ltd which promotes infant nutrition among health professionals and the public.

Local public health offices often provide pamphlets and brochures on infant feeding which might be appropriate for class handouts.

HIGHLIGHT 17 - FETAL ALCOHOL SYNDROME

The National Guidelines for Nutrition in Pregnancy addresses the question of alcohol[34]. No minimum safe level for alcohol intake is identified. The guidelines suggest that reduction in drinking during pregnancy could be beneficial.

Canadian Information 67

TEACHING CANADIAN INFORMATION: CHAPTER 18
LIFE CYCLE NUTRITION: CHILDHOOD, ADOLESCENCE, AND THE LATER YEARS

18.1 DIETARY FAT AND CHILDREN

The Nutrition Recommendations Update... Dietary Fat and Children[19] which were discussed in Chapter 5, The Lipids: Triglycerides, Phospholipids, and Sterols. These should be discussed here in the context of the importance of young children meeting their energy needs to support normal growth and development.

18.2 SCHOOL FOOD POLICY

Canada has no national policy or program for feeding school children. Some provinces or local boards of education are developing school food policies which address availability and quality of food in schools and nutrition curriculum. The Canadian Education Association collected information from schools across Canada to prepare the report: Food For Thought: School Board Nutrition Policies and Programs for Hungry Children[35]. Teacher associations are showing great concern for the hungry children in classrooms. Instructors could check with the local board of education to get details on local programs and policies.

18.3 CHILD HUNGER

Poverty is a problem affecting the health and nutritional status of many Canadian children. An overview of this problem was presented by Davis in *Nutrition Quarterly*[36]. For courses with students who will be involved with teaching or providing social services for children, some attention should be given to the barriers to nutritional health and normal behavioral development. Health Canada has identified children as a priority area for health promotion. Instructors should watch for local programs which support this priority at either the federal or provincial level.

18.4 PROGRAMS FOR THE ELDERLY

As with other target groups, there are no national programs focused on nutrition for the elderly. However many of the provinces or municipalities have meals-on-wheels programs or education programs aimed at the aging population. Instructors could check with social service agencies in their community to provide examples of these programs for students.

The January 1991 issue of *NIN Rapport* addressed risks, challenges and programs related to nutrition and the elderly in Canada.

Readings and Resources

CHILDHOOD:
Brown, H. Canadian guidelines on preschool nutrition. *NIN Rapport* 5(1):1-3, 1990.

Campbell, M.L. Nutrient intake, growth and eating patterns of preschool children with single, employed mothers. *J Can Diet Assoc* 54(3):151-6, 1993.

National Institute of Nutrition. *Sub-optimal Zinc Status during Infancy and Childhood* NIN Review No. 11, October 1989.

National Institute of Nutrition. *Nutritional Needs of Young Athletes*. NIN Review No. 14, July 1990.

Promoting Nutritional Health during the Preschool Years: Canadian Guidelines. Network of the Federal/Provincial/Territorial Group on Nutrition and the National Institute of Nutrition, Ottawa: 1989.

Sauve, R.S. Nutrition in preschoolers. *NIN Rapport* 5(1):4-5, 1990.

AGING:
Beaton, G.H. Geriatric nutrition: Issues in perspective. *NIN Rapport* 3(4):5, 1988.

Mathews, A.M. Trends in Population Aging in Canada. *NIN Review* 3(4):1-2, 1988.

Ness, K., Elliott, P., Wilbur, V. A peer educator program for seniors in a community development context. *J Nutr Ed* 24(1992):91-94.

Yeung, D.L. and Imbach, A. Geriatric practice in Canada - A review. *J. Nutr. Elderly* 7:27-46, 1988.

Canadian Information 69

HIGHLIGHT 18 - CAFFEINE: THE BREWING CONTROVERSY

The Canadian perspective on the caffeine issue is presented in the section on caffeine in *Nutrition Recommendations*[8]. Information about the caffeine for consumers is included in Food Guide Facts 6: A Closer Look at Other Foods (A fact sheet to support Canada's Food Guide for Healthy Eating, 1992.)

HIGHLIGHT 19 - DIET AND HEALTH

Nutrition Recommendations

The 1990 Nutrition Recommendations address the role of nutrition in chronic disease and disease prevention[8]. An overview is provided in Nutrition and Disease, pp.13-18. The relationship of specific nutrients with diseases are discussed in the sections for the individual nutrients. Alcohol and caffeine are addressed in Part III. This information may be helpful to Canadian instructors planning lectures on the topic of nutrition and disease.

Canadian Consensus Conference on Cholesterol

The Canadian Consensus Conference on Cholesterol: Final Report identified the following priority groups of patients for determining lipid risk factors:[37]
- patients known to have coronary heart disease;
- patients with a family history of hyperlipidemia or early onset of coronary heart disease; and

- patients with hypertension, diabetes mellitus, renal failure or obesity, especially abdominal obesity.

Intensive dietary intervention comparable to the American Heart Association phase II diet and with the assistance of a dietitian was recommended for:
- adults 30 years and over with blood cholesterol level above 6.2 mmol/L (240 mg/dl);
- adults 18 to 29 years with blood cholesterol level above 5.7 mmol/L (220 mg/dl); and
- children and adolescents under age 18 years with blood cholesterol level above the 90th percentile for their group in the population.

Dietary advice approximating the American Heart Association phase I diet was recommended for:
- adults 30 years and over with blood cholesterol level 5.2 to 6.2 mmol/L (200 to 240 mg/dl) and
- adults 18 to 29 years with blood cholesterol level 4.6 to 5.7 mmol/L (180 to 200 mg/dl)

More intensive dietary counselling and therapy were indicated for:
- adults 30 years and over if LDL cholesterol level is greater than 3.4 mmol/L (130 mg/dl), the HDL cholesterol level is less than 0.9 mmol/L (35 mg/dl) or the triglyceride level is above 2.3 mmol/L (200 mg/dl) and
- adults 18 to 29 if the LDL cholesterol level is greater than 3.0 mmol/L (115 mg/dl), the HDL cholesterol is less than 0.9 mmol/L (35 mg/dl) or the triglyceride level is above 2.3 mmol/L (220 mg/dl).

Consensus was not reached about guidelines for the treatment of mild to moderate hypercholesterolemia among children and adolescents under 18 years.

Health Promotion

Canada has shown some political commitment to health promotion through the release of papers starting in 1974 with *A New Perspective on the Health of Canadians*[38] and followed in 1986 by the discussion paper, *Achieving Health for All: A Framework for Health Promotion*[39]. Many of the provincial governments developed statements or strategies to incorporate the concept of health promotion in their health policies. Instructors could consult with the provincial health ministry for their documents supporting health promotion.

In 1992, Health and Welfare Canada published *Heart Health Equality: Mobilizing Communities for Action*[40]. This presents on approach for applying the concept of community development to health promotion. This publication also presents a comparison of the health promotion and disease prevention approaches.

Canadian Readings

Connolly, C. A commentary on Achieving Health for All: A Framework for Health Promotion. *J Can Diet Assoc* 50(1989):89-97.

Harvey, D.A.A. Trends in health concepts and health promotion: A discussion paper. *J Can Diet Assoc* 49(1988):42-47.

Nielsen H. Achieving health for All: A Framework for Nutrition in Health Promotion. *J Can Diet Assoc* 50(1989):77-80.

Stachtchenko, S. and Jenicek, M. Conceptual differences between prevention and health promotion: Research implications for community health programs. *Can J Public Health* 81(1990):53-59.

TEACHING CANADIAN INFORMATION: CHAPTER 26
NUTRITION, DIABETES, AND HYPOGLYCEMIA

26.1 CANADIAN FOOD CHOICE SYSTEM

The Canadian exchange system is called the *Good Health Eating Guide*, published by the Canadian Diabetes Association[13]. This system is described in chapter 2 of this Canadian Information Section. The complete lists for the Good Health Eating Guide are in Appendix G of the textbook. Canadian students should use this system when developing meals patterns and food plans in this chapter. Educational materials to support teaching this section can be ordered from the Canadian Diabetes Association. (See Resource Groups for the mailing address).

TEACHING CANADIAN INFORMATION: CHAPTER 29
NUTRITION AND WASTING DISORDERS: CANCER AND AIDS

Canadian Resource and Readings

Healthy Eating Makes a Difference: Food Resource Kit for People Living with HIV is a useful resource for teaching about nutrition and AIDS. It can be ordered from National AIDS Clearinghouse, Canadian Public Health Association, 400-1565 Carling Avenue, Ottawa, ON K1Z 8R1.

Cossette, M. Nutrition and aids: A challenge for the '90s. *NIN Rapport* 5(1990):1-3.

Murphy, J., Cameron, D.W., Garber, G., Conway, B., Denomme, N. Dietary counselling and nutritional supplementation in HIV infection. *J Can Diet Assoc* 53(1992):205-208.

Walters, D. A public health approach to nutrition problems in HIV disease. *NIN Rapport* 5(1990):7

Canadian Information

HIGHLIGHT 29 - HEALTH CARE REFORM, COST CONTAINMENT, AND NUTRITION SERVICES

Canada's health care system is under considerable pressure because of the high financial cost. Federal and provincial governments are searching for ways to provide needed services at lower costs. Several provincial governments are trying to shift health care services from institutions to the community. When teaching this section, refer to the current activities in the media related to health care in your community. Changes could have an important impact on the careers of students.

RESOURCE GROUPS

Please note that offices may move or phone numbers may change from the date printing. Check with the Telephone Information if you are unable to contact these offices.

GOVERNMENT

HEALTH CANADA

Health Protection Branch:
Bureau of Nutritional Sciences, Food Directorate, Health Protection Branch, Health Canada, Banting Building, Tunney's Pasture, Ottawa, Ontario K1A 0L2

Regional Offices:
Atlantic Region: Health Protection Branch, Ralston Building, 1557 Hollis Street, Halifax, Nova Scotia B3J 1V5 - (902)426-2160

Quebec Region: Health Protection Branch, 1001 rue St. Laurent ouest, Longeuil, Quebec J4K 1C7 - (514)283-5488

Ontario Region: Health Protection Branch, 2301 Midland Avenue, Scarborough, Ontario M1P 4R7 - (416)973-1600

Central Region: Health Protection Branch, 310-269 Main Street, Winnipeg, Manitoba R3C 1B2 - (204)949-5490

78   Canadian Information: Resource Groups

Western Region: Health Protection Branch, 3155 Willingdon Green, Burnaby, British Columbia V5G 4T2 - (604)666-3359

Health Services and Promotion Branch:

Nutrition Programs Unit, Health Promotion Directorate, Health Canada, 4th Floor, Jeanne Mance Building, Tunney's Pasture, Ottawa, Ontario K1A 1B4

Medical Services Branch

Epidemiology and Community Health Specialties, Indian and Northern Health Services, Health Canada, 11th Floor, Jeanne Mance Building, Tunney's Pasture, Ottawa, Ontario K1A 0L3

Regional Offices:
Regional Nutritionist, Pacific Region, Suite 540, 740 West Hastings Street, Vancouver, British Columbia V6C 3E6

Regional Nutritionist, Alberta Region, Suite 730, 9700 Jasper Avenue, Edmonton, Alberta T5J 4C3

Regional Nutritionist, Saskatchewan Region, 1855 Smith Street, Regina, Saskatchewan S4P 2N5

Regional Nutritionist, Manitoba Region, Room 500, 303 Main Street, Winnipeg, Manitoba R3C 0H4

Regional Nutritionist, Ontario Region, 3rd Floor, 1547 Merivale Road, Nepean, Ontario K1A 0C3

Nutritionniste Regionale, Region Du Québec, Suite 202, 2nd floor, East Tower, Place Guy Favreau, 200 Ouest, boul. René Lévesque, Montreal, Quebec H2Z 1X3

Regional Nutritionist, Atlantic Region, Room 4391 Ralston Bldg, 1557 Hollis Street, Halifax, Nova Scotia B3J 1V6

Regional Nutritionist, Yukon Region, No. 5 Hospital Road, Whitehorse, Yukon Territory, Y1A 3H8

Network of the Federal/Provincial/Territorial Group on Nutrition

Chief, Nutrition Programs Unit, Health Promotion Directorate, Health Canada, Room 456, Jeanne Mance Building, Tunney's Pasture, Ottawa, Ontario K1A 1B4

Director, Bureau of Nutritional Sciences, Food Directorate, Health Protection Branch, Health Canada, Banting Building, Tunney's Pasture, Ottawa, Ontario K1A 0L2

Nutrition Specialist, Epidemiology and Community Health Specialities, Indian and Northern Health Services, Health Canada, 11th Floor, Jeanne Mance Building, Tunney's Pasture, Ottawa, Ontario K1A 0L3

Coordinator Nutrition Programs, Department of Health and Social Services, P.O. Box 2000, Charlottetown, Prince Edward Island C1A 7J9

Provincial Nutrition Consultant, Health Promotion and Nutrition Division, Department of Health, Box 4750, St. John's, Newfoundland A1C 5T7

Senior Nutrition Consultant, Public Health Services, Department of Health and Community Services, P.O. Box 5100, Fredericton, New Brunswick E3B 5G8

Nutrition Coordinator, Department of Health and Fitness, P.O. Box 488, Halifax, Nova Scotia B3J 2R8

Responsable des programmes de nutrition, Direction de la santé, Ministère de la Santé et des Services sociaux, 10e étage, 1075 chemin Saint-Foy, Québec, Québec G1S 2M1

Senior Nutrition Consultant, Public Health Branch, Ministry of Health, 5th Floor, 15 Overlea Boulevard, Toronto, Ontario M4H 1A9

Program Specialist Nutrition, Health and Wellness Branch, Healthy Public Policy Program Division, Manitoba Health, 303 - 800 Portage Avenue, Winnipeg, Manitoba R3G 0N4

Provincial Nutritionist, Community Services, Saskatchewan Health, 3475 Albert Street, Regina, Saskatchewan S4S 6X6

Community Nutrition Program, Family Health Services, Public Health Division, Alberta Health, Seventh Street Plaza, South Tower, 10030-107 Avenue, Edmonton, Alberta T5J 3E4

Director Nutrition, Family Health Division, Ministry of Health, 5th Floor, 1515 Blanshard Street, Victoria, British Columbia V8W 3C8

A/Director Dietetics, Department of Health and Human Resources, #5 Hospital Road, Whitehorse, Yukon Y1A 2C6

Nutritionist, Community Health, Department of Health, 7th Floor, Lahm Ridge Tower, Box 1320, Yellowknife, Northwest Territories X1A 2L9

AGRICULTURE AND AGRI-FOOD CANADA

Food Production and Inspection Branch, Agriculture and Agri-Food Canada, 151 Cleopatra Drive, Nepean, Ontario

DIETETIC ASSOCIATIONS

The Canadian Dietetic Association, 480 University Avenue, Suite 601, Toronto, Ontario M5G 1V2 - (416)596-0857

Newfoundland Dietetic Association, P.O. Box 1756, Station "C", St. John's, Newfoundland A1C 5P5

Prince Edward Island Dietetic Association, P.O. Box 2575, Charlottetown, Prince Edward Island C1A 8C2

Nova Scotia Dietetic Association, P.O. Box 8841, Stn A, Halifax, Nova Scotia B3K 5M5

New Brunswick Dietetic Association, P.O. Box 4102, Moncton, New Brunswick E1A 6E7

Corporation professionnelle des diététistes du Québec, 1425 Boulevard René Lévesque, bureau 402, Montreal, Québec H3G 1T7 (514)393-3733

The Ontario Dietetic Association, 480 University Avenue, Suite 604, Toronto, Ontario M5G 1V2 - (416)599-7289

Manitoba Association of Registered Dietitians, 320 Sherbrooke Street, Winnipeg, Manitoba R3B 2W6

Saskatchewan Dietetic Association, P.O. Box 3894, Regina Saskatchewan S4P 3R8

Alberta Registered Dietitians' Association, 370 Terrace Plaza Tripple 45, Edmonton, Alberta T6H 5R7

British Columbia Dietitians' and Nutritionists' Association, Suite 306, 1037 West Broadway, Vancouver, British Columbia V6H 1E3

OTHER ORGANIZATIONS

AGCare (Agricultural Groups Concerned About Resources and the Environment), 90 Woodlawn Rd. W., Guelph, Ontario N1H 1B2.

Canadian Diabetes Association, National Office, Toronto Street, Suite 1001, Toronto, Ontario M5C 2E3 - (416)363-3373.

Canadian Living Foundation for Families, 50 Holly Street, Toronto, Ontario M4S 3B3.

Canadian Public Health Association, Publications, Suite 400, 1565 Carling Ave. Ottawa, Ontario K1Z 8R1 (613)725-3769.

Canadian Restaurant and Foodservices Association, 80 Bloor Street West, Suite 1201, Toronto, Ontario M5S 2V1 - (416)923-8416 or 1-800-387-5649.

Consumer's Association of Canada, 307 Gilmour St., Ottawa, Ontario K2P 0P7 (613) 238-2533

Fresh for Flavour Foundation, 310-1101 Prince of Wales Dr., Ottawa, Ontario K2C 3W7 - (613)226-4187

National Eating Disorder Information Centre, 200 Elizabeth St., College Wing 1-328, Toronto, Ontario M5G 2C4 - (416)340-4156.

Canadian Information: Resource Groups 81

National Institute of Nutrition, 302 - 265 Carling Avenue, Ottawa, Ontario K1S 2E1 - (613)235-3355

Organization for Nutrition Education, P.O. Box 818, Guelph, Ontario N1H 6L6

Sports Medicine and Science Council of Canada, 1600 James Naismith Drive, Suite 502, Gloucester, Ontario K1B 5N4

For Canadian Cancer Society and Canadian Heart and Stroke Foundation, information and publications are available from local or provincial offices.

Educational material is also available from many of the food manufacturers, food producer organizations, provincial ministries of agriculture, and provincial or local health departments.

REFERENCES

1. Health and Welfare Canada. *Departmental Consolidation of the Food and Drugs Act and Regulations*. Ottawa: Health Protection Branch, Nov. 1988.

2. Health and Welfare Canada. *Health Protection and Food Laws*. Ottawa: Health Protection Branch, 1987.

3. Consumer and Corporate Affairs Canada. *Guide for Food Manufacturers and Advertisers,* Rev. 1988. Ottawa: Consumer Products Branch, 1988.

4. Robbins, L.G. and Robichon-Hunt, L. The Agriculture Canada Nutritious Food Basket and Thrifty Nutritious Food Basket. *Food Market Commentary* 11(1989):31-41.

5. Robbins, L. Comparison of the cost of a nutritious food basket in border cities in Canada and the United States. *Food Market Commentary* 13(1991):23-31.

6. Agriculture Canada. *Consumer Trends for the 1990s*. Ottawa: Food Development Division, 1990.

7. Health and Welfare Canada. *Recommended Nutrient Intakes for Canadians*. Ottawa:Bureau of Nutritional Sciences 1983, p.18.

8. Health and Welfare Canada. *Nutrition Recommendations*. Ottawa: Minister of Supply and Services Canada, 1990.

9. Murray, T.K. and Beare-Rogers, J.L. Nutrition recommendations, 1990. *J Can Diet Assoc* 51(1990):391-395.

10. Health and Welfare Canada. *Action Towards Healthy Eating...Canada's Guidelines for Healthy Eating and Strategies for Implementation*. The Report of the Communications/Implementation Committee. Ottawa: Minister of Supply and Services Canada, 1990.

11. Woolcott, D.M. Canada's Guidelines for Healthy Eating: Strategies for communicating and implementing Nutrition Recommendations. *J Can Diet Assoc* 51(1990):396-399.

12. Health and Welfare Canada. *Action Towards Healthy Eating... Technical Report*. Ottawa: Supply and Services Canada, 1990.

13. Canadian Diabetes Association. *Good Health Eating Guide*. Toronto, 1982.

14. Health and Welfare Canada. *Nutrient Value of Some Common Foods,* Rev. 1988. Ottawa: Canadian Government Publishing Centre, 1988.

15. Verdier, P. and Beare-Rogers, J.L. The Canadian nutrient file. *J Can Diet Assoc* 45(1984):52-55.

16. Verdier, P.C. The Canadian nutrient file: How Canadian are the data? *J Can Diet Assoc* 49(1987):21-23.

Canadian Information: References

17. Crane, N.T., Behlen, P.M., Yetley, E.A., Vanderveen, J.E. Nutrition labelling of foods: A global perspective. *Nutrition Today* July/August 1990.

18. Health and Welfare Canada. *Report of the Expert Committee on Dietary Fibre to the Health Protection Branch Health and Welfare Canada.* Ottawa: Minister of National Health and Welfare, 1985.

19. The Joint Working Group of the Canadian Paediatric Society and Health Canada. *Nutrition Recommendations Update... Dietary Fat and Children.* Ottawa: Minister of Supply and Services Canada, 1993.

20. National Institute of Nutrition. Red Meats in the Canadian Diet *NIN Review No. 11*, July, 1989.

21. Sarwar, G., Ujiie, M., Botting, H.G. Protein and amino acid analyses of some protein/amino acid preparations sold in Canada. *J Can Diet Assoc* 53(1992):159-163.

22. Health and Welfare Canada. *Canadian Guidelines for Healthy Weights.* Ottawa: Minister of Supply and Services, 1988.

23. The Canadian Dietetic Association. *Healthy Eating Is... A Resource Manual for Health Professionals.* Toronto: The Canadian Dietetic Association, 1988, p.20.

24. Health and Welfare Canada. *Promoting Healthy Weights in Canada.* Ottawa: Minister of Supply and Services, 1988.

25. Stephens, T. and Craig, C.L. *The Well-Being of Canadians: Highlights of the 1988 Campbell's Survey.* Ottawa: Canada Fitness and Lifestyle Research Institute, 1990.

26. Fresh for Flavour Foundation. Pesticide Registration and Regulation. *Fresh Fact Finder,* 1989.

27. *Food Allergies and the Foodservice Industry.* Toronto: Canadian Restaurant and Foodservices Association, 1989.

28. Sahasrabudhe, M.R. Food irradiation: Current status, concerns, limitations and future prospects. *J Can Diet Assoc* 51(1990):329-334.

29. Palin, D. and Rankine, D. Nutrition in pregnancy - National guidelines: A summary. *J Can Diet Assoc* 48(1987):209-210.

30. Higgins, A.C. Nutritional status and the outcome of pregnancy. *J Can Diet Assoc* 37(1976):17-35.

31. Mendelson, R., Dollard, D., Hall, P., Zarrabi, S.Y., Desjardin, E. The impact of the Healthiest Babies Possible Program on maternal diet and pregnancy outcome in underweight and overweight clients. *J Can Diet Assoc* 52(1991):229-234.

32. Greene-Finestone, L., Feldman, W., Heick, H., Luke B. Prevalence and risk factors of iron depletion and iron deficiency anemia among infants in Ottawa-Carleton. *J Can Diet Assoc* 52(1991):20-23.

33. Nutrition Committee, Canadian Paediatric Society. Position Statement: Meeting the iron needs of infants and young children: an update. *Can Med Assoc J* 144(1991):1451-1454.

34. Federal-Provincial Subcommittee on Nutrition. *Nutrition in Pregnancy - National Guidelines*. Ottawa: Minister of Supply and Services, 1987.

35. Canadian Education Association. *Food for Thought: School Board Nutrition Policies and Programs for Hungry Children.* CEA Information Note, Suite 8-200, 252 Bloor St. W., Toronto, Ontario. M5S 1V5.

36. Davis, B.A. Children, poverty, and nutrition: a Canadian overview. *Nutrition Quarterly*. 15 (1991):34-39.

37. Canadian Consensus Conference on the Prevention of Heart and Vascular Disease by Altering Serum Cholesterol and Lipoprotein Risk Factors. Canadian Consensus Conference on Cholesterol: final report. *Can Med Assoc J* 139(Supplement) (1988):1-8.

38. Health and Welfare Canada. *A New Perspective on the Health of Canadians: a Working Document,* by Marc Lalonde. Ottawa: Supply and Services Canada, 1974.

39. Epp, J. *Achieving Health for All: A Framework for Health Promotion.* Ottawa: Health and Welfare Canada, 1986.

40. Health and Welfare Canada. *Heart Health Equality: Mobilizing Communities for Action.* Ottawa: Supply and Services Canada, 1992.

TEST BANK

CHAPTER 1
AN OVERVIEW OF NUTRITION

MULTIPLE CHOICE

1. By chemical analysis, most foods contain which nutrient in highest amounts?

K   A. Fats
      B. Water
      C. Proteins
      D. Carbohydrates
ANSWER: B   p. 3

2. Which of the following is an organic compound?

K   A. Salt
      B. Water
      C. Calcium
      D. Vitamin C
ANSWER: D   p. 3

3. What is the residue that remains when a food is burned?

K   A. Ash
      B. Fiber
      C. Water
      D. Carbon
ANSWER: A   p. 4

Chapter 1   An Overview of Nutrition

4. Which of the following is characteristic of an essential nutrient?

AP
A. Cannot be found in food
B. Cannot be degraded by the body
C. Cannot be made in sufficient quantities by the body
D. Cannot be used to synthesize other compounds in the body
ANSWER: C   p. 3

5. Which of the following most accurately describes the term organic?

AP
A. Products sold at health food stores
B. Products grown without use of pesticides
C. Foods possessing superior nutrient qualities
D. Substances possessing carbon-carbon or carbon-hydrogen bonds
ANSWER: D   p. 3

6. Which of the following is NOT one of the six classes of nutrients?

K
A. Fiber
B. Protein
C. Minerals
D. Vitamins
ANSWER: A   p. 3

7. Which nutrient is usually consumed in greatest quantity from the diet?

K
A. Fat
B. Water
C. Protein
D. Carbohydrate
ANSWER: B   p. 3

8. Which of the following nutrients does NOT yield energy on being oxidized during metabolism?

K
A. Fat
B. Proteins
C. Vitamins
D. Carbohydrates
ANSWER: C   p. 4

9. Which of the following results from oxidation of energy nutrients?

AP
A. Energy is released
B. Body fat increases
C. Energy is destroyed
D. Body water decreases
ANSWER: A   p. 4

10. International units of energy are expressed in

K   A. newtons.
    B. calories.
    C. kilojoules.
    D. kilocalories.
    ANSWER: C   p. 4

11. How much energy is required to raise the temperature of one <u>liter</u> of water 1°C?

AP   A. 10 calories
    B. 1 kilocalorie
    C. 10,000 calories
    D. 1000 kilocalories
    ANSWER: B   p. 4

12. Which of the following nutrient sources yield <u>more</u> than 4 kcalories per gram?

AP   A. Plant fats
    B. Plant proteins
    C. Animal proteins
    D. Plant carbohydrates
    ANSWER: A   p. 4

13. Which of the following <u>CANNOT</u> be "fattening" to the body?

AP   A. Alcohol
    B. Proteins
    C. Carbohydrates
    D. Inorganic nutrients
    ANSWER: D   p. 4

14. A diet provides a total of 2,200 kcalories of which 40% of the <u>energy</u> is from fat and 20% from protein. How many <u>grams</u> of carbohydrate are contained in the diet?

AP   A. 220
    B. 285
    C. 440
    D. 880
    ANSWER: A   p. 5

4   Chapter 1   An Overview of Nutrition

15. A weight reduction regimen calls for a daily intake of 1400 kcal and 30g of fat. Approximately what percentage of the total energy is contributed by fat?

AP   A. 19
     B. 15
     C. 8.5
     D. 25.5
     ANSWER: A   p. 5

16. What is the kcalorie value of a meal supplying 110 g of carbohydrates, 25 g of protein, 20 g of fat, and 5 g of alcohol?

AP   A. 160
     B. 345
     C. 560
     D. 755
     ANSWER: D   p. 5

17. Which statement most accurately describes the composition of most foods?

AP   A. Contain only one of the three energy nutrients although a few contain all of them.
     B. Contain mixtures of the three energy nutrients, although only one or two may predominate.
     C. Contain equal amounts of the three energy nutrients although only one or two may predominate.
     D. Contain only two of the three energy nutrients although there are numerous foods that contain only one.
     ANSWER: B   p. 5

18. Gram for gram, which provides the most energy?

K   A. Fats
     B. Alcohol
     C. Proteins
     D. Carbohydrates
     ANSWER: A   p. 5

19. Which of the following is NOT a characteristic shared by minerals?

AP   A. Yield no energy
     B. Stable in cooked foods
     C. Metabolized in the body
     D. Structurally smaller than vitamins
     ANSWER: C   p. 5

Chapter 1   An Overview of Nutrition   5

20. A normal half-cup vegetable serving weighs approximately how many grams?

K
    A.   5
    B.   50
    C.   100
    D.   200
    ANSWER: C   p. 6

21. A teaspoonful of sugar or salt weighs about how many grams?

K
    A.   5
    B.   9
    C.   15
    D.   20
    ANSWER: A   p. 6

22. Approximately how many milliliters are contained in a half-cup of milk?

K
    A.   50
    B.   85
    C.   125
    D.   200
    ANSWER: C   p. 6

23. Which of the following is NOT a characteristic of the vitamins?

K
    A.   Organic
    B.   Essential
    C.   Inorganic
    D.   Destructible
    ANSWER: C   p. 7

24. Which of the following is/are NOT fat-soluble?

K
    A.   Vitamin A
    B.   Vitamin K
    C.   Vitamin D
    D.   B vitamins
    ANSWER: D   p. 7

25. How many vitamins are known to exist for human beings?

K
    A.   5
    B.   8
    C.   10
    D.   13
    ANSWER: D   p. 7

Chapter 1   An Overview of Nutrition

26. Overcooking a food is LEAST likely to affect the value of which group of nutrients?

AP
A. Vitamins
B. Minerals
C. Proteins
D. Carbohydrates
ANSWER: B   p. 8

27. Which of the following is NOT a source of water for the body?

K
A. Foods
B. Vitamins
C. Water itself
D. Metabolic reactions
ANSWER: B   p. 8

28. How many minerals are known to be required in the diet of human beings?

K
A. 6
B. 12
C. 16
D. 24
ANSWER: C   p. 8

29. Recommended Dietary Allowances may be used to

AP
A. measure nutrient balance.
B. assess dietary nutrient adequacy.
C. treat persons with diet related illness.
D. calculate exact food requirements for most individuals.
ANSWER: B   p. 9

30. The RDA (Recommended Dietary Allowances) for nutrients are generally

K
A. more than twice as high as anyone needs.
B. the minimum amounts that average people need.
C. designed to be adequate for almost all normal people.
D. designed to prevent deficiency disease in half the population.
ANSWER: C   p. 9

31. Which of the following groups is charged with producing the standards known as the Recommended Dietary Allowances?

AP
A. U.S. Public Health Service
B. Food and Drug Administration
C. Committee on Diet and Health
D. Committee on Dietary Allowances
ANSWER: D   p. 9

32. RDA exist for all of the following EXCEPT

K
A. fiber.
B. energy.
C. protein.
D. most vitamins.
ANSWER: A   p. 10

33. According to the Committee on Diet and Health, what percentage of the daily energy intake should be derived from carbohydrate?

AP
A. Over 50
B. Over 75
C. Less than 20
D. Between 25 and 45
ANSWER: A   p. 11

34. Approximately what level of fat in the diet is considered to promote optimal health for most people?

AP
A. 10-25% of energy intake
B. 30% of energy intake
C. 45% of energy intake
D. 50-60% of energy intake
ANSWER: B   p. 11

35. The quantity of a nutrient that will just prevent the appearance of specific deficiency signs is known as the

K
A. quota.
B. ration.
C. allowance.
D. requirement.
ANSWER: D   p. 11

8 Chapter 1 An Overview of Nutrition

36. If a group of people consumed an amount of protein equal to the average requirement, what percentage would receive insufficient amounts?

AP   A. 2
B. 33
C. 50
D. 98
ANSWER: C   p. 12

37. Which of the following represents a rationale for setting the RDA for energy?

AP   A. Since protein is an energy nutrient, the figures for energy intake are set in proportion to protein intake
B. Since a large number of people are overweight, the figures are set to induce a gradual weight loss in most individuals
C. Since the energy needs within each population group show little variation, the figures are set to meet the needs of almost all individuals
D. Since a margin of safety would result in excess energy intake for a large number of people, the figures are set at the average energy intake
ANSWER: D   p. 12

38. In setting Recommended Dietary Allowances (RDA) for nutrients, the Committee makes all of the following assumptions EXCEPT

K   A. people are generally healthy.
B. people generally consume protein of good quality.
C. people generally consume diets adequate in kcalories.
D. people buy their foods exclusively at health food stores.
ANSWER: D   p. 14

39. Which of the following is NOT a feature of the RDA?

AP   A. Designed for the restoration of health
B. Useful to measure the adequacy of diets in groups of people
C. Useful to formulate menus for government food programs
D. Designed as approximate, flexible and generous guidelines
ANSWER: A   p. 14

40. All of the following are features of the FAO/WHO nutrient recommendations EXCEPT

K   A. they are superior to the RDA.
B. they are usually lower than the RDA.
C. they are stated in terms of high quality protein.
D. they are followed by most countries of the world.
ANSWER: A   p. 14

Chapter 1   An Overview of Nutrition   9

41. How are the RDA figures for nutrient intakes set?

K A. Low, so as not to risk toxicity
   B. Extremely high, to cover every single person
   C. At the mean, to cover most healthy individuals
   D. High, to cover virtually all healthy individuals
   ANSWER: D   p. 14

42. Which of the following is used to detect nutrient deficiencies?

K A. Overt symptoms
   B. Nutrient stages
   C. Assessment techniques
   D. Outward manifestations
   ANSWER: C   p. 15

43. Which of the following is used to determine the presence of abnormal functions inside the body due to a nutrient deficiency?

K A. Diet history
   B. Body weight loss
   C. Laboratory tests
   D. Physical examination
   ANSWER: C   p. 16-17

44. Inspection of hair, eyes, skin, and posture is part of the nutrition assessment component known as

K A. diet history.
   B. anthropometrics.
   C. biochemical testing.
   D. physical examination.
   ANSWER: D   p. 16

45. Which of the following is an overt symptom of iron deficiency?

K A. Anemia
   B. Headaches
   C. Skin dryness
   D. Decreased red blood cell count
   ANSWER: B   p. 17

10 Chapter 1 An Overview of Nutrition

46. What type of deficiency is caused by inadequate absorption of a nutrient?

K
- A. Primary
- B. Clinical
- C. Secondary
- D. Subclinical

ANSWER: C   p. 17

47. Which of the following changes would NOT lead to a secondary nutrient deficiency?

A
- A. Inadequate nutrient intake
- B. Reduced nutrient absorption
- C. Increased nutrient excretion
- D. Increased nutrient destruction

ANSWER: A   p. 17

48. One of the recommendations of the Committee on Diet and Health is for all people to decrease their intake of salt to prevent or delay the onset of disease. This intervention concept is an example of the

AP
- A. medical approach.
- B. individual approach.
- C. population approach.
- D. risk-factor approach.

ANSWER: C   p. 19

49. Which of the following is NOT a valid recommendation to remedy nutrition problems in the United States?

- A. Consume less fat, sugar, and salt
- B. Take vitamin supplements twice weekly
- C. Choose more foods high in fiber and nutrients relative to their kcalorie content
- D. Exercise regularly to afford a food energy intake sufficient to provide the required amounts of nutrients

ANSWER: B   p. 20-21

50. Who would be the most appropriate person to consult regarding nutrition information?

AP
- A. Chiropractor
- B. Medical doctor
- C. Registered dietitian
- D. Health food store manager

ANSWER: C   p. 24

51. All of the following are recognized, credible sources of nutrition information EXCEPT

    A. Who's Who in Nutrition.
    B. Food and Drug Administration.
    C. American Dietetic Association.
    D. United States Department of Agriculture.
    ANSWER: A   p. 26

Essay Questions

2-3   52. What is the meaning and significance of the phrase "You are what you eat?"

3,4,7,8   53. Define the term organic. How do the properties of vitamins relate to their organic nature? Contrast these points with the properties of inorganic compounds such as minerals.

9   54. List important criteria in formulating recommendations to support sound nutritional health. How close does the Committee on Dietary Allowances and the Committee on Diet and Health come to meeting these criteria?

9-11   55. Describe the criteria used to establish the RDA for most nutrients. What types of recommendations are made for nutrients that do not have RDA?

12   Chapter 1   An Overview of Nutrition

12   56.   What approach is taken in setting allowances for energy intakes? Why is this approach taken? How does this approach differ from that taken for other nutrients?

15-17   57.   List and discuss four methods used to assess nutritional status. What types of individuals are qualified to evaluate nutritional health of individuals?

23-26   58.   List techniques that help identify nutrition quackery. Where can you find reliable sources of nutrition information?

24   59.   a. Explain the requirements for education and training associated with obtaining registration as a dietitian.

                    b. List several career areas in which registered dietitians are often employed.

CHAPTER 2
FOOD CHOICES AND DIET-PLANNING GUIDES

MULTIPLE CHOICE

1. What are the principles of the "ABCDMV" diet?

K A. Abundance, B vitamins, calories, diet control, minerals, and variety
   B. Abundance, balance, conservative, diversity, moderation, and vitamins
   C. Adequacy, bone development, correction, vitamin density, master, and variety
   D. Adequacy, balance, calorie control, nutrient density, moderation, and variety
   ANSWER: D   p. 30

2. Which of the following is the most nutrient dense food relative to calcium content?

AP A. Whole milk
   B. Non-fat milk
   C. Low-fat milk
   D. Cheddar cheese
   ANSWER: B   p. 31

3. Nutrient density refers to foods that

K A. carry the USDA nutrition labeling.
   B. are higher in weight relative to volume.
   C. contain a mixture of carbohydrate, fat, and protein.
   D. provide more nutrients than kcalories relative to the RDA.
   ANSWER: D   p. 31

2   Chapter 2   Food Choices and Diet-Planning Guides

4. The concept of nutrient density is most helpful in achieving what principle of diet planning?

K A. Variety
  B. Balance
  C. Moderation
  D. Calorie control
  ANSWER: D p. 31

5. Which of the following is NOT a feature of a food group plan?

K A. Excludes some foods
  B. Considered a tool for diet-planning
  C. Sorts foods of similar water content
  D. Specifies the number of servings from each group
  ANSWER: C p. 32

6. Which of the following foods would be placed in the "miscellaneous" category of food group plans?

AP A. Jam
  B. Watermelon
  C. Raw carrots
  D. Brussels sprouts
  ANSWER: A p. 32

7. Applying the principle of variety in food planning also applies the principle of

AP A. dilution.
  B. moderation.
  C. vegetarianism.
  D. nutrient density.
  ANSWER: A p. 32

8. Which of the following is NOT a diet-planning guide widely used by nutrition-conscious people?

  A. Food group plans
  B. Exchange patterns
  C. The rice diet plan
  D. Dietary guidelines
  ANSWER: C p. 32-36

9. Which of the following is a valid criticism of the Four Food Group Plan?

K A. Difficult to learn and to teach
  B. Overemphasizes animal products
  C. Underemphasizes animal products
  D. Does not provide guidance on energy intakes
  ANSWER: D p. 33

Chapter 2 Food Choices and Diet-Planning Guides 3

10. Which of the following is NOT characteristic of the Daily Food Guide?

AP
    A. Most foods can be placed into one of the five groups
    B. It can be used with great flexibility once its intent is understood
    C. It specifies that a certain quantity of food must be consumed from each group
    D. Following all of the plan's rules ensures that the day's needs for all nutrients are met
ANSWER: D   p. 33

11. What are two major nutrients supplied by the fruit and vegetable group?

K
    A. Vitamins D and E
    B. Vitamins A and C
    C. Protein and calcium
    D. B vitamins and iron
ANSWER: B   p. 34

12. Consider the following menu from the point of view of the Daily Food Guide.

Breakfast	Lunch	Supper
2 eggs	2 oz tuna fish	3 oz hamburger meat
1 tsp margarine	lettuce	1 oz cheese
2 slices enriched white bread	1 tbsp mayonnaise	2 slices enriched white bread
coffee	1 c whole milk	1/2 c cooked rice
	1 apple	1/2 c carrots
		coffee

Which of the following describes the nutritional value of the fruits and vegetables in this menu?

AP
    A. They are missing a vitamin A source
    B. They are missing a vitamin C source
    C. They meet the Four Food Group recommendations
    D. They exceed the Four Food Group recommendations
ANSWER: B   p. 34

13. Which of the following is an alternative choice for meats in the Daily Food Guide?

AP
    A. Nuts
    B. Bacon
    C. Baked potatoes
    D. Sweet potatoes
ANSWER: A   p. 34

Chapter 2 Food Choices and Diet-Planning Guides

14. Which of the following is descriptive of the USDA Food Pyramid?

K
- A. A three-dimensional structure designed to assist the average consumer in the use of the Food Exchange System
- B. An education tool for teaching nutrition to children which consists of food blocks that require stacking in a specific order
- C. A graphic representation of the Dietary Guidelines that displays complex carbohydrates at the base and fats and sweets at the very top
- D. A system of specialized containers of several different sizes which allows for better storage and preservation of perishable food items

ANSWER: C   p. 35

15. The availability of orange juice containing added calcium is an example of the process of

AP
- A. pH control.
- B. enrichment.
- C. fortification.
- D. flavor enhancements.

ANSWER: C   p. 36

16. Exchange patterns for meal planning were originally developed for people with

K
- A. obesity.
- B. diabetes.
- C. hypertension.
- D. renal disease.

ANSWER: B   p. 36

17. In an exchange list, which nutrients are NOT found in approximately the same amounts in all food portions?

AP
- A. Calories
- B. Proteins
- C. Vitamins and minerals
- D. Fats and carbohydrates

ANSWER C: p. 36

18. The addition of liberal amounts of calcium to some commercially available orange juice products by juice processors is most properly termed nutrient

AP
- A. restoration.
- B. enrichment.
- C. fortification.
- D. mineralization.

ANSWER: C   p. 36

Chapter 2 Food Choices and Diet-Planning Guides   5

19. Which of the following items would NOT be found on the Food Exchange lists?

AP
A. Olives
B. Brown sugar
C. Salad dressing
D. Evaporated milk
ANSWER: B   p. 37

20. Mr. Jones ate 1 fruit exchange, 2 starch/bread exchanges, 1 medium-fat meat exchange, and 1 fat exchange for breakfast. Approximately how many kcalories did he consume?

AP
A. 120
B. 230
C. 340
D. 450
ANSWER: C   p. 37

21. Which of the following provides the most energy?

AP
A. 4 fruit exchanges
B. 3 bread exchanges
C. 2 lean meat exchanges
D. 2 whole milk exchanges
ANSWER: D   p. 37

22. What is the approximate kcalorie content of the following menu?

2 oz lean roast beef   1 small pear
2 slices bread   1 nonfat milk
2 tsp butter

AP
A. 240
B. 450
C. 500
D. 800
ANSWER: C   p. 37-39

23. How many grams of carbohydrates are supplied by the following meal?

3 oz skinned chicken
1/2 c brussels sprouts
1 small baked potato
1 slice whole-wheat bread

AP
A. 10
B. 25
C. 35
D. 45
ANSWER: C   p. 37-38

6   Chapter 2 Food Choices and Diet-Planning Guides

24. Which of the following foods is NOT found in the meat exchange list?

    A. Eggs
    B. Fish
    C. Bacon
    D. Cheese
    ANSWER: C   p. 37-39

25. Which of the following foods is NOT considered to be a lean meat in the exchange system of meal planning?

K   A. Canned tuna
    B. Low-fat cheese
    C. Skinned chicken
    D. Hard-boiled egg
    ANSWER: D   p. 38

26. Using the exchange system for meal planning, how many ounces of meat are in one meat exchange?

AP   A. 1
    B. 3
    C. 5
    D. 7
    ANSWER: A   p. 38

27. Which of the following is NOT listed on the vegetable group of the exchange system?

K   A. Tomato
    B. Carrots
    C. Spinach
    D. Avocado
    ANSWER: D   p. 38

28. Which of the following exchange lists is separated into three categories?

K   A. Fruit
    B. Meat
    C. Vegetable
    D. Starch/bread
    ANSWER: B   p. 38

29. Which of the following foods is listed in the high-fat meat exchange category?

AP   A. Egg
    B. Pork loin
    C. Cheddar cheese
    D. Creamed cottage cheese
    ANSWER: C   p. 39

30. Which of the following foods is NOT considered to be a fat in the exchange system of meal planning?

AP   A. Bacon
      B. Olives
      C. Salad dressing
      D. Country-style ham
ANSWER: D   p. 39

31. On what Food Exchange list would American cheese be placed?

AP   A. Fats
      B. Milks
      C. Meats
      D. Starches/breads
ANSWER: C   p. 41

32. All of the following are features of the Food Exchange System EXCEPT

K   A. it can be used to regulate fat intake.
     B. it can be used to guide and control energy intake.
     C. it was originally developed for treatment of diabetes.
     D. it virtually guarantees adequate vitamin and mineral intakes.
ANSWER D: p. 42

33. Which of the following is a disadvantage of the Food Exchange System?

K   A. It is used primarily by diabetics
     B. It defines food portions according to energy content
     C. The groupings are made without regard to micronutrient content
     D. It subdivides the milk group and meat group based on fat content
ANSWER: C   p. 42

34. Which of the following is a characteristic of enriched grain products?

K   A. They have all of the added nutrients listed on the label
     B. They have the fiber restored from the refining procedure
     C. They have 4 vitamins and 4 minerals added by the food processor
     D. They have virtually all the nutrients restored from refining procedure
ANSWER: A   p. 45

35. What federal law mandated the addition of thiamin, riboflavin, niacin, and iron to white flour?

K   A. Fortification Mandate
     B. Enrichment Act of 1942
     C. Nutritification Mandate
     D. Restoration Act of 1910
ANSWER: B   p. 45

Chapter 2 Food Choices and Diet-Planning Guides

36. What nutrient makes up most of the endosperm section of grains such as wheat and rice?

K
A. Fat
B. Fiber
C. Starch
D. Protein
ANSWER: C   p. 48

37. Which of the following breads has the highest fiber content?

AP
A. White
B. Refined
C. Enriched
D. Whole-grain
ANSWER: D   p. 49

38. What are foodways?

K
A. Techniques of food preparation for ethnic cuisine
B. Very large supermarkets that carry a variety of ethnic foods
C. The dietary food habits, customs, beliefs and preferences of a particular culture
D. Lists of imitation and substitute foods to help meet dietary planning guidelines of at-risk individuals
ANSWER: C   p. 50

39. To meet the recommendations promulgated in the work Diet and Health, which of the following adjustments is necessary for northern European cuisine?

AP
A. Reduce meat intake
B. Reduce fiber intake
C. Increase iron intake
D. Increase meat intake
ANSWER: A   p. 51

40. Which of the following ethnic diets is noted for its dish of red beans and rice?

AP
A. Cajun
B. Chinese
C. West African
D. Southern European
ANSWER: A   p. 51

41. Features of Chinese cuisine include all of the following EXCEPT

AP
A. it is low in fat.
B. it is high in fiber.
C. it is low in sodium.
D. it includes soup with each meal.
ANSWER: C   p. 54

Chapter 2 Food Choices and Diet-Planning Guides   9

42. Which of the following foods could be subjected to kosher preparation?

AP   A. Steak
     B. Bagels
     C. Pickles
     D. Noodles
     ANSWER: A   p. 54

43. Which of the following is a feature of the 1990 Nutrition Labeling and Education Act?

K   A. Restaurant foods will be required to provide nutrient content on the menu
     B. The term "fresh" can be used only for raw and moderately processed food
     C. Nutrition labeling will be required to appear on virtually all processed as well as fresh foods
     D. Health claims will not be permitted if a standard serving size contains more than 11.5 g fat or more than 45 mg cholesterol
     ANSWER: D   p. 58-62

44. Information that must be lawfully provided on food labels includes all of the following EXCEPT

K   A. the amount recommended for ingestion each day.
     B. the amounts of specified nutrients and food components.
     C. the net contents expressed by weight, measure, or count.
     D. the name and address of the manufacture, packer, or distributor.
     ANSWER: A   p. 58

45. Which of the following ingredient lists conforms to the newest FDA food label laws?

AP   A. Corn, sweeteners, salt....
     B. Flour, sugar, soybean and/or coconut oil...
     C. Chocolate (sugar, coconut or palm oil), salt...
     D. Water, orange concentrate, sucrose, fructose, glucose....
     ANSWER: D   p. 59

46. Which of the following groups represents the most frequently eaten raw fruit, vegetable, and seafood in the U.S.?

K   A. Apple, tomato, cod
     B. Orange, carrot, scallop
     C. Banana, potato, shrimp
     D. Grape, lettuce, flounder
     ANSWER: C   p. 59

Chapter 2 Food Choices and Diet-Planning Guides

47. Under the new food labeling regulations, food companies are permitted to list all of the following health claims regarding nutrition and disease EXCEPT

K   A.   sugar and diabetes.
       B.   sodium and hypertension.
       C.   calcium and osteoporosis.
       D.   lipids and cancer and cardiovascular disease.
ANSWER: A   p. 62

48. According to the FDA, which of the following diet-health messages would NOT be approved for use on food labels?

K   A.   Fiber and cancer
       B.   Lipids and obesity
       C.   Calcium and osteoporosis
       D.   Sodium and high blood pressure
ANSWER: B   p. 62

Essay Questions

49. List and discuss the significance of six diet-planning principles.

50. What is meant by the term nutrient-dense food? Give 3 examples of foods with high nutrient density and low nutrient density.

51. List the five food groups and describe how foods are classified. What are the advantages and disadvantages of the Daily Food Guide?

36 52. Present the 6 exchange lists and explain how foods are classified.

50 53. Discuss ways in which dietary guidelines can be applied to ethnic diets.

58-61 54. Describe the major regulations of the Nutrition Labeling and Education Act of 1990. List the information that must be displayed on food labels.

60 55. Explain the meaning, significance, and purpose of the two sets of reference values: Reference Daily Intakes and Daily Reference Values.

CHAPTER 3
DIGESTION, ABSORPTION, AND TRANSPORT

MULTIPLE CHOICE

1. What structure prevents food from entering the trachea when you swallow?

K   A.   Tongue
       B.   Esophagus
       C.   Epiglottis
       D.   Cardiac sphincter
ANSWER: C   p. 68

2. A bolus that is conducted past the diaphragm must pass through what structure?

K   A.   Stomach
       B.   Esophagus
       C.   Epiglottis
       D.   Large intestine
ANSWER: B   p. 68

3. What is one function of the pyloric sphincter?

K   A.   Secretes acid into the stomach
       B.   Secretes hormones into the stomach
       C.   Prevents the contents of the intestines from backing up into the stomach
       D.   Prevents the contents of the intestine from emptying too quickly into the colon
ANSWER: C   p. 68

Chapter 3 Digestion, Absorption, and Transport

4. What structure separates the colon from the small intestine?

K   A. Pylorus
     B. Ileocecal valve
     C. Gastric retainer
     D. Rectal sphincter
     ANSWER: B   p. 68

5. Into what region of the intestinal tract does the stomach empty?

K   A. Ileum
     B. Cecum
     C. Jejunum
     D. Duodenum
     ANSWER: D   p. 68

6. What is a bolus?

K   A. Enzyme that hydrolyzes starch
     B. Portion of food swallowed at one time
     C. Device used to analyze the contents of the stomach
     D. Sphincter muscle separating the stomach from the small intestine
     ANSWER: B   p. 68

7. Which of the following is a description of chyme?

K   A. The semisolid mass of undigested food which passes through the ileocecal valve
     B. A semiliquid mass of partially digested food released by the stomach into the intestines
     C. The mixture of pancreatic juices containing enzymes for digestion of the macronutrients
     D. A thick, viscous material synthesized by mucosal cells for protection against digestive juices
     ANSWER: B   p. 68

8. After swallowing, in what order does food pass through the GI tract?

AP A. Jejunum, duodenum, colon, ileum, rectum
     B. Jejunum, ileum, duodenum, rectum, colon
     C. Stomach, duodenum, jejunum, ileum, colon
     D. Stomach, jejunum, duodenum, colon, ileum
     ANSWER: C   p. 68-69

9. What structure functions to prevent entrance of food into the trachea?

K   A. Tongue
     B. Epiglottis
     C. Cardiac sphincter
     D. Trachea sphincter
     ANSWER: B   p. 68

10. What structure controls the passage of material from the small intestines to the large intestines?

K   A. Pyloric valve
      B. Ileocecal valve
      C. Jejunal sphincter
      D. Colonic sphincter
      ANSWER: B   p. 68

11. What is the primary function of the rectum?

K   A. Controls functioning of the colon
      B. Absorbs minerals from waste materials
      C. Stores waste materials prior to evacuation
      D. Absorbs excess water from waste materials
      ANSWER: C   p. 68

12. What is the name given to partially digested food expelled by the stomach into the duodenum?

K   A. Chyme
      B. Liquid food
      C. Gastric mucus
      D. Semiliquid mass
      ANSWER: A   p. 68

13. Which of the following body organs does **NOT** secrete digestive enzymes?

K   A. Liver
      B. Stomach
      C. Pancreas
      D. Salivary glands
      ANSWER: A   p. 69

14. Where does peristalsis begin?

K   A. Back of the mouth
      B. Top of the esophagus
      C. Bottom of the stomach
      D. Beginning of small intestine
      ANSWER: B   p. 71

15. Where does peristalsis begin?

K   A. Mouth
      B. Stomach
      C. Top of intestines
      D. Top of esophagus
      ANSWER: D   p. 71

4   Chapter 3   Digestion, Absorption, and Transport

16. Which of the following is a function of sphincter muscles?

K A. Control peristalsis
   B. Grind large food particles
   C. Secrete digestive juices into the GI tract
   D. Control the passage of food through the GI tract
   ANSWER: D   p. 72

17. Which of the following is NOT a sphincter muscle?

K A. Anus
   B. Cardiac
   C. Duodenum
   D. Ileocecal valve
   ANSWER: C   p. 72

18. Which of the following best describes the normal pH of the stomach?

K A. Slightly acidic
   B. Very acidic
   C. Neutral
   D. Slightly alkaline
   ANSWER: B   p. 73

19. What is the function of mucus in the stomach?

K A. Emulsifies fats
   B. Neutralizes stomach acid
   C. Activates pepsinogen to pepsin
   D. Protects stomach cells from gastric juices
   ANSWER: D   p. 73

20. What is a function of hydrochloric acid of the stomach?

K A. Absorbs water
   B. Inhibits hydrolysis
   C. Neutralizes the food mass
   D. Creates an optimum acidity
   ANSWER: D   p. 73

21. Why is there little or no digestion of starch in the stomach?

AP A. Stomach enzymes are dysfunctional
   B. Starch should not be eaten with protein
   C. Gastric juice contains inactive amylase
   D. Salivary amylase does not work in an acid environment
   ANSWER: D   p. 73

Chapter 3 Digestion, Absorption, and Transport   5

22. What is the fate of any enzymes that are present in the foods we eat?

AP
A. Hydrolyzed in the GI tract
B. Absorbed intact by the stomach
C. Absorbed intact by the small intestine
D. Passed through the GI tract and excreted in the stool
ANSWER: A   p. 73-74

23. Which part of the GI tract contains very acidic digestive juices?

K
A. Colon
B. Ileum
C. Stomach
D. Duodenum
ANSWER: C   p. 73

24. What substance protects the stomach lining from damage due to digestive juices?

K
A. Water
B. Mucus
C. Pepsinogen
D. Dietary fats
ANSWER: B   p. 73

25. Which of the following is NOT a component of pancreatic juice?

K
A. Bile
B. Water
C. Protease
D. Sodium bicarbonate
ANSWER: A   p. 74

26. After the pancreatic juices have mixed with chyme in the intestine, which of the following describes the pH of the resulting mixture?

AP
A. Very acidic
B. Slightly alkaline
C. Strongly alkaline
D. Approximately neutral
ANSWER: D   p. 74

27. What is one function of the gallbladder?

K
A. Stores bile
B. Produces bile
C. Reabsorbs water and salts
D. Performs enzymatic digestion
ANSWER: A   p. 74

Chapter 3 Digestion, Absorption, and Transport

28. What is the function of bile?

K
A. Emulsifies fats
B. Initiates digestion of protein
C. Enhances absorption of complex carbohydrates
D. Protects the stomach and small intestine from the action of hydrochloric acid
ANSWER: A   p. 74

29. Which of the following is NOT a component of pancreatic juice?

K
A. Lipase
B. Maltase
C. Amylase
D. Bicarbonate
ANSWER: B   p. 74

30. Which of the following would NOT be acted upon by pancreatic juice secreted into the intestinal tract?

AP
A. Fats
B. Fiber
C. Proteins
D. Carbohydrates
ANSWER: B   p. 74-75

31. Which of the following is NOT a typical component of stools?

AP
A. Water
B. Fiber
C. Starch
D. Bacteria
ANSWER: C   p. 74-75

32. What is the primary role of the normal, thriving intestinal bacterial population?

AP
A. Helps degrade meat and dairy proteins
B. Helps prevent infectious bacteria from attacking the system
C. Synthesizes most vitamins which can be absorbed into the body
D. Synthesizes several amino acids which can be absorbed into the body
ANSWER: B   p. 75

33. Which of the following is known to be produced by small intestinal bacteria?

K
A. Mucus
B. Chyme
C. Glucose
D. Vitamins
ANSWER: D   p. 75

34. Which of the following is generally NOT digested but does stimulate intestinal muscle contractions?

K A. Bile
  B. Fiber
  C. Starch
  D. Amylase
  ANSWER: B p. 75

35. Which of the following is a property of dietary fiber?

AP A. Inhibits intestinal motility
  B. Inhibits gastrointestinal peristalsis
  C. Promotes water retention of stools
  D. Promotes vitamin excretion in stools
  ANSWER: C p. 75

36. Which of the following classes of nutrients requires the least amount of digestion?

K A. Lipids
  B. Proteins
  C. Vitamins
  D. Carbohydrates
  ANSWER: C p. 75

37. Which of the following nutrients requires the least amount of digestion?

AP A. Starch
  B. Calcium
  C. Animal fats
  D. Animal proteins
  ANSWER: B p. 75

38. Which of the following nutrients requires the greatest amount of digestion?

AP A. Fats
  B. Water
  C. Minerals
  D. Vitamins
  ANSWER: A p. 75

39. What is the name of the projections on the inner surface of the small intestine?

K A. Villi
  B. Lymphatic cilia
  C. Mesenteric vessels
  D. Vascular projectiles
  ANSWER: A p. 76

8   Chapter 3 Digestion, Absorption, and Transport

40. Which of the following is a function of the intestinal microvilli?

K   A. Secretion of bile salts
     B. Secretion of digestive acid
     C. Transport of nutrient molecules
     D. Transport of pancreatic enzymes
     ANSWER: C   p. 76

41. An example of an important function of the colon would be its absorption of

AP A. bile.
     B. fats.
     C. fiber.
     D. sodium chloride.
     ANSWER: D   p. 76

42. What is the primary site for absorption of nutrients?

K   A. Crypt
     B. Villus
     C. Microvillus
     D. Macrovillus
     ANSWER: C   p. 76

43. Which of the following are found on the microvilli and function to break apart small nutrients to the final products of digestion?

K   A. Cells
     B. Micelles
     C. Enzymes
     D. Hormones
     ANSWER: C   p. 78

44. To assist the process of digestion and absorption, it is best to

AP A. eat several snacks per day so the system is not overwhelmed.
     B. combine different food types to enhance the absorption process.
     C. avoid eating meat and fruit at the same meal to prevent competition.
     D. take enzyme pills or powder periodically so the system can rest and rejuvenate.
     ANSWER: B   p. 78

45. Blood leaving the digestive system goes by way of a vein to what organ?

K   A. Heart
     B. Liver
     C. Lungs
     D. Kidneys
     ANSWER: B   p. 79

Chapter 3 Digestion, Absorption, and Transport 9

46. When nutrients are transported from intestinal epithelial cells to the vascular system, what organ is first to receive them?

AP
A. Liver
B. Heart
C. Lungs
D. Kidneys
ANSWER: A   p. 79

47. When alcohol and barbiturates are ingested, they are absorbed from the gastrointestinal tract and transported first to the

AP
A. heart.
B. liver.
C. spleen.
D. kidneys.
ANSWER: B   p. 80

48. Which of the following products of digestion is NOT normally released directly into the bloodstream?

K
A. Minerals
B. Vitamin C
C. Monoglycerides
D. Monosaccharides
ANSWER: C   p. 82

49. After absorption, the fat soluble vitamins and large fats are first carried through which circulatory system?

K
A. Vascular
B. Mesentery
C. Lymphatic
D. Subclavian vein
ANSWER: C   p. 82

50. What structure conducts lymph into the vascular system?

K
A. Villi
B. Mesentery
C. Subclavian vein
D. Common bile duct
ANSWER: C   p. 82

10   Chapter 3 Digestion, Absorption, and Transport

51. Which of the following hormones regulates pH of the stomach?

K   A. Gastrin
B. Insulin
C. Secretin
D. Cholecystokinin
ANSWER: A   p. 83

52. Which of the following substances controls the release of hydrochloric acid to prevent excessive acidity, which could lead to damage of the GI tract lining?

AP   A. Fiber
B. Gastrin
C. Secretin
D. Bicarbonate
ANSWER: B   p. 83

53. Which of the following hormones stimulates the pancreas to release its juices?

K   A. Gastrin
B. Glucagon
C. Secretin
D. Gastric-inhibitory polypeptide
ANSWER: C   p. 84

54. The presence of fat in the intestine stimulates cells of the intestinal wall to release

K   A. gastrin.
B. secretin.
C. enterogastrone.
D. cholecystokinin.
ANSWER: D   p. 84

55. Which of the following is associated with the presence of fat in the GI?

K   A. Inhibition of mucosal enzyme activities
B. Stimulation and hastening of digestion and absorption
C. Slowing down the process of digestion and absorption
D. Inhibition of thiamin, riboflavin, and niacin absorption
ANSWER: C   p. 84

56. What is the very first thing you should do if you suspect someone is choking on food?

AP   A. Perform the Heimlich maneuver
B. Strike the person sharply on the back
C. Ask the person to make sounds from the throat
D. Attempt to dislodge the food with your fingers
ANSWER: C   p. 86

Chapter 3 Digestion, Absorption, and Transport 11

57. Choking occurs when a piece of food becomes firmly lodged in what structure?

AP   A. Larynx
B. Trachea
C. Esophagus
D. Epiglottis
ANSWER: B   p. 86

58. Which of the following involves reverse peristalsis?

K   A. Gas
B. Choking
C. Vomiting
D. Diarrhea
ANSWER: C   p. 88

59. Chronic diarrhea may result in which of the following?

AP   A. Dehydration
B. Constipation
C. Peptic ulcers
D. Heimlich's disease
ANSWER: A   p. 88

60. People are said to be constipated when they experience

AP   A. painful or difficult bowel movements.
B. more than a day without a bowel movement.
C. more than three days without a bowel movement.
D. soft or watery bowel movements with little notice.
ANSWER: A   p. 89

61. Therapy for constipation would include all of the following EXCEPT

AP   A. increasing water intake.
B. decreasing fiber intake.
C. increasing physical activity.
D. responding promptly to the defecation signal.
ANSWER: B   p. 89

62. Which of the following is most likely to result from insufficient intake of fibers?

AP   A. Diarrhea
B. Bloating
C. Constipation
D. Pancreatitis
ANSWER: C   p. 89

12   Chapter 3 Digestion, Absorption, and Transport

63. Which of the following is known to irritate a heartburn condition?

AP
- A. Low-fat foods
- B. High-fat foods
- C. Low-carbohydrate foods
- D. High-carbohydrate foods

ANSWER: B   p. 90-91

64. The use of an antacid is indicated primarily for which condition?

AP
- A. Excessive gas
- B. Acid indigestion
- C. Excessive belching
- D. Active ulcer in the stomach

ANSWER: D   p. 90-91

Essay Questions

70,72   65. Name and describe the functions of the four major sphincter muscles that divide the GI tract into its principal divisions.

73-74   66. What is the function of hydrochloric acid and why is it necessary in the process of digestion?

75-76   67. What is the primary function of the colon? What are the effects on colonic function from insufficient fluid intake, insufficient fiber intake, and intestinal infection?

76-79   68. Describe features of the small intestine that facilitate absorption.

86-91   69. Describe four common digestive problems and their recommended treatments or therapies.

CHAPTER 4
THE CARBOHYDRATES: SUGARS, STARCH, AND FIBERS

MULTIPLE CHOICE

1. Which of the following is <u>NOT</u> a characteristic shared by all carbohydrates?

K   A.   Their primary role is to supply energy
        B.   They appear in virtually all animal foods
        C.   They include sugars, starches, and most fibers
        D.   Their secondary role is to spare protein from being used as energy
ANSWER: B   p. 93

2. In which of the following are carbohydrates almost always found?

AP   A.   Plant foods
        B.   Health foods
        C.   Animal products
        D.   Protein-rich foods
ANSWER: A   p. 93

3. What type of nutrient is starch?

K   A.   Fiber
        B.   Gluten
        C.   Simple carbohydrate
        D.   Complex carbohydrate
ANSWER: D   p. 93

Chapter 4   The Carbohydrates: Sugars, Starch, and Fibers

4. How many carbon atoms are found in the ring structure of the most common monosaccharides in nutrition?

K A. 5
  B. 6
  C. 8
  D. 12
  ANSWER: B p. 93

5. Which of the following is NOT a simple carbohydrate?

K A. Starches
  B. White sugar
  C. Disaccharides
  D. Monosaccharides
  ANSWER: A p. 94

6. The types of atoms found in a glucose molecule include all of the following EXCEPT

K A. carbon.
  B. oxygen.
  C. nitrogen.
  D. hydrogen.
  ANSWER: C p. 94

7. Which of the following is NOT a characteristic of glucose?

AP A. Monosaccharide
  B. Soluble in water
  C. Part of the sucrose molecule
  D. Sweeter tasting than sucrose
  ANSWER: D p. 94,97

8. Milk that has been treated with a commercially available lactase preparation undergoes which of the following changes?

AP A. Increase in sweetness
  B. Decrease in sweetness
  C. Increase in carbohydrate content
  D. Decrease in carbohydrate content
  ANSWER: A p. 94,97,100,104

9. Which of the following is known as grape sugar or dextrose?

K A. Glucose
  B. Maltose
  C. Sucrose
  D. Fructose
  ANSWER: A p. 94

Chapter 4 Carbohydrates: Sugars, Starch, and Fibers   3

10. What component accounts for the usually sweet taste of fruits?

K
    A. Fats
    B. Fiber
    C. Simple sugars
    D. Complex carbohydrates
    ANSWER: C   p. 95

11. What is the sweetest tasting simple carbohydrate in the diet?

K
    A. Glucose
    B. Lactose
    C. Fructose
    D. Sucrose
    ANSWER: C   p. 95

12. Which of the following is a component of all three dietary disaccharides?

K
    A. Sucrose
    B. Glucose
    C. Fructose
    D. Galactose
    ANSWER: B   p. 95

13. Which of the following is known as fruit sugar or levulose?

K
    A. Maltose
    B. Glucose
    C. Fructose
    D. Galactose
    ANSWER: C   p. 95

14. What is the reaction that links two monsaccharides together?

K
    A. Hydrolysis
    B. Absorption
    C. Disaccharide
    D. Condensation
    ANSWER: D   p. 96

15. Which of the following is a byproduct from the condensation of two molecules of glucose?

AP
    A. Water
    B. Oxygen
    C. Hydrogen
    D. Carbon dioxide
    ANSWER: A   p. 96-97

4   Chapter 4 The Carbohydrates: Sugars, Starch, and Fibers

16. What is the principle carbohydrate of milk?

K   A. Lactose
      B. Sucrose
      C. Maltose
      D. Glycogen
      ANSWER: A   p. 97

17. What is the composition of sucrose?

K   A. Two fructose units
      B. One glucose and one fructose unit
      C. One glucose and one galactose unit
      D. One galactose and one fructose unit
      ANSWER: B   p. 97

18. What is the composition of lactose?

K   A. Two fructose units
      B. One glucose and one fructose unit
      C. One glucose and one galactose unit
      D. One galactose and one fructose unit
      ANSWER: C   p. 97

19. What is another name for lactose?

K   A. Milk sugar
      B. Table sugar
      C. Fruit sugar
      D. Artificial sugar
      ANSWER: A   p. 97

20. What is the composition of maltose?

K   A. Two glucose units
      B. Two fructose units
      C. One glucose and one fructose unit
      D. One glucose and one galactose unit
      ANSWER: A   p. 97

21. Which of the following sugars is NOT found in plants?

K   A. Glucose
      B. Lactose
      C. Sucrose
      D. Fructose
      ANSWER: B   p. 97

Chapter 4 Carbohydrates: Sugars, Starch, and Fibers   5

22. What is the name of the animal polysaccharide composed of glucose units?

K A. Fiber
   B. Enzyme
   C. Dextrin
   D. Glycogen
   ANSWER: D   p. 98

23. Glycogen is stored mainly in which of the following tissues?

K A. Muscle and liver
   B. Pancreas and kidneys
   C. Stomach and intestine
   D. Brain and red blood cells
   ANSWER: A   p. 98

24. Which of the following is NOT a rich source of dietary starch?

AP A. Grains
   B. Fruits
   C. Tubers
   D. Legumes
   ANSWER: B   p. 98

25. Which of the following is a feature of glycogen?

K A. Found in plants
   B. Absent from animal meats
   C. Unimportant as a dietary nutrient
   D. Plays an insignificant role in the body
   ANSWER: C   p. 98

26. What is the primary storage form of carbohydrate in the body?

K A. Fiber
   B. Starch
   C. Glucose
   D. Glycogen
   ANSWER: D   p. 98

27. What is the staple grain of Canada, the United States, and Europe?

K A. Oats
   B. Rice
   C. Corn
   D. Wheat
   ANSWER: D   p. 99

Chapter 4 The Carbohydrates: Sugars, Starch, and Fibers

28. What is the name of the short chains of glucose units that result from starch breakdown?

K   A. Sucrose
     B. Lignins
     C. Pectins
     D. Dextrins
     ANSWER: D   p. 100

29. Digestion of starches takes place in the small intestines and in what other organ?

K   A. Mouth
     B. Colon
     C. Stomach
     D. Pancreas
     ANSWER: A   p. 100

30. What is the primary organ that converts fructose to glucose following absorption?

K   A. Liver
     B. Pancreas
     C. Skeletal muscle
     D. Small intestines
     ANSWER: A   p. 100

31. Which of the following enzymes does NOT act on simple sugars?

K   A. Lactase
     B. Sucrase
     C. Amylase
     D. Maltase
     ANSWER: C   p. 100

32. What is the first organ to receive carbohydrates absorbed from the intestine?

K   A. Heart
     B. Liver
     C. Pancreas
     D. Skeletal muscle
     ANSWER: B   p. 100

33. Where is the location of enzymes that digest dietary sugars?

K   A. Mouth
     B. Stomach
     C. Pancreas
     D. Small intestines
     ANSWER: D   p. 100

34. What is the primary absorption site for digestible carbohydrates?

K   A. Mouth
      B. Stomach
      C. Large intestines
      D. Small intestines
      ANSWER: D   p. 100

35. Which of the following is NOT a symptom of lactose intolerance?

K   A. Nausea
      B. Cramping
      C. Diarrhea
      D. Constipation
      ANSWER: D   p. 103

36. Which of the following sweeteners contains a significant amount of iron?

K   A. Molasses
      B. Brown sugar
      C. Maple sugar
      D. Invert sugar
      ANSWER: A   p. 103

37. Which of the following is NOT a symptom of lactose intolerance?

K   A. Nausea
      B. Diarrhea
      C. Cramping
      D. Constipation
      ANSWER: D   p. 103

38. For most of the world's population, what is the effect of aging on the activity of lactase?

AP   A. Rapid decline
      B. Rapid increase
      C. Gradual decline
      D. Gradual increase
      ANSWER: C   p. 103

39. Which of the following would LEAST likely be associated with the development of lactose intolerance?

AP   A. Medicines
      B. Milk allergy
      C. Prolonged diarrhea
      D. Inherited lactase deficiency
      ANSWER: B   p. 103

8   Chapter 4   The Carbohydrates: Sugars, Starch, and Fibers

40. Which of the following ingredients listed on food labels would be acceptable to the person who is highly intolerant to lactose in the diet?

AP
   A.   Whey
   B.   Casein
   C.   Dextrins
   D.   Milk solids
ANSWER: C   p. 104

41. When blood glucose concentrations fall, what is the primary source of glucose to replenish the level?

AP
   A.   Blood lipids
   B.   Liver glycogen
   C.   Blood fructose
   D.   Muscle glycogen
ANSWER: B   p. 105

42. What is the minimum daily amount of dietary carbohydrate necessary to spare body protein from excessive breakdown?

K
   A.   10-25 g
   B.   50-100 g
   C.   150-175 g
   D.   200-400 g
ANSWER: B   p. 106

43. Gluconeogenesis would describe the synthesis of which of the following?

   A.   Amino acids from glucose
   B.   Lactose from a source of sucrose
   C.   Fat from excess carbohydrte intake
   D.   Glucose from a noncarbohydrte substance
ANSWER: D   p. 106

44. When you are under physical stress, what hormone is released quickly to stimulate an increase in blood glucose concentration?

AP
   A.   Insulin
   B.   Secretin
   C.   Glucogen
   D.   Epinephrine
ANSWER: D   p. 107

Chapter 4 Carbohydrates: Sugars, Starch, and Fibers 9

45. What is the primary function of insulin?

K
A. Raise blood glucose levels
B. Lower blood glucose levels
C. Stimulate glycogen breakdown
D. Stimulate intestinal carbohydrate absorption
ANSWER: B   p. 107

46. Which of the following is a typical response of the body to changes in blood glucose?

AP
A. Blood glucose levels that fall too low signal the release of insulin
B. Blood glucose levels that fall too low signal the release of glucagon
C. Blood glucose levels that rise too high signal the release of glycogen
D. Blood glucose levels that rise too high signal the release of epinephrine
ANSWER: B   p. 107

47. What is the first organ to respond to an increase in blood glucose concentration?

AP
A. Brain
B. Liver
C. Muscle
D. Pancreas
ANSWER: D   p. 107

48. When blood glucose concentration falls, what pancreatic hormone is secreted to stimulate release of stored glucose?

AP
A. Insulin
B. Glucagon
C. Epinephrine
D. Cholecystokinin
ANSWER: B   p. 107

49. Which of the following statements best describes the glycemic effect of foods?

K
A. A measure of how fast and high the food causes the blood glucose to rise
B. The newest, most practical means of planning diets for people with diabetes
C. A well-utilized, highly valued mechanism to control the intake of simple sugars
D. A measure of the percentage of digestible carbohydrates in relation to total energy content of the food
ANSWER: A   p. 108

10   Chapter 4   The Carbohydrates: Sugars, Starch, and Fibers

50.   Approximately how many pounds of refined sugars are consumed by the average United States resident each year?

K   A.   25
      B.   65
      C.   100
      D.   200
      ANSWER: B   p. 109

51.   What is the appropriate term to describe a food that contributes energy but is virtually devoid of protein, vitamins, and minerals?

AP   A.   Nutrient-dense food
      B.   Calorie-devoid food
      C.   Empty-kcalorie food
      D.   Nutrient-selective food
      ANSWER: C   p. 109

52.   What is the leading food additive?

K   A.   Fat
      B.   Sugar
      C.   Fiber
      D.   Vitamins
      ANSWER: B   p. 109

53.   What is the name of the sweetener consisting of a mixture of glucose and fructose formed by chemical hydrolysis of sucrose?

AP   A.   Molasses
      B.   Invert sugar
      C.   Turbinado sugar
      D.   High-fructose syrup
      ANSWER: B   p. 110

54.   What is the predominant sweetener used in formulating beverages?

K   A.   Glucose
      B.   Sucrose
      C.   Invert sugar
      D.   High-fructose corn syrup
      ANSWER: D   p. 110

Chapter 4 Carbohydrates: Sugars, Starch, and Fibers 11

55. Which of the following is known to result from regular ingestion of sugar?

AP
    A. Ulcers
    B. Diabetes
    C. Dental caries
    D. Cardiovascular disease
    ANSWER: C   p. 111-112

56. Which of the following most closely correlates with deaths from heart disease?

K
    A. Obesity
    B. Low fiber intake
    C. High sugar intake
    D. High blood lipids
    ANSWER: D   p. 111

57. Dietary guidelines recommend that carbohydrates contribute what percentage of total energy intake?

K
    A. 25-35
    B. 55-60
    C. 65-75
    D. 85-90
    ANSWER: B   p. 113

58. According to the current dietary recommendations for consumers, what is the maximum percentage of sugar in the diet that should be contributed toward total energy intake?

K
    A. 5
    B. 10
    C. 15
    D. 20
    ANSWER: B   p. 113

59. According to most dietary guidelines, what percentage of the day's total energy intake should be furnished by carbohydrates?

K
    A. 10-15%
    B. 30-35%
    C. 55-60%
    D. 90-95%
    ANSWER: C   p. 113

12   Chapter 4   The Carbohydrates: Sugars, Starch, and Fibers

60. Dietary guidelines recommend that concentrated sweets contribute what percentage of total energy intake?

K A. 10-20
  B. 20-30
  C. up to 10
  D. less than 40
  ANSWER: C p. 113

61. Most estimates of the energy value of foods are rough approximations. What is a reasonable range of energy content for a medium-size apple listed as 100 kcal?

AP A. 25-175 kcal
  B. 50-150 kcal
  C. 80-120 kcal
  D. 95-105 kcal
  ANSWER: C p. 115

62. Which of the following is an example of the difference between the chemical bonds in starch and those in cellulose?

AP A. Starch bonds are single
  B. Starch bonds are fatty acids
  C. Cellulose bonds release energy
  D. Cellulose bonds are not hydrolyzed by human enzymes
  ANSWER: D p. 117

63. What are cellulose, pectin, hemicellulose, and lignin?

K A. Fibers
  B. Starches
  C. Sugar alcohols
  D. Artificial sweeteners
  ANSWER: A p. 117

64. Which of the following fibers is water insoluble?

K A. Gums
  B Pectins
  C. Cellulose
  D. Mucilages
  ANSWER: C p. 118

Chapter 4 Carbohydrates: Sugars, Starch, and Fibers 13

65. With few exceptions, which of the following characteristics are shared by water-soluble and water-insoluble fibers?

K   A. Neither can be used as an energy source by the body
       B. Neither has an appreciable affect on intestinal transit time
       C. Both lower blood cholesterol levels in people with high blood cholesterol concentrations
       D. Both slow the breakdown of starch and retard absorption of glucose from the intestines
ANSWER: D   p. 118-119

66. What is the source of enzymes that act on several types of dietary fiber reaching the large intestines?

K   A. Pancreas
       B. Bacteria
       C. Colonic cells
       D. Small intestinal villus cells
ANSWER: B   p. 118

67. Which of the following is a characteristic of dietary fiber?

K   A. Causes diverticulosis
       B. Usually found in high fat foods
       C. Raises blood cholesterol levels
       D. Classified according to solubility in water
ANSWER: D   p. 119

68. Which of the following is NOT a characteristic of dietary phytic acid?

K   A. Classified as a fiber
       B. Found in the husks of grains
       C. Synonymous with the term phytate
       D. Inhibits absorption of several minerals
ANSWER: A   p. 119

69. Which of the following describes the compound phytic acid?

K   A. Product of starch digestion
       B. Nonnutrient component of plant seeds
       C. Found in gastric juice and helps to lower pH of chyme
       D. Found in high concentrations in the blood of people with diabetes
ANSWER: B   p. 119

70. Which of the following is NOT a feature of high-fiber foods?

K   A. Effective in weight control
       B. Provide feeling of fullness
       C. Usually lower in fat and simple sugars
       D. Provide more energy per pound than processed foods
ANSWER: D   p. 120

14   Chapter 4 The Carbohydrates: Sugars, Starch, and Fibers

71.   Which of the following contains the LEAST amount of fiber?

AP   A.   Apples
      B.   Prunes
      C.   Potatoes
      D.   White rice
      ANSWER: D   p. 122-123

72.   Which of the following would NOT describe a diet consisting of a decrease in the amount of pure sugars and an increase in the level of complex carbohydrates?

AP   A.   Lower in fat
      B.   Lower in fiber
      C.   Lower in energy
      D.   Lower in refined foods
      ANSWER: B   p. 122

73.   What is the recommended daily intake of dietary fiber?

K   A.   20-35 g
      B.   40-50 g
      C.   55-70 g
      D.   75-100 g
      ANSWER: A   p. 122

74.   What is the average intake of fiber in the United States?

K   A.   1 g
      B.   5 g
      C.   10 g
      D.   25 g
      ANSWER: C   p. 122

75.   All of the following are features of artificial sweeteners EXCEPT

K   A.   there is an Acceptable Daily Intake which provides a wide margin of safety.
      B.   there is a lack of scientific consensus on their benefits for weight reduction.
      C.   they provide about one-half the energy of carbohydrates plus small amounts of vitamins and minerals.
      D.   if used, the American Dietetics Association advises moderate intake and only in a well-balanced, nutritious diet.
      ANSWER: C   p. 126

Chapter 4 Carbohydrates: Sugars, Starch, and Fibers 15

76. Which of the following is NOT a classification for the food additives mannitol, sorbitol, and xylitol?

K   A. Carbohydrates
B. Sugar alcohols
C. Artificial sweeteners
D. Alternative sweeteners
ANSWER: C   p. 130

77. Which of the following is a characteristic of the sugar alcohols?

K   A. Not sweet
B. Not metabolized
C. Contain kcalories
D. Promote dental caries
ANSWER: C   p. 130

78. Which of the following is found to inhibit the growth of mouth bacteria?

K   A. Sucrose
B. Xylitol
C. Fructose
D. Sorbitol
ANSWER: B   p. 130

79. What is the energy content of most sugar alcohols?

K   A. 0 kcal/g
B. 2 kcal/g
C. 4 kcal/g
D. 7 kcal/g
ANSWER: C   p. 130

Essay Questions

108-109   80. Discuss the actions of the hormones insulin and glucagon and the relationship between them in the regulation of blood glucose.

Chapter 4 The Carbohydrates: Sugars, Starch, and Fibers

108-109   81.   List six common accusations of dietary sugar. What is the evidence for and against these accusations?

115-122   82.   Give several examples of soluble and insoluble dietary fibers. List food sources of these fibers. Contrast the physical characteristics and features of these two types of fiber and their effects on gastrointestinal tract function.

120-121,118   83.   List and discuss 7 benefits of fiber.

120-121,118   84.   How is fiber thought to exert an influence over carcinogenesis of the colon?

121-122   85.   What are potential hazards of consuming too much fiber? Give examples of the circumstances, conditions, and forms under which a person might ingest large amounts of fiber.

CHAPTER 5
THE LIPIDS: TRIGLYCERIDES, PHOSPHOLIPIDS, AND STEROLS

MULTIPLE CHOICE

1. Satiety in the diet is provided primarily by which of the following nutrients?

K   A. Water
       B. Lipids
       C. Proteins
       D. Carbohydrates
       ANSWER: B   p. 132

2. Which of the following does NOT describe a function of fat?

AP   A. Adds flavor to food
        B. Carrier of fat-soluble vitamins
        C. Best source of energy for the brain
        D. Essential constituent of body tissues
        ANSWER: C   p. 132

3. Which of the following is the most desirable quality that fat adds to foods?

K   A. Color
       B. Sweetness
       C. Palatability
       D. Hydrogenation
       ANSWER: C   p. 132

2   Chapter 5 The Lipids: Triglycerides, Phospholipids, and Sterols

4.   What is the composition of fats?

K   A.   Hexose polymers
      B.   Glycogen granules
      C.   Fatty acids and glycerol
      D.   Combinations of long chain fatty acids
      ANSWER: C   p. 132

5.   A compound composed of carbon, hydrogen, and oxygen with 3 fatty acids attached to a molecule of glycerol would be known as a

AP   A.   diglyceride.
      B.   triglyceride.
      C.   phospholipid.
      D.   monoglyceride.
      ANSWER: B   p. 132

6.   What compound is composed of 3 fatty acids and glycerol?

K   A.   Steroid
      B.   Lecithin
      C.   Triglyceride
      D.   Monoglyceride
      ANSWER: C   p. 132

7.   What percentage of stored body fat is in the form of triglycerides?

K   A.   2
      B.   50
      C.   78
      D.   99
      ANSWER: D   p. 132

8.   What is the simplest fatty acid found in the diet?

K   A.   Oleic acid
      B.   Acetic acid
      C.   Linoleic acid
      D.   Palmitic acid
      ANSWER: B   p. 133

9.   In which form are most dietary lipids found?

K   A.   Sterols
      B.   Glycerols
      C.   Triglycerides
      D.   Monoglycerides
      ANSWER: C   p. 133

Chapter 5   The Lipids: Triglycerides, Phospholipids, and Sterols   3

10. Which of the following describes a fatty acid that has one double bond?

K   A. Saturated
     B. Hydrogenated
     C. Monounsaturated
     D. Polyunsaturated
ANSWER: C   p. 134

11. Lipids differ in their degree of saturation or unsaturation due to their number of

K   A. amino acids.
     B. double bonds.
     C. saccharide units.
     D. peptide linkages.
ANSWER: B   p. 134

12. What is the most common polyunsaturated fatty acid in foods?

K   A. Oleic acid
     B. Stearic acid
     C. Linoleic acid
     D. Linolenic acid
ANSWER: C   p. 134

13. Olive oil contains abundant amounts of which type of fatty acid?

K   A. Saturated
     B. Monounsaturated
     C. Polyunsaturated
     D. Partially hydrogenated
ANSWER: B   p. 134,138

14. Which of the following is a common dietary saturated fatty acid?

K   A. Oleic acid
     B. Stearic acid
     C. Linolenic acid
     D. Arachidonic acid
ANSWER: B   p. 134

15. Which one of the following compounds is missing 4 or more hydrogen atoms?

AP A. Monounsaturated fatty acid
     B. Polyunsaturated fatty acid
     C. Long chain saturated fatty acid
     D. Short chain saturated fatty acid
ANSWER: B   p. 136

Chapter 5 The Lipids: Triglycerides, Phospholipids, and Sterols

16. How many carbons are contained in a medium-chain fatty acid?

K A. 2-4
  B. 6-10
  C. 12-22
  D. 24-26
  ANSWER: B p. 136

17. Which of the following is a source of medium-chain fatty acids?

AP A. Fish oils
  B. Beef products
  C. Vegetable oils
  D. Dairy products
  ANSWER: D p. 136

18. Which of the following are characteristics shared by olive oil and canola oil?

AP A. Neither is liquid at room temperature
  B. Neither contains saturated fatty acids
  C. Both contain high levels of monounsaturated fatty acids
  D. Both contain high levels of polyunsaturated fatty acids
  ANSWER: C p. 137

19. Which of the following is considered a major source of polyunsaturated fat?

K A. Corn oil
  B. Palm oil
  C. Peanut oil
  D. Chicken fat
  ANSWER: A p. 137

20. When stored at room temperature in loosely capped containers, which of the following dietary lipids would turn rancid in the shortest time?

AP A. Lard
  B. Peanut oil
  C. Soybean oil
  D. Coconut oil
  ANSWER: C p. 138

21. Which of the following is a factor that determines the hardness of a fat at a given temperature?

AP A. Origin of the fat
  B. Degree of saturation
  C. Number of acid groups
  D. Number of oxygen atoms
  ANSWER: B p. 138

Chapter 5 The Lipids: Triglycerides, Phospholipids, and Sterols 5

22. Which of the following fats would be the softest at room temperature?

AP A. Lard
    B. Beef fat
    C. Pork fat
    D. Chicken fat
    ANSWER: D   p. 138

23. Which of the following is a feature of the polyunsaturated fats?

AP A. Low melting point
    B. High melting point
    C. Solid at room temperature
    D. Solid at refrigerator temperature
    ANSWER: A   p. 138

24. Which of the following is NOT a rich source of polyunsaturated fatty acid?

AP A. Palm oil
    B. Fish oils
    C. Soybean oil
    D. Safflower oil
    ANSWER: A   p. 138

25. Which of the following is NOT of concern regarding hydrogenation of oils?

AP A. Products become rancid sooner, contributing to a shorter shelf life
    B. The body absorbs, metabolizes, and incorporates trans-fatty acids into its tissues
    C. The long-term health consequences of trans-fatty acids in the body remain unknown
    D. The configuration changes from cis to trans and trans-fatty acids are not made by the body's cells
    ANSWER: A   p. 138

26. Of the following foods, which has the highest percentage of its fat in saturated form?

AP A. Butter
    B. Soybean
    C. Coconut
    D. Beef tallow
    ANSWER: C   p. 138

27. Of the following foods, which has the highest percentage of its fat in polyunsaturated form?

AP A. Butter
    B. Soybean
    C. Coconut
    D. Beef tallow
    ANSWER: B   p. 138

Chapter 5 The Lipids: Triglycerides, Phospholipids, and Sterols

28. In the process of fat hydrogenation, hydrogen atoms are added to which part of the molecule?

AP A. Oxygen
    B. Carbon
    C. Glycerol
    D. Other hydrogens
    ANSWER: B   p. 138

29. Which of the following chemical characteristics of fatty acids determines their susceptibility to spoilage by oxygen?

AP A. Chain length
    B. Number of double bonds
    C. Position of first saturated bond
    D. Size of adjacent fatty acids on the triglyceride molecule
    ANSWER: B   p. 138

30. Which of the following is NOT a method used by food processors to stabilize the lipids in food products?

AP A. Refrigeration
    B. Hydrogenation
    C. Tightly sealed packaging
    D. Addition of oxidizing chemicals
    ANSWER: D   p. 138

31. Which of the following would be LEAST effective at preventing oxidation of the polyunsaturated fatty acids in processed foods?

AP A. Refrigeration
    B. Addition of BHT
    C. Partial hydrogenation
    D. Addition of phosphorus
    ANSWER: D   p. 138

32. A major cause of rancidity of lipids in foods is exposure to

AP A. heat and oxygen.
    B. freezer temperatures.
    C. fluorescent lighting.
    D. enrichment additives.
    ANSWER: A   p. 138

Chapter 5 The Lipids: Triglycerides, Phospholipids, and Sterols 7

33. An oil that is partially hydrogenated sometimes changes one or more of its double bond configurations from

AP
A. cis to trans.
B. solid to liquid.
C. covalent to ionic.
D. saturated to unsaturated.
ANSWER: A   p. 139

34. A primary function of fat in the body is to

K
A. build muscle tissue.
B. protect vital organs.
C. regulate body processes.
D. provide precursors for glucose synthesis.
ANSWER: B   p. 140

35. Which of the following lipids is an essential nutrient?

K
A. Lecithin
B. Cholesterol
C. Stearic acid
D. Linoleic acid
ANSWER: D   p. 140

36. Why does the essentiality of certain fatty acids remain an unresolved issue?

AP
A. Researchers disagree regarding criteria for essentiality
B. The composition of some dietary fatty acids has not yet been determined
C. Essential fatty acids can be synthesized by the liver when intake is low
D. Essential fatty acids cannot be found in vegetarian diets although vegetarians remain healthy
ANSWER: A   p. 140-141

37. Which of the following is used by the body to synthesize arachidonic acid?

K
A. Oleic acid
B. Linoleic acid
C. Palmitic acid
D. Linolenic acid
ANSWER: B   p. 140

38. What are the building blocks in the body's synthesis of fatty acids?

K
A. 1-carbon fragments
B. 2-carbon fragments
C. 4-carbon fragments
D. 7-carbon fragments
ANSWER: B   p. 140

8   Chapter 5 The Lipids: Triglycerides, Phospholipids, and Sterols

39. What fatty acid plays a prominent role in both the retina of the eye and cerebral cortex of the brain?

K
A. Acetic acid
B. Arachidonic acid
C. Docosahexaenoic acid
D. Eicosahexaenoic acid
ANSWER: C   p. 140

40. Which of the following is a likely explanation for the imbalance between omega-6 and omega-3 lipids in the diet?

AP
A. High intakes of vegetable oils and low intakes of fish
B. Low intakes of vegetable oils and high intakes of fish
C. High intakes of beef fat and low intakes of vegetable oils
D. Low intakes of beef fat and high intakes of vegetable oils
ANSWER: A   p. 140-141,155

41. Where can essential fatty acids be found?

AP
A. Fish only
B. Beef only
C. Plants only
D. Fish, beef, and plants
ANSWER: D   p. 140

42. What is the immediate precursor for the eicosanoids?

AP
A. Glucose
B. Hormones
C. Fatty acids
D. Cholesterol
ANSWER: C   p. 142

43. Which of the following vegetable oils is a good source of omega-3 fatty acids?

AP
A. Corn
B. Sesame
C. Canola
D. Coconut
ANSWER: C   p. 142

44. Which of the following is a good source of eicosapentanoic acid?

AP
A. Tuna
B. Butter
C. Salad oil
D. Shortening
ANSWER: A   p. 142

Chapter 5 The Lipids: Triglycerides, Phospholipids, and Sterols   9

45.   Which of the following is NOT a component of lecithin?

K   A.   Choline
      B.   Phosphate
      C.   Magnesium
      D.   Fatty acids
      ANSWER: C   p. 142

46.   Which of the following fatty acids is known to reduce the tendency of blood to clot?

K   A.   Oleic acid
      B.   Stearic acid
      C.   Arachidonic acid
      D.   Eicosapentaenoic acid
      ANSWER: D   p. 142

47.   What are the precursors for synthesis of the thromboxanes?

K   A.   Steroids
      B.   Short-chain fatty acids
      C.   Medium-chain saturated fatty acids
      D.   Long-chain polyunsaturated fatty acids
      ANSWER: D   p. 142

48.   Which of the following is a feature of the lipid content of foods?

K   A.   Omega-3 fats are in fish
      B.   Cholesterol is in peanuts
      C.   Essential fatty acids are in olestra
      D.   Low-density lipoproteins are in coconut oil
      ANSWER: A   p. 142,155

49.   Which of the following characteristics are shared by cholesterol and lecithin?

AP   A.   Both are sterols
      B.   Both are phospholipids
      C.   Both are essential nutrients
      D.   Both are synthesized in the body
      ANSWER: D   p. 142-145

50.   What type of compound is lecithin?

K   A.   Bile salt
      B.   Glycolipid
      C.   Lipoprotein
      D.   Phospholipid
      ANSWER: D   p. 143

10 Chapter 5 The Lipids: Triglycerides, Phospholipids, and Sterols

51. Which of the following is NOT a feature of lecithin?

AP A. Widespread in foods
    B. Found in cell membranes
    C. Manufactured by the body
    D. Dietary supplements inhibit fat absorption
    ANSWER: D   p. 143

52. What is the usual fate of dietary lecithin?

AP A. Unabsorbed and passes out in the feces
    B. Absorbed intact and broken down by the liver
    C. Absorbed intact and incorporated into tissues
    D. Hydrolyzed by the intestinal enzyme lecithinase
    ANSWER: D   p. 143

53. Which of the following does NOT act as an emulsifier in the intestinal tract?

AP A. Lecithin
    B. Bile salts
    C. Bile acids
    D. Pancreatic lipase
    ANSWER: D   p. 143,146

54. Which of the following foods contains cholesterol?

AP A. Corn
    B. Olives
    C. Roasted turkey
    D. Roasted peanuts
    ANSWER: C   p. 144-145

55. Which of the following foods contains the least amount of cholesterol per serving?

K   A. Liver
    B. Shrimp
    C. Hot dog
    D. Veal cutlet
    ANSWER: B   p. 144-145

56. What is the approximate cholesterol content of an egg?

K   A. 200 mg
    B. 310 mg
    C. 490 mg
    D. 900 mg
    AMSWER: A   p. 144

Chapter 5   The Lipids: Triglycerides, Phospholipids, and Sterols   11

57. What is the major steroid in the diet?

K
   A. Palm oil
   B. Lecithin
   C. Cholesterol
   D. Arachidonic acid
ANSWER: C   p. 144

58. Which of the following CANNOT be found in plants?

AP
   A. Cholesterol
   B. Triglycerides
   C. Essential fatty acids
   D. Nonessential fatty acids
ANSWER: A   p. 144

59. Which of the following foods has the lowest cholesterol content per serving?

AP
   A. Eggs
   B. Liver
   C. Kidneys
   D. Lobster
ANSWER: D   p. 144

60. Which of the following contains the LEAST cholesterol per serving size?

AP
   A. Steamed fish
   B. Steamed corn
   C. Broiled chicken
   D. Very lean steak
ANSWER: B   p. 144

61. Which of the following is a feature of cholesterol?

AP
   A. Synthesized by the body
   B. No relation to heart disease
   C. Recommended intake is zero
   D. No function in the human body
ANSWER: A   p. 145

62. Which of the following is NOT a destination for cholesterol?

AP
   A. Converted into fiber
   B. Synthesized into bile
   C. Excreted in the feces
   D. Accumulates in arteries
ANSWER: A   p. 146,151

12   Chapter 5 The Lipids: Triglycerides, Phospholipids, and Sterols

63.   Which of the following is a characteristic of cholesterol?

K   A.   It is 90-95% absorbed from the diet
     B.   It is a precursor for bile and vitamin D
     C.   It is not formed in the body when provided by the diet
     D.   It is found in abundance in tropical fats such as palm oil
     ANSWER: B   p. 145

64.   Which of the following compounds may NOT be synthesized from cholesterol?

K   A.   Bile
     B.   Glucose
     C.   Vitamin D
     D.   Sex hormones
     ANSWER: B   p. 145

65.   Which of the following is NOT a feature of the bile acids?

K   A.   Stored in the gallbladder
     B.   Synthesized from cholesterol
     C.   Manufactured by the gallbladder
     D.   Released into the intestines whenever fat is present
     ANSWER: C   p. 146

66.   Bile is known to assist in the absorption of which of the following?

AP   A.   Fat only
     B.   All macronutrients only
     C.   Carbohydrate and fat only
     D.   All macronutrients and micronutrients
     ANSWER: A   p. 146

67.   What is the storage site of bile?

K   A.   Liver
     B.   Pancreas
     C.   Gallbladder
     D.   Intestinal epithelial cells
     ANSWER: C   p. 146

68.   What term may be used to describe a substance that is hydrophobic?

K   A.   Lipophilic
     B.   Lipophobic
     C.   Glycerophilic
     D.   Glycerophobic
     ANSWER: A   p. 146

Chapter 5   The Lipids: Triglycerides, Phospholipids, and Sterols   13

69. Which part of the gastrointestinal tract is the predominant site of dietary fat hydrolysis?

K A. Mouth
  B. Stomach
  C. Large intestines
  D. Small intestines
  ANSWER: D p. 146

70. After a meal, most of the fat that eventually empties into the blood is in the form of particles known as

K A. micelles.
  B. chylomicrons.
  C. low-density lipoproteins.
  D. very-low-density lipoproteins.
  ANSWER: B p. 147

71. Which of the following substances CANNOT be absorbed directly into the blood?

AP A. Glycerol
  B. Long-chain fatty acids
  C. Short-chain fatty acids
  D. Medium-chain fatty acids
  ANSWER: B p. 147

72. In comparison to a low-density lipoprotein, a high-density lipoprotein contains

AP A. less lipid.
  B. less protein.
  C. more cholesterol.
  D. more carbohydrate.
  ANSWER: A p. 151

73. How is soluble fiber in the diet thought to lower blood cholesterol level?

AP A. It denatures cholesterol in the stomach
  B. It hydrolyzes cholesterol in the intestinal tract
  C. It binds cholesterol in the intestinal tract and prevents its absorption
  D. It enhances recycling of bile and thereby increases cholesterol turnover
  ANSWER: C p. 151

74. Which of the following lipoproteins contains the highest percentage of cholesterol?

K A. Chylomicron
  B. Low-density lipoprotein
  C. High-density lipoprotein
  D. Very-low-density lipoprotein
  ANSWER: B p. 151

14   Chapter 5   The Lipids: Triglycerides, Phospholipids, and Sterols

75. What tissue contains special receptors for removing low-density lipoproteins from the circulation?

AP
A. Liver
B. Adipose
C. Arterial walls
D. Skeletal muscle
ANSWER: A   p. 151

76. High levels of which of the following blood constituents correlate to a lower risk of cardiovascular disease?

K
A. Triglycerides
B. Free fatty acids
C. High-density lipoproteins
D. Very-low-density lipoproteins
ANSWER: C   p. 151

77. What lipoprotein is responsible for transporting cholesterol back to the liver from the periphery?

K
A. Chylomicron
B. Low-density lipoprotein
C. High-density lipoprotein
D. Very-low density lipoprotein
ANSWER: C   p. 151

78. Which of the following would be the LEAST effective method to control blood cholesterol levels?

AP
A. Control weight
B. Eat more insoluble fiber
C. Consume less saturated fat
D. Exercise intensely and frequently
ANSWER: B   p. 153

79. What is the function of lipoprotein lipase?

K
A. Synthesizes lipoproteins in liver cells
B. Synthesizes triglycerides in adipose cells
C. Assembles lipid particles into chylomicrons
D. Hydrolyzes blood triglycerides for incorporation into cells
ANSWER: D   p. 153

Chapter 5 The Lipids: Triglycerides, Phospholipids, and Sterols 15

80. Approximately what percentage of the body's energy needs at rest is supplied by fat?

AP A. 5
    B. 25
    C. 40
    D. 60
    ANSWER: D   p. 153

81. What is the function of adipose cell hormone-sensitive lipase?

K   A. Hydrolyzes hormones involved in fat breakdown
    B. Synthesizes new adipose cells from simple fatty acids
    C. Hydrolyzes triglycerides to provide fatty acids for other cells
    D. Synthesizes long-chain fatty acids to provide precursors for other cells
    ANSWER: C   p. 153

82. The results of blood tests that reveal a person's total cholesterol and triglycerides is called a
K   A. lipid profile.
    B. circulating fat count.
    C. fasting blood glucose test.
    D. glucose intolerance profile.
    ANSWER: A   p. 154

83. Approximately how many kcalories are contained in a pound of body fat?

K   A. 1,000
    B. 2,500
    C. 3,500
    D. 4,000
    ANSWER: C   p. 154

84. What nutrient is used to form ketones?

AP A. Fats
    B. Protein
    C. Simple carbohydrates
    D. Complex carbohydrate
    ANSWER: A   p. 154

85. Which of the following is NOT known to be linked to excessive intake of fats?

AP A. Cancer
    B. Obesity
    C. Diabetes
    D. Lactose intolerance
    ANSWER: D   p. 154

16   Chapter 5 The Lipids: Triglycerides, Phospholipids, and Sterols

86. According to the report Diet and Health, what is the upper limit of fat that should be consumed by a healthy person requiring 3,000 kcalories per day?

AP
A. 33 grams
B. 50 grams
C. 60 grams
D. 100 grams
ANSWER: D   p. 155-156

87. According to the Diet and Health report, what should be the total fat intake as a percent of energy intake?

K
A. 10
B. 20
C. 30
D. 40
ANSWER: C   p. 156

88. According to the Diet and Health report, what should be the maximum daily intake of cholesterol?

K
A. 50 mg
B. 150 mg
C. 300 mg
D. 1,000 mg
ANSWER: C   p. 156

89. Approximately how many grams of fat would be contained in a 800 kcalorie meal which provides 50% of the energy from carbohydrate, 20% from protein, and the remainder from fat?

AP
A. 15
B. 22
C. 27
D. 35
ANSWER: C   p. 156

90. A meal providing 1200 kcalories contains 10 g of saturated fats, 14 g of monounsaturated fats and 20 g of polyunsaturated fats. What is the percentage of energy supplied by the lipid?

AP
A. 22
B. 33
C. 44
D. 55
ANSWER: B   p. 156

Chapter 5 The Lipids: Triglycerides, Phospholipids, and Sterols 17

91. All of the following lists in the exchange system include foods containing appreciable amounts of fat EXCEPT the

K   A. milk list.
B. meat list.
C. vegetable list.
D. miscellaneous list.
ANSWER: C   p. 160-162

92. The milk list is divided into three parts based on the amount of which nutrient?

K   A. Fat
B. Protein
C. Calcium
D. Carbohydrate
ANSWER: A   p. 160

93. How many kcalories are contributed by oen serving on the Fat Exchange List?

A. 5
B. 20
C. 35
D. 45
ANSWER: D   p. 160

94. Which of the following foods is NOT found in the fat exchange list?

K   A. Nuts
B. Cheese
C. Olives
D. Avocados
ANSWER: B   p. 162

95. Food that represents invisible fat in the diet would be

AP   A. nuts.
B. butter.
C. salad dressing oil.
D. fat trimmed from meat.
ANSWER: A   p. 162

96. Food that represents visible fat in the diet would be

AP   A. nuts.
B. butter.
C. avocados.
D. chocolate.
ANSWER: B   p. 162

18   Chapter 5   The Lipids: Triglycerides, Phospholipids, and Sterols

97. Which of the following is NOT a feature of the artificial fat Simplesse?

AP
A. Composed of proteins
B. Digested and absorbed
C. Contains about 1.3 kcalories per gram
D. Stable to ordinary cooking temperatures
ANSWER: D   p. 166

98. Which of the following is a drawback of olestra consumption?

K
A. Yields 9 kcalories per gram
B. Imparts off-flavors to foods
C. Inhibits absorption of vitamin E
D. Increases blood cholesterol concentration
ANSWER: C   p. 167

Essay Questions

138   99. Describe the process of fat hydrogenation and discuss its advantages and disadvantages.

138-139   100. What methods are used by the food industry to inhibit rancidity of the unsaturated lipids in foods?

139-140,   101. Discuss the functions of lipids in the body. What is the role of
143,145-146   the liver in metabolizing and processing of fats?
150-151,153

Chapter 5 The Lipids: Triglycerides, Phospholipids, and Sterols

140-142 102. List the essential fatty acids (EFA) for human beings. What are the signs of essential fatty acid deficiency? What is the minimum amount of EFA required to prevent a deficiency? What foods are rich sources of EFA?

146-149 103. Compare and contrast the digestion-absorption mechanisms for long-chain vs. short-chain fatty acids.

146-151 104. Discuss in detail the digestion, absorption, and transport of dietary fats, including the sterols.

150-151 105. Discuss the composition and function of the major circulating lipoproteins.

154-155 106. Discuss the relationship of dietary fats to atherosclerosis. Which dietary changes bring about the greatest reductions in blood lipids?

Chapter 5 The Lipids: Triglycerides, Phospholipids, and Sterols

155 107. Explain the chemical differences between fish oil and corn oil. Discuss the health benefits of fish oil. What are some of the possible disadvantages of increasing the consumption of fish?

162 108. What is meant by invisible fat? List 3 common sources in the diet.

166-168 109. Discuss the benefits and possible hazards of dietary fat alternative substances that are currently in use or are under consideration for use.

CHAPTER 6
PROTEIN: AMINO ACIDS

MULTIPLE CHOICE

1. What element is found in proteins but <u>NOT</u> in carbohydrates and fats?

K   A. Carbon
      B. Oxygen
      C. Calcium
      D. Nitrogen
ANSWER: D   p. 170

2. How many different kinds of amino acids make up proteins?

K   A. 8
      B. 10
      C. 14
      D. 20
ANSWER: D   p. 170

3. In comparison to the composition of carbohydrates and fats, which element found in proteins makes then unique?

K   A. Carbon
      B. Oxygen
      C. Nitrogen
      D. Hydrogen
ANSWER: C   p. 170

Chapter 6 Protein: Amino Acids

4. What is the simplest amino acid?

K
A. Valine
B. Glycine
C. Alanine
D. Methionine
ANSWER: B p. 170

5. Approximately how many different amino acids are used in the synthesis of body proteins?

AP
A. 5
B. 10
C. 20
D. 35
ANSWER: C p. 170

6. Which of the following compounds does NOT contain nitrogen?

AP
A. Urea
B. Enzymes
C. Ammonia
D. Cholesterol
ANSWER: D p. 170

7. Which of the following is NOT an essential amino acid in human nutrition?

K
A. Proline
B. Threonine
C. Methionine
D. Tryptophan
ANSWER: A p. 171

8. Which of the following is a feature of an essential amino acid?

K
A. It is not necessary in the diet
B. It must be supplied by the diet
C. It can be made from fat in the body
D. It can be made from glucose in the body
ANSWER: B p. 171

9. What is the composition of a tripeptide?

K
A. One amino acid with three carbons
B. Three amino acids bonded together
C. One amino acid with three acid groups
D. Three small protein chains bonded together
ANSWER: B p. 172

Chapter 6 Protein: Amino Acids   3

10. Which of the following elements is found in certain amino acids?

K
A. Iron
B. Sulfur
C. Calcium
D. Potassium
ANSWER: B   p. 172

11. What is meant by the amino acid sequence of a protein?

K
A. Number of side chains in the protein
B. Folding arrangement of the peptide chain
C. Order of appearance of amino acids in the peptide chain
D. Order of appearance of only the essential amino acids in the protein
ANSWER: C   p. 172

12. What type of reaction is required to bind two molecules of glycine together and release a molecule of water?

AP
A. Hydrolysis
B. Deamination
C. Denaturation
D. Condensation
ANSWER: D   p. 172

13. When two amino acids are chemically joined together, the resulting structure is called a

K
A. dipeptide.
B. diglyceride.
C. polypeptide.
D. polysaccharide.
ANSWER: A   p. 172

14. What is the process by which heat or acidity disrupts the normal shape of a protein chain?

K
A. Digestion
B. Condensation
C. Denaturation
D. Hydrogenation
ANSWER: C   p. 173

15. In comparison to the well-defined structure of starch, which of the following is the most important factor that allows for the synthesis of thousands of different proteins?

AP
A. Number of cell ribosomes
B. Number of different amino acids
C. Availability of amino acids containing sulfur
D. Availability of amino acids containing hydroxyl groups
ANSWER: B   p. 173

4   Chapter 6   Protein: Amino Acids

16. The application of heat or acid to a protein which causes a change in shape is known as

K
A. stiffening.
B. condensation.
C. denaturation.
D. destabilization.
ANSWER: C   p. 173

17. What is the process that results in the hardening of an egg when it is exposed to heat?

AP
A. Condensation
B. Denaturation
C. Solidification
D. Protein interaction
ANSWER: B   p. 173

18. Upon eating a hamburger, in what organ is the hydrolysis of its proteins initiated?

AP
A. Mouth
B. Stomach
C. Small intestine
D. Large intestine
ANSWER: B   p. 174

19. What is the usual fate of orally ingested enzyme supplements?

AP
A. Digested by gastrointestinal proteases
B. Rapidly degraded by salivary secretions
C. Mostly absorbed in original form from stomach
D. Completely absorbed in original form from jejunum
ANSWER: A   p. 174

20. In which organ is pepsin active?

K
A. Stomach
B. Pancreas
C. Small intestine
D. Large intestine
ANSWER: A   p. 174

21. What digestive enzyme would be most affected in people who are unable to produce hydrochloric acid?

AP
A. Pepsin
B. Transaminase
C. Pancreatic protease
D. Intestinal peptidase
ANSWER: A   p. 174

22. What is the name given to the inactive form of the protein splitting enzyme in the stomach?

K   A. Peptidase
      B. Pepsinogen
      C. Propeptidase
      D. Propepsinogen
      ANSWER: B   p. 174

23. Of the following sources of amino acids, which would show the highest absorption in normal, healthy people?

AP   A. Whole proteins
       B. Raw protein foods
       C. Predigested proteins
       D. Mixture of free amino acids
       ANSWER: A   p. 174

24. Which of the following describes the structure of pepsin?

AP   A. Lipid
       B. Protein
       C. Carbohydrate
       D. Nucleic acid
       ANSWER: B   p. 174

25. What percentage of dietary protein is hydrolyzed in the mouth?

AP   A. 0
       B. 5-10
       C. 15-20
       D. 25-30
       ANSWER: A   p. 174

26. After digestion of proteins, what products are absorbed into the circulation?

AP   A. Free amino acids only
       B. Free amino acids and oligopeptides
       C. Free amino acids and dipeptides only
       D. Free amino acids, dipeptides and tripeptides only
       ANSWER: C   p. 174

27. Which of the following statements is NOT characteristic of enzymes?

K   A. They are all catalysts
      B. They have a protein structure
      C. They can be destroyed by heat
      D. They are involved in synthesis reactions only
      ANSWER: D   p. 174-178

6   Chapter 6 Protein: Amino Acids

28.   What is the structure of an enzyme?

K   A.   Lipid
      B.   Protein
      C.   Carbohydrate
      D.   Nucleic acid
      ANSWER: B   p. 176

29.   Which of the following does NOT function as a transport protein?

K   A.   Collagen
      B.   Hemoglobin
      C.   Transferrin
      D.   Lipoproteins
      ANSWER: A   p. 176,180

30.   What protein is intimately involved in the formation of scar tissue in wound healing?

K   A.   Albumin
      B.   Thrombin
      C.   Collagen
      D.   Hydroxyproline
      ANSWER: C   p. 176

31.   What type of protein would the body make to heal a wound?

AP   A.   Albumin
      B.   Ferritin
      C.   Collagen
      D.   Hemoglobin
      ANSWER: C   p. 176

32.   What function does a buffer perform?

K   A.   Emulsifies fats
      B.   Maintains a constant pH
      C.   Facilitates chemical reactions
      D.   Protects against plaque buildup
      ANSWER: B   p. 178-179

33.   Proteins, because they attract hydrogen ions, can act as

AP   A.   acids.
      B.   buffers.
      C.   enzymes.
      D.   antibodies.
      ANSWER: B   p. 178

Chapter 6 Protein: Amino Acids 7

34. Which of the following processes is regulated primarily by the buffering action of proteins?

K   A.   pH balance
      B.   Fluid balance
      C.   Blood clotting
      D.   Synthesis of visual pigments
      ANSWER: A   p. 178

35. What is the relationship between body proteins and water?

AP   A.   Proteins attract water
       B.   Water attracts proteins
       C.   Water degrades proteins
       D.   Proteins form polymers of water
       ANSWER: A   p. 178

36. Which of the following are proteins that inactivate foreign bacteria and viruses?

K   A.   Enzymes
      B.   Collagen
      C.   Hormones
      D.   Antibodies
      ANSWER: D   p. 179

37. Which of the following proteins inactivates foreign bacteria and viruses?

K   A.   Enzymes
      B.   Hormones
      C.   Antibodies
      D.   Lipoproteins
      ANSWER: C   p. 179

38. Which of the following describes the structure of an antibody?

K   A.   Tripeptide
      B.   Small nucleic acid
      C.   Huge protein molecule
      D.   Large peptide molecule
      ANSWER: C   p. 179

39. Which of the following is a characteristic of hormones?

K   A.   Act as messenger molecules
      B.   Coordinate visual response
      C.   Capable of inactivating bacteria
      D.   Act as buffers in the bloodstream
      ANSWER: A   p. 179

8   Chapter 6   Protein: Amino Acids

40. Which of the following is NOT involved in the clotting of blood?

K
A. Opsin
B. Fibrin
C. Thrombin
D. Fibrinogen
ANSWER: A   p. 181

41. Which of the following illustrates a deamination reaction?

AP
A. Removal of the amino group from an amino acid
B. Separation of an amino acid from a peptide chain
C. Addition of an amino group to form a new amino acid
D. Addition of an amino acid to form a larger peptide chain
ANSWER: A   p. 182

42. What amino acid is used to synthesize the important neurotransmitter serotonin and the vitamin niacin?

K
A. Glycine
B. Tyrosine
C. Methionine
D. Tryptophan
ANSWER: D   p. 182

43. Protein-sparing in the body is best achieved under which of the following circumstances?

AP
A. Ingesting proteins of animal origin only
B. Ingesting proteins of plant origin only
C. Ingesting mixed protein sources on alternate days
D. Ingesting adequate levels of carbohydrate and fat
ANSWER: D   p. 182

44. Which of the following are precursors of urea synthesis?

AP
A. All amino acids
B. Animal proteins only
C. Essential amino acids only
D. Nonessential amino acids only
ANSWER: A   p. 182

45. What is the primary site for synthesis of the body's major nitrogen waste product?

K
A. Liver
B. Kidney
C. Stomach
D. Skeletal muscle
ANSWER: A   p. 182

Chapter 6 Protein: Amino Acids 9

46. What is the primary organ for production of urea?

K
   A. Liver
   B. Pancreas
   C. Small intestines
   D. Large intestines
ANSWER: A   p. 182

47. What is the fate of excess intake of dietary protein?

AP
   A. After absorption, the liver will store the extra amino acids
   B. After absorption, the extra amino acids will be rapidly degraded
   C. Digestion will be decreased by 30-60% resulting in less absorption
   D. After absorption, extra proteins will be synthesized and stored for use when protein intake returns to normal
ANSWER: B   p. 182

48. What cell structure is involved directly in the synthesis of proteins?

K
   A. Golgi
   B. Ribosomes
   C. Mitochondria
   D. Endoplasmic reticulum
ANSWER: B   p. 184

49. What is the abnormality involved in sickle-cell anemia?

K
   A. Decreased synthesis of myoglobin
   B. Impaired synthesis of transferrin protein
   C. Altered amino acid sequence of hemoglobin
   D. Excessive chelation of iron by hepatic proteins
ANSWER: C   p. 184

50. If the diet is lacking an essential amino acid, what will be the course of action?

AP
   A. Body cells will synthesize it
   B. Protein synthesis will be limited
   C. Health will not be affected as long as other nutrients are adequate
   D. Proteins will be made but they will lack that particular amino acid
ANSWER: B   p. 184

51. Which of the following foods has the best assortment of essential amino acids for the human body?

AP
   A. Eggs
   B. Fish
   C. Corn
   D. Rice
ANSWER: A   p. 185

10   Chapter 6 Protein: Amino Acids

52. Which of the following is related to the quality of a food protein?

AP
A. Essential amino acid balance
B. Nonessential amino acid balance
C. Total amino acids per gram of food
D. Quantity of nonessential amino acids that can be converted to glucose
ANSWER: A   p. 185

53. Which of the following is NOT considered to be a source of complete protein in human nutrition?

AP
A. Soy
B. Egg
C. Corn
D. Fish
ANSWER: C   p. 185

54. In the study of protein nutrition, what is the term given to the amount of amino acids absorbed as a percentage of the amount of protein consumed?

K
A. Digestibility
B. Completeness
C. Biological Value
D. Comparative Equivalence
ANSWER: A   p. 185

55. What is the chief factor that governs the quality of a food protein?

K
A. Fat content
B. Essential amino acid content
C. Complex carbohydrate content
D. Nonessential amino acid content
ANSWER: B   p. 185

56. What is a "limiting" amino acid in a protein?

K
A. A nonessential amino acid present in high amounts which inhibits protein synthesis
B. An amino acid of the wrong structure to be utilized for protein synthesis efficiently
C. An essential amino acid present in insufficient quantity for body protein synthesis to take place
D. An amino acid that limits the absorption of other essential amino acids by competing with them for transport sites within the GI tract
ANSWER: C   p. 185

Chapter 6 Protein: Amino Acids   11

57. Which of the following is NOT a common measure of protein quality?

K   A. Chemical score
    B. Biological value
    C. Metabolic utilization
    D. Protein efficiency ratio
ANSWER: C   p. 186

58. Which of the following is a common measure of protein quality?

K   A. Metabolic value
    B. Biological value
    C. Protein excretion score
    D. Protein complementation index
ANSWER: B   p. 186

59. Which of the following is a feature of malnutrition?

K   A. Dysentery is a common occurrence and leads to diarrhea and nutrient depletion
    B. Intestinal villi grow slightly larger to provide additional absorptive surfaces for nutrients
    C. Digestive enzyme production increases in order to extract as much of the ingested nutrients as possible
    D. Infections are uncommon due to insufficient availability of nutrients in the body to support growth of bacteria and viruses
ANSWER: A   p. 188

60. What is the usual initial therapy for the treatment of kwashiorkor?

AP A. Fat replacement
    B. Energy replacement
    C. Protein replacement
    D. Fluid balance restoration
ANSWER: D   p. 188

61. Which of the following conditions is associated with edema?

K   A. Excessive use of certain drugs which causes high excretion of water and amino acids
    B. Above-normal concentration of blood protein which causes fluid to leak from the blood vessels
    C. Below-normal concentration of blood protein which causes fluid to leak from the blood vessels
    D. Excessive protein in the diet leading to increased retention of fluid, especially in the extravascular spaces
ANSWER: C   p. 188

12   Chapter 6 Protein: Amino Acids

62. What term describes the following quote: "The evil spirit that infects the first child when the second child is born"?

K
A. Marasmus
B. Kwashiorkor
C. Psychomalnutrition
D. Postbirth malnutrition
ANSWER: B   p. 188

63. What is the most likely explanation for the fatty liver that develops from protein deficiency?

AP
A. Increased uptake of circulating fats
B. Increased absorption of dietary fats
C. Inability of adipose tissue to remove circulating fats
D. Inability of the liver to synthesize lipoproteins for fat export
ANSWER: D   p. 188

64. Which of the following would you NOT expect to see in a person with kwashiorkor?

AP
A. Edema
B. Dysentery
C. Increased infection rate
D. Increased physical activity
ANSWER: D   p. 188

65. Which of the following is associated with the presence of tissue edema in kwashiorkor?

AP
A. Inadequate intake of water
B. Low concentration of blood protein
C. High concentration of blood protein
D. Excessive intake of dietary protein
ANSWER: B   p. 188

66. Which of the following is a feature of kwashiorkor?

K
A. It makes the child appear grossly dehydrated
B. It usually occurs prior to the onset of marasmus
C. It is absent in communities where marasmus is present
D. It may be precipitated in the undernourished child by exposure to moldy grain
ANSWER: D   p. 189

67. Which of the following is NOT a characteristic of marasmus?

K
A. Results in a low resistance to disease
B. Affects brain development only minimally
C. Occurs most commonly in children from 6 to 18 months of age
D. Results in little or no fat under the skin to insulate against cold
ANSWER: B   p. 189

68. According to recommendations in the report <u>Diet and Health</u>, what would be the highest safe level of protein intake for a 60 kg adult?

AP   A.   48 g
       B.   60 g
       C.   96 g
       D.   120 g
ANSWER: C   p. 190

69. Which of the following is a known consequence of excess protein intake in animals or human beings?

K   A.   Increased excretion of water
    B   Decreased excretion of calcium
    C.   Decreased size of the liver and kidneys
    D.   Increased protein storage by the liver and kidneys
ANSWER: A   p. 190

70. Which of the following may be used to determine protein utilization?

AP   A.   Calorimetry
       B.   Nitrogen balance
       C.   Supplementary value
       D.   Basal metabolic rate
ANSWER: B   p. 191

71. When nitrogen taken into the body exceeds nitrogen losses, we say the person is

AP   A.   healthy.
       B.   in nitrogen equilibrium.
       C.   in positive nitrogen balance.
       D.   in negative nitrogen balance.
ANSWER: C   p. 191

72. How many grams of nitrogen are contained in a 2,500 kcal diet that provides 15% of the energy as protein?

AP   A.   2.5
       B.   5
       C.   10
       D.   15
ANSWER: D   p. 191

14 Chapter 6 Protein: Amino Acids

73. Which of the following describes the state of nitrogen balance for a normal, healthy 35-year-old person who weighs 60 kg and consumes a diet that provides 75 g of protein and adequate energy?

AP
    A. Equilibrium
    B. Positive balance
    C. Negative balance
    D. Endogenous balance
    ANSWER: A   p. 191

74. What is the nitrogen balance of a person who consumed a 3,500 kilocalorie diet containing 10% protein and excreted a total of 12 grams of nitrogen?

AP
    A. 0 g
    B. -3 g
    C. -1 g
    D. +2 g
    ANSWER: D   p. 191

75. Which of the following would describe the state of nitrogen balance of a person who ingested 16 g of food nitrogen and lost 19 g of nitrogen?

AP
    A. Equilibrium
    B. Negative balance
    C. Positive balance
    D. Exogenous balance
    ANSWER: B   p. 191

76. What would be the usual state of nitrogen balance for healthy infants, children, and pregnant women?

AP
    A. Equilibrium
    B. Metabolic
    C. Positive
    D. Negative
    ANSWER: C   p. 191

77. What is the percentage of total energy derived from protein in a diet containing 50 grams of protein and 2,000 kcal?

AP
    A. 2.5
    B. 5
    C. 10
    D. 20
    ANSWER: C   p. 191

78. If a man consumes 65 grams of protein and a total of 2,700 kcal per day, approximately what percentage of energy would be derived from protein?

AP   A.   7
       B.   10
       C.   14
       D.   20
ANSWER: B   p. 191

79. Which of the following is an assumption made in the formulation of the RDA for protein?

K   A.   Dietary protein is of high quality only
     B.   Dietary protein is of animal origin only
     C.   Dietary carbohydrate and fat intakes are adequate
     D.   Dietary protein should represent 12% of total energy
ANSWER: C   p. 191-192

80. Which of the following is a feature of the protein RDA?

AP   A.   The recommendations are generous
      B.   It is highest proportionately for adult males
      C.   It is established at 8 grams per kilogram of ideal body weight
      D.   An assumption is made that dietary protein is from animal sources only
ANSWER: A   p. 192

81. What is the RDA for protein for a 48 kg woman?

AP   A.   24 g
      B.   34 g
      C.   38 g
      D.   40 g
ANSWER: C   p. 192

82. All of the following assumptions are made by the committee in setting the RDA for protein EXCEPT

K   A.   adequate kcalories will be consumed.
     B.   protein eaten will be of mixed quality.
     C.   the fat content of the diet will be high.
     D.   other nutrients in the diet will be adequate.
ANSWER: C   p. 192

16   Chapter 6 Protein: Amino Acids

83. If proteins needs are expressed per kilogram of body weight, which of the following describes the requirements of infants?

AP
A. Less than adults
B. Similar to adults
C. Greater than adults
D. Less than adolescents
ANSWER: C   p. 192

84. What exchange list contributes zero protein?

K
A. Milk
B. Meat
C. Fruit
D. Vegetable
ANSWER: C   p. 193

85. A breakfast meal consists of the following.

1 boiled egg   2 teaspoons butter
1/2 cup grits   1/2 cup orange juice
1 slice whole-wheat toast   1 cup nonfat milk

How many meat exchanges does this meal include?

AP
A. 0
B. 1
C. 2
D. 3
ANSWER: B   p. 193

86. Using the exchange system, how many grams of protein would be provided by the following meal.

3 ounces chicken   1 fresh peach
1/2 cup green beans   1 cup nonfat milk
1 slice whole-wheat bread

AP
A. 22
B. 28
C. 34
D. 43
ANSWER: C   p. 193

Chapter 6 Protein: Amino Acids   17

87. In the Food Exchange System, all of the following would provide approximately 7 to 8 grams of protein EXCEPT

K   A.   1 cup milk.
     B.   1 ounce meat.
     C.   1 slice bread.
     D.   1/2 cup legumes.
ANSWER: C   p. 193

88. What would be the primary principle of wise diet planning as related to protein nutrition?

K   A.   Variety
     B.   Moderation
     C.   Nutrient density
     D.   Calorie control
ANSWER: B   p. 195

89. Which of the following are allowed in the diet of a lactovegetarian?

AP   A.   Plant foods only
      B.   Eggs and plant foods only
      C.   Meat, eggs, and plant foods only
      D.   Milk products and plant foods only
ANSWER: D   p. 195

90. What amino acid has recently been linked to the development of the rare blood disorder eosinophilia myalgia in people taking it as a supplement?

K   A.   Glycine
     B.   Arginine
     C.   Tryptophan
     D.   Phenylalanine
ANSWER: C   p. 196

91. Which of the following ingredients found on a food label is a protein?

AP   A.   BHT
      B.   Tofu
      C.   Corn starch
      D.   Diglycerides
ANSWER: B   p. 197

Chapter 6 Protein: Amino Acids

92. What is protein mutual supplementation?

K   A. A dietary program involving consumption of vegetable and animal proteins on alternating days
    B. A strategy combining plant proteins in the same meal to improve the balance of essential amino acids
    C. A technique developed specifically for the elderly which involves optimizing protein intake to energy intake
    D. A body process involving synthesis of crucial proteins from amino acids made available by breakdown of storage proteins
ANSWER: B   p. 197

93. All of the following are advantages of vegetarian diets EXCEPT

K   A. fat content is lower.
    B. vitamin B_{12} intake is higher.
    C. fiber content is often higher.
    D. vitamins A and C are found in liberal quantities.
ANSWER: B   p. 198, 204

94. All of the following are documented benefits for people practicing vegetarianism EXCEPT

K   A. lower blood pressure.
    B. better digestive function.
    C. lower blood cholesterol levels.
    D. lower rates of certain kinds of cancer.
ANSWER: A   p. 198, 200

Essay Questions

184   95. Describe the processes involved in cellular protein synthesis. How would synthesis be affected by intake of an otherwise adequate diet which is very low in glycine or tryptophan? How would synthesis be affected by a diet that is low in energy?

186   96. Compare and contrast the characteristics of the common protein quality evaluation methods.

190	97.	What are the possible consequences of consuming too much protein?

191	98.	What is meant by nitrogen balance and how are nitrogen balance studies conducted?

195-200	99.	List the advantages of a vegetarian diet. What nutrient requirements are more difficult to meet on this diet, and what precautions are needed to prevent insufficient intakes?

CHAPTER 7
METABOLISM: TRANSFORMATIONS AND INTERACTIONS

MULTIPLE CHOICE

1. Which of the following describes the sum of all chemical reactions that go on in living cells?

K   A. Digestion
      B. Metabolism
      C. Absorption
      D. Catabolism
ANSWER: B   p. 205

2. What term is specific to reactions in which simple compounds are combined into more complex molecules?

K   A. Anabolic
      B. Catabolic
      C. Ergogenic
      D. Gluconeogenic
ANSWER: A   p. 205

3. Which of the following reactions is an example of an anabolic reaction?

AP   A. Formation of pyruvate from glucose
       B. Formation of carbon dioxide from citric acid
       C. Formation of cholesterol from acetyl-CoA molecules
       D. Formation of acetyl-CoA molecules from cholesterol
ANSWER: C   p. 205

Chapter 7 Metabolism: Transformations and Interactions

4. The formation of glycogen by the liver cell is an example of

AP
   A. oxidation.
   B. anabolism.
   C. catabolism.
   D. glycolysis.
ANSWER: B   p. 205

5. Which of the following is a feature of catabolic reactions?

K
   A. Involve release of energy
   B. Occur only in mitochondria
   C. Involve consumption of energy
   D. Occur only during loss of body weight
ANSWER: A   p. 206

6. What is the major energy carrier molecule in most cells?

K
   A. ATP
   B. Glucose
   C. Pyruvate
   D. A kcalorie
ANSWER: A   p. 206

7. Which of the following metabolic reactions occurs when a cell needs energy?

AP
   A. ATP gains a phosphate group and becomes ADP
   B. ADP gains a phosphate group and becomes ATP
   C. ATP releases a phosphate group and becomes ADP
   D. ADP releases a phosphate group and becomes ATP
ANSWER: C   p. 206

8. Which of the following is an example of a catabolic reaction?

AP
   A. Formation of glucose from glycerol
   B. Formation of urea from an amino acid
   C. Formation of albumin from amino acids
   D. Formation of palmitic acid from acetate
ANSWER: B   p. 206

9. Which of the following defines a coenzyme?

K
   A. A unit consisting of an enzyme bound to reactants plus ATP
   B. The small, active part of an enzyme that binds to the organic reactants
   C. A small organic molecule required for the functioning of an enzyme
   D. An inactive enzyme that becomes functional upon contact with specific cofactors
ANSWER: C   p. 208

Chapter 7 Metabolism: Transformations and Interactions

10. All of the following are among the functions of the liver EXCEPT

K   A. synthesis of urea.
      B. formation of lymph.
      C. production of red blood cells.
      D. conversion of fructose to glucose.
      ANSWER: C   p. 209

11. Glycolysis is the conversion of

K   A. glycogen to fat.
      B. glucose to glycogen.
      C. glucose to pyruvate.
      D. glycogen to protein.
      ANSWER: C   p. 210

12. The series of reactions involving the conversion of glucose to pyruvate is known as

K   A. pyrolysis.
      B. glycolysis.
      C. beta-oxidation.
      D. coupled reaction.
      ANSWER: B   p. 210

13. Which of the following can NOT be formed from acetyl-CoA molecules?

K   A. Glucose
      B. Cholesterol
      C. Stearic acid
      D. Carbon dioxide
      ANSWER: A   p. 210

14. Which of the following can NOT be formed from pyruvate?

AP   A. Glucose
      B. Fructose
      C. Lactic acid
      D. Linoleic acid
      ANSWER: D   p. 210,213

15. Which of the following is NOT an aspect of glycolysis?

K   A. It generates ATP
      B. It is irreversible
      C. It occurs in the absence of oxygen
      D. It generates two molecules of pyruvate
      ANSWER: B   p. 210-211

4   Chapter 7 Metabolism: Transformations and Interactions

16. The Cori cycle involves the interconversion of

K A. lactic acid and glucose.
  B. glucose and amino acids.
  C. pyruvate and citric acid.
  D. fatty acids and acetyl-CoA.
  ANSWER: A p. 212

17. When a person is performing intense physical exercise and begins to feel fatigue and a stinging or burning pain in the muscles, it is most likely due to the muscle's accumulation of

AP A. ammonia.
  B. citric acid.
  C. lactic acid.
  D. pyruvic acid.
  ANSWER: C p. 212

18. Which of the following is a possible fate of acetyl CoA?

AP A. Degradation to urea
  B. Synthesis to glycerol
  C. Synthesis to fatty acids
  D. Degradation to ammonia
  ANSWER: C p. 213,224

19. Which of the following dietary components CANNOT be used to synthesize and store glycogen?

AP A. Lactose
  B. Animal fats
  C. Wheat starch
  D. Plant protein
  ANSWER: B p. 217-218

20. What is the first product of fatty acid catabolism?

AP A. Glycerol
  B. Pyruvate
  C. Acetyl CoA
  D. Triglycerides
  ANSWER: C p. 217

Chapter 7 Metabolism: Transformations and Interactions

21. Which of the following nutrients can be made from compounds composed of 2-carbon skeletons?

AP
A. Glucose
B. Fructose
C. Glycogen
D. Fatty acids
ANSWER: D   p. 218

22. In a triglyceride that contains 54 carbon atoms, how many can become part of glucose?

AP
A. 3
B. 9
C. 54
D. 108
ANSWER: A   p. 218

23. Which of the following compounds CANNOT be formed from fatty acids?

K
A. Ketones
B. Glucose
C. Acetyl CoA
D. Carbon dioxide
ANSWER: B   p. 218

24. Which portion of protein, fat, and carbohydrate molecules is NOT convertible to glucose?

AP
A. Fructose
B. Glycerol
C. Amino acids
D. Fatty acids
ANSWER: D   p. 218

25. Approximately what percentage of triglycerides fat CANNOT be converted to glucose?

K
A. 70
B. 80
C. 90
D. 95
ANSWER: D   p. 218

26. What is the immediate fate of excess dietary protein in the body?

AP
A. Stored
B. Reduced
C. Oxidized
D. Deaminated
ANSWER: D   p. 218

6   Chapter 7 Metabolism: Transformations and Interactions

27. Which of the following CANNOT be used to make body proteins?

AP
    A. Glucose
    B. Glycerol
    C. Fatty acids
    D. Amino acids
    ANSWER: C   p. 218-220

28. After digestion and absorption, an amino acid not used to build protein will first be subjected to

AP
    A. removal of its amino group.
    B. removal of its carboxyl group.
    C. hydrolysis of its peptide bond.
    D. condensation of its peptide bond.
    ANSWER: A   p. 218

29. When protein consumption is in excess of body needs and energy needs are met, the excess amino acids are metabolized and the energy in the molecules is

AP
    A. stored as fat only.
    B. excreted in the feces.
    C. stored as amino acids only.
    D. stored as glycogen and fat.
    ANSWER: D   p. 218-222

30. When energy yielding nutrients are consumed in excess, which one(s) can lead to storage of fat?

AP
    A. Fat only
    B. Carbohydrate only
    C. Fat and carbohydrate only
    D. Fat, carbohydrate, and protein
    ANSWER: D   p. 220

31. If the carbohydrate content of the diet is insufficient to meet the body's needs for glucose, which of the following can be converted to glucose?

AP
    A. Acetyl-CoA
    B. Fatty acids
    C. Amino acids
    D. Carbon dioxide
    ANSWER: C   p. 220

Chapter 7 Metabolism: Transformations and Interactions

32. Which of the following leads to the production of urea?

AP A. Oxidation of glucose
    B. Oxidation of amino acids
    C. Incomplete oxidation of fatty acids
    D. Synthesis of protein from amino acids
    ANSWER: B   p. 221

33. In the metabolism of amino acids for energy, what is the fate of the amino group?

K   A. Excreted as urea
    B. Burned for energy
    C. Stored in the liver
    D. Converted to glucose
    ANSWER: A   p. 221

34. Which of the following is NOT a possible fate of metabolized glucose?

AP A. Urea
    B. Acetyl CoA
    C. Amino acids
    D. Muscle glycogen
    ANSWER: A   p. 221

35. Which of the following products is NOT generated via TCA cycle or electron transport chain?

AP A. Water
    B. Energy
    C. Ammonia
    D. Carbon dioxide
    ANSWER: C   p. 221

36. The body's need for water increases on a diet high in

K   A. protein.
    B. carbohydrate.
    C. saturated fat.
    D. unsaturated fat.
    ANSWER: A   p. 221

37. What is the process whereby an amino group is combined with a keto acid to form an amino acid?

K   A. Deamination
    B. Ureagenesis
    C. Transamination
    D. Ammononiogensis
    ANSWER: C   p. 221

8   Chapter 7   Metabolism: Transformations and Interactions

38. What is the most likely cause for a person to have abnormally high blood ammonia levels?

AP
A. Liver dysfunction
B. Kidney dysfunction
C. Protein intake of twice the RDA
D. Protein intake of one-tenth the RDA
ANSWER: A   p. 221

39. What is the most likely reason for having an abnormally high blood urea level?

AP
A. Liver dysfunction
B. Kidney dysfunction
C. Protein intake of twice the RDA
D. Protein intake of one-tenth the RDA
ANSWER: B   p. 221

40. In addition to energy, what are principal end products of cellular oxidation of carbohydrates?

K
A. Water and carbon dioxide
B. Carbon, hydrogen, and urea
C. Indigestible fiber and nitrogen
D. Monosaccharides and amino acids
ANSWER: A   p. 222

41. What are the products from the complete oxidation of fatty acids?

K
A. Urea and acetone
B. Fatty acids and glycerol
C. Carbon, hydrogen, and oxygen
D. Water, carbon dioxide, and energy
ANSWER: D   p. 222-223

42. Which of the following outlines the overall sequence of events in the complete oxidation of glucose?

AP
A. Cori cycle-TCA cycle-glycolysis
B. Glycolysis-TCA cycle-electron transport chain
C. Electron transport chain-TCA cycle-Cori cycle
D. TCA cycle-electron transport chain-glycolysis
ANSWER: B   p. 222-224

Chapter 7 Metabolism: Transformations and Interactions

43. Which of the following accounts for the higher energy density of a fatty acid compared with the other energy-yielding nutrients?

K
A. Fatty acids have a greater percentage of hydrogen-carbon bonds
B. Fatty acids have a lower percentage of hydrogen-carbon bonds
C. Other energy-yielding nutrients have a lower percentage of oxygen-carbon bonds
D. Other energy-yielding nutrients undergo fewer metabolic reactions thereby lowering the energy yield
ANSWER: A   p. 225

44. The number of ATP's that can be produced from a molecule of protein, fat, or carbohydrate is generally related to the number of atoms of

AP
A. carbon.
B. oxygen.
C. nitrogen.
D. hydrogen.
ANSWER: D   p. 225

45. After the first day or so of fasting, which of the following is most depleted in the body?

AP
A. Glycogen
B. Fatty acids
C. Amino acids
D. Triglycerides
ANSWER: A   p. 228

46. If a normal person expends 1500 kcal while at rest, approximately how many are used by the brain?

AP
A. 40
B. 100
C. 200
D. 300
ANSWER: D   p. 228

47. Which of the following is used to supply some of the fuel needed by the brain only after the body has been fasting for a while?

AP
A. Ketones
B. Glycerol
C. Fatty acids
D. Amino acids
ANSWER: A   p. 229

10   Chapter 7 Metabolism: Transformations and Interactions

48. How are ketones formed?

K   A.   Condensing of acetyl CoA molecules
     B.   Condensing of lactic acid molecules
     C.   Hydrolysis of excess glycerol fragments
     D.   Hydrolysis of excess pyruvate fragments
     ANSWER: A   p. 229

49. Which of the following is a feature of ketosis?

AP   A.   Occurs when fats are partially oxidized
     B.   Results from lack of protein in the diet
     C.   Occurs when fats are completely oxidized
     D.   Results from excess carbohydrate in the diet
     ANSWER: A   p. 229

50. During the first few days of a fast, what energy source provides about 90% of the glucose needed to fuel the body?

K   A.   Ketones
     B.   Protein
     C.   Glycogen
     D.   Triglycerides
     ANSWER: B   p. 229

51. How soon would death occur from starvation if the body was unable to shift to a state of ketosis?

AP   A.   Within 3 weeks
     B.   Less than 2 weeks
     C.   Between 5 and 6 weeks
     D.   Between 2 and 3 months
     ANSWER: A   p. 229

52. Which of the following is a side effect of a high-protein, low-carbohydrate diet?

K   A.   Edema
     B.   Diarrhea
     C.   Dehydration
     D.   Nitrogen toxicity
     ANSWER: C   p. 230-231

53. Which of the following is a characteristic of ketosis?

K   A.   It may lead to a lowering of blood pH
     B.   It leads to increased appetite in most individuals
     C.   It may be alleviated quickly by ingestion of some dietary fat
     D.   It is a necessary physiological adjustment for maximum weight loss
     ANSWER: A   p. 230

Chapter 7 Metabolism: Transformations and Interactions

54. Which of the following dietary nutrients would most rapidly reverse a state of ketosis in a starving person?

AP   A. Fat
       B. Protein
       C. Amino acids
       D. Carbohydrate
       ANSWER: D   p. 230

55. All of the following are general features of starvation in people EXCEPT

AP   A. a decrease in metabolic rate.
       B. a decrease in immune function.
       C. a decrease in body temperature.
       D. a decrease in mental alertness.
       ANSWER: D   p. 230

56. Which of the following are consequences of low-carbohydrate diets?

AP   A. Increases in bowel movements
       B. Minimal losses of muscle and high losses of fat
       C. Increases in energy level of body and mental alertness
       D. High losses of water and protein and lower losses of fat
       ANSWER: D   p. 231

57. Which of the following is a feature of the protein-sparing fast for weight loss?

K   A. It has a low long-term success rate
       B. It has a high long-term success rate
       C. It is more effective than diets containing both protein and carbohydrate
       D. It is much less effective than diets containing both protein and carbohydrate
       ANSWER: A   p. 231

58. What is the percentage of ethanol in 120-proof scotch whiskey?

AP   A. 5
       B. 30
       C. 60
       D. 95
       ANSWER: C   p. 233

59. Which of the following is/are best suited for slowing alcohol absorption?

AP   A. Not eating
       B. Protein snacks
       C. Caffeine drinks
       D. Carbohydrate snacks
       ANSWER: D   p. 234-235

12   Chapter 7   Metabolism: Transformations and Interactions

60. Which of the following defines a moderate level of alcohol intake per day for the average-sized woman?

AP   A.   Up to 1 drink
     B.   Up to 2 drinks
     C.   Up to 3 drinks
     D.   Up to 5 drinks
     ANSWER: A   p. 234

61. Which of the following defines a moderate level of alcohol intake per day for the average-sized man?

K   A.   Up to 1 drink
     B.   Up to 2 drinks
     C.   Up to 3 drinks
     D.   Up to 5 drinks
     ANSWER: B   p. 234

62. What organ is first to absorb the alcohol after taking a drink?

AP   A.   Colon
     B.   Stomach
     C.   Jejunum
     D.   Duodenum
     ANSWER: B   p. 234

63. One average-sized can of beer contains about the same amount of alcohol as

K   A.   ½ ounce of rum.
     B.   ½ quart of wine.
     C.   1 ounce of vodka.
     D.   1 quart of wine cooler.
     ANSWER: C   p. 234

64. What is the sequence of stages that brings about advanced liver disease caused by chronic alcohol toxicity?

K   A.   Fibrosis-gout-cirrhosis
     B.   Fibrosis-cirrhosis-fat depletion
     C.   Cirrhosis-fat accumulation-fibrosis
     D.   Fat accumulation-fibrosis-cirrhosis
     ANSWER: D   p. 234-236

Chapter 7 Metabolism: Transformations and Interactions

65. What is the primary organ that oxidizes alcohol for fuel?

K   A. Brain
      B. Liver
      C. Pancreas
      D. Digestive tract
      ANSWER: B   p. 235

66. Which of the following plays a major role in regulating the elimination of alcohol from the body?

K   A. Lung respiratory rate
      B. Kidney antidiuretic hormone
      C. Liver alcohol dehydrogenase
      D. Brain acetaldehyde dehydrogenase
      ANSWER: C   p. 235

67. Which of the following statements is NOT characteristic of alcohol metabolism?

K   A. There are gender differences in the rate of breakdown
      B. It is metabolized primarily by muscle cells and liver
      C. The average person needs about 3 hours to metabolize two drinks
      D. The amount in the breath is proportional to the amount in the blood
      ANSWER: B   p. 235,237,240

68. Excess alcohol intake leads to a reduction in the synthesis rate of

K   A. liver fat.
      B. lipoproteins.
      C. ketone bodies.
      D. acetyl CoA molecules.
      ANSWER: B   p. 236

69. What is MEOS?

K   A. An advanced liver disorder
      B. A waste product of alcohol metabolism
      C. A drug that inhibits alcohol absorption
      D. A system of enzymes that oxidizes alcohol and drugs
      ANSWER: D   p. 236

70. What minimum concentration of alcohol in the blood is usually fatal?

K   A. 0.5%
      B. 1%
      C. 5%
      D. 50%
      ANSWER: A   p. 238

14 Chapter 7 Metabolism: Transformations and Interactions

71. Approximately how many kcal from <u>ethanol</u> are contained in one alcoholic drink?

K
A. 25
B. 50
C. 100
D. 200
ANSWER: C   p. 239

72. Which of the following represents the changes in the blood lipoprotein profile from regular consumption of alcohol?

AP
A. Reduction in all forms of lipoproteins resulting in increased risk for heart disease
B. Reduction in one form of low-density lipoproteins resulting in increased risk of heart disease
C. Rise in one type of high-density lipoproteins that is associated with lower risk of heart disease
D. Rise in one type of high-density lipoproteins that is <u>NOT</u> associated with lower risk of heart disease
ANSWER: D   p. 240

Essay Questions

205-208   73. Compare and contrast the various ways in which the body uses carbohydrate, fat, and amino acids.

211-214   74. What are the major differences between aerobic and anaerobic metabolism? Give an example of an aerobic reaction and an anaerobic reaction.

221   75. What is urea? How and where is it synthesized and how is it removed from the body?

Chapter 7 Metabolism: Transformations and Interactions

226-230   76.   Discuss ways in which the body's metabolism adapts to conditions of fasting/starvation. How do these adaptations affect the rate of weight loss when dieting?

228-230   77.   Explain the roles of protein and fat as nutrients for gluconeogenesis. What are the circumstances that favor low and high rates of gluconeogenesis?

229-230   78.   What is ketosis and how can it be identified? What conditions typically induce a state of ketosis? What are the adverse effects of this abnormality?

231   79.   Describe the protein-sparing fast and its limitations for use in obese individuals.

233-241   80.   Discuss ways in which alcohol interferes with metabolism of proteins, fats, carbohydrates, vitamins, minerals, and water.

235-238   81.   Describe the two major pathways for metabolism of alcohol in the liver. How does the liver adapt when forced to metabolize high quantities of alcohol on a daily basis?

235   82.   Describe the differences between men and women in the metabolism of alcohol.

CHAPTER 8
ENERGY BALANCE AND WEIGHT CONTROL

MULTIPLE CHOICE

1. What is the recommended rate of weight loss per week for a 250-pound obese individual?

AP   A.   1 lb
        B.   5 lbs
        C.   1 % of body weight
        D.   5 % of body weight
        ANSWER: C   p. 243

2. To provide satiety in a balanced weight reduction diet, approximately what percentage of total energy should be derived from fat?

AP   A.   5
        B.   10
        C.   20
        D.   40
        ANSWER: C   p. 243

3. What instrument is used to measure the energy content of foods?

K   A.   Energy chamber
       B.   Exothermic meter
       C.   Bomb calorimeter
       D.   Combustion chamber
       ANSWER: C   p. 244

2   Chapter 8   Energy Balance and Weight Control

4. What would be the approximate weight gain of a person who consumes an excess of 500 kcal daily for one month?

AP
- A. 0.5 lb
- B. 2 lbs
- C. 3 lbs
- D. 4 lbs

ANSWER: D   p. 243

5. Which of the following identifies a specific food intake behavior?

K
- A. The absence of appetite is called anorexia
- B. A physiological need to eat is called satiety
- C. A pleasurable desire for food is called hunger
- D. An intense feeling of hunger is called insatiable nervosa

ANSWER: A   p. 245

6. After consuming a very large meal, the desire to eat a slice of chocolate cake is an example of behavior known as

AP
- A. hunger.
- B. satiety.
- C. anorexia.
- D. appetite.

ANSWER: D   p. 245

7. Research on "cafeteria rats" found they would eat

K
- A. very little food and lose weight.
- B. large quantities of food and become obese.
- C. large quantities of food yet maintain weight.
- D. moderate amounts of food and maintain weight.

ANSWER: B   p. 245

8. An emotionally insecure person might eat for all of the following reasons EXCEPT

AP
- A. to relieve boredom.
- B. to ward off depression.
- C. in preference to socializing.
- D. to satisfy energy needs only.

ANSWER: D   p. 246

Chapter 8 Energy Balance and Weight Control

9. External cues that may cause an obese person to respond helplessly to food typically include all of the following EXCEPT

K   A.   TV commercials.
     B.   outdoor exercises.
     C.   availability of food.
     D.   "time of day" patterns.
     ANSWER: B   p. 246

10. Which of the following describes the process of thermogenesis?

K   A.   Burning of fat
     B.   Synthesis of fat
     C.   Generation of heat
     D.   Generation of water
     ANSWER: C   p. 247

11. What is the overall efficiency of the human body in converting food energy to work?

K   A.   10%
     B.   25%
     C.   50%
     D.   75%
     ANSWER: B   p. 247

12. What method is used to measure the amount of heat given off by the body?

K   A.   Bomb calorimetry
     B.   Basal calorimetry
     C.   Direct calorimetry
     D.   Indirect calorimetry
     ANSWER: C   p. 247

13. What fraction of the day's energy expenditure of the average person is represented by the basal metabolism?

AP   A.   about 1/10
     B.   up to 1/2
     C.   at least 2/3
     D.   over 9/10
     ANSWER: C   p. 247

14. What are endogenous opiates?

K   A.   Circulating purines
     B.   Over-the-counter diet pills
     C.   Illegal drugs used for weight loss
     D.   Morphine-like compounds produced in the brain
     ANSWER: D   p. 247

4   Chapter 8   Energy Balance and Weight Control

15. If a 60 kg woman expends 750 kcal in her daily activities, approximately how many kcal are needed to maintain energy equilibrium?

AP   A.   1950
     B.   2250
     C.   2400
     D.   2600
     ANSWER: B   p. 247-252

16. Which of the following is used to calculate the amount of energy expended by the body?

K   A.   Oxygen consumed
     B.   Total air exchanged
     C.   Intestinal gas expelled
     D.   Carbon dioxide consumed
     ANSWER: A   p. 247

17. Which of the following is a feature of the basal metabolic rate (BMR)?

K   A.   Fever decreases the BMR
     B.   Fasting increases the BMR
     C.   Pregnancy increases the BMR
     D.   Females have higher BMR's than males on a body weight basis
     ANSWER: C   p. 247-248

18. For every decade beyond the age of 30, what is the percentage decrease in the need for kcalories?

K   A.   2
     B.   5
     C.   10
     D.   15
     ANSWER: B   p. 248

19. Which of the following groups has the highest metabolic rate?

K   A.   Females
     B.   Older individuals
     C.   Younger individuals
     D.   People with smaller surface areas
     ANSWER: C   p. 248

20. What is the major factor that determines metabolic rate?

K   A.   Age
     B.   Gender
     C.   Amount of fat tissue
     D.   Amount of lean body tissue
     ANSWER: D   p. 248

21. Which of the following does NOT decrease the metabolic rate?

K
- A. Fever
- B. Fasting
- C. Inactivity
- D. Malnutrition

ANSWER: A   p. 248

22. If a normal 30 year-old woman has a daily energy expenditure of 2,200 kcal, what would be her expected output when she reaches 60 years of age?

AP
- A. 1210 kcal
- B. 1450 kcal
- C. 1885 kcal
- D. 2275 kcal

ANSWER: C   p. 248

23. If a dancer and a typist are the same height and have the exact same body build, the dancer will be heavier because she has

AP
- A. more body fat.
- B. stronger bones.
- C. stronger muscles.
- D. more muscle mass.

ANSWER: D   p. 248

24. If a normal 60 kg person has a resting energy expenditure of 1300 kcal/day, about how many extra kcal are needed to sustain 4 hours of studying?

AP
- A. 50
- B. 120
- C. 260
- D. 400

ANSWER: A   p. 248

25. What is the approximate value for the thermic effect of a 2,500 kcal diet?

AP
- A. 25 kcal
- B. 250 kcal
- C. 400 kcal
- D. 500 kcal

ANSWER: B   p. 250

Chapter 8 Energy Balance and Weight Control

26. What is the term that describes the increase in energy expenditure that occurs in a person who fractures a leg?

AP
- A. Febrile hyperthermia
- B. Physical hyperthermia
- C. Specific thermogenesis
- D. Adaptive thermogenesis

ANSWER: D   p. 250

27. To estimate the basal metabolic rates of individuals, which of the following was used in the equations by the Committee on Dietary Allowances?

K
- A. Weight
- B. Surface area
- C. Activity level
- D. Fat-fold thickness

ANSWER: A   p. 251

28. How does the metabolic rate of males compare with that of females of the same body weight?

AP
- A. About 5% lower
- B. About 5% higher
- C. About 10% lower
- D. About 10% higher

ANSWER: D   p. 252

29. What is the approximate basal metabolism of a 110 pound woman?

AP
- A. 850 kcal/day
- B. 960 kcal/day
- C. 1080 kcal/day
- D. 1240 kcal/day

ANSWER: C   p. 252

30. According to the Dietary Guidelines for Americans, "healthy weight" is defined by all of the following criteria EXCEPT

K
- A. a body mass index figure between 20 and 25.
- B. a weight within the ranges suggested by the U.S.D.A.
- C. a fat distribution pattern unrelated to high risk of illness.
- D. the absence of any medical condition associated with weight loss.

ANSWER: A   p. 253

Chapter 8 Energy Balance and Weight Control   7

31. An index of a person's weight in relation to height is called

K
- A. body mass index.
- B. height to weight index.
- C. ideal body weight index.
- D. desirable body weight index.

ANSWER: A   p. 255

32. Which of the following is a feature of the body mass index?

K
- A. It correlates with disease risks
- B. It decreases by 1 unit for every 10 years of life
- C. It provides an estimate of the fat level of the body
- D. It is defined as the person's height divided by the square of the weight

ANSWER: A   p. 255

33. What is the approximate body mass index of a woman who is 5'5" and 125 lbs?

AP
- A. 21
- B. 26
- C. 31
- D. 36

ANSWER: A   p. 255

34. Which of the following is NOT a feature of the fatfold test?

K
- A. Can be self-administered
- B. Correlates with risk of heart disease
- C. Provides a direct estimate of the amount of body fat
- D. Considered a practical diagnostic tool for trained users

ANSWER: A   p. 256

35. Which of the following is a characteristic associated with using weight measures to assess risk of disease?

K
- A. They are expensive to perform
- B. They are complicated to perform
- C. They are subject to inaccuracies
- D. They fail to quantitate total body fat

ANSWER: D   p. 256

36. All of the following are features of using weight measures to assess risk of disease EXCEPT

K
- A. they are inexpensive.
- B. they are very accurate.
- C. they are easy to perform.
- D. they provide information on body composition.

ANSWER: D   p. 256

8   Chapter 8   Energy Balance and Weight Control

37. Which of the following is a disadvantage of using weight measures for the assessment of disease risk?

K   A. Cost
      B. Accuracy
      C. Complexity
      D. Amount of body composition data
ANSWER: D   p. 256

38. In what region of the body is the storage of excess body fat associated with highest risks for cardiovascular disease and diabetes?

K   A. Neck
      B. Abdomen
      C. Hips and thighs
      D. Arms and shoulders
ANSWER: B   p. 256

39. Which of the following defines central obesity?

K   A. Accumulation of fat during the mid-years of life
      B. Storage of excess fat around the central part of the body
      C. Overfatness due to a large number of interacting behavioral problems
      D. Overfatness due to reliance on high fat foods as a central part of the diet
ANSWER: B   p. 256

40. Research in obese people seems to show that there is no increase in the risks for strokes and hypertension provided that the excess body fat is distributed around the

AP   A. stomach.
      B. arms and chest.
      C. hips and thighs.
      D. neck and shoulders.
ANSWER: C   p. 256

41. Which of the following is a feature of fatfold <u>assessment</u> techniques?

K   A. The device to measure fatfold thickness is called a lipidometer
      B. The folds of fat increase in size in proportion to the gain in body fat
      C. Measures taken from upper body sites are more precise than those from the lower-body sites
      D. The principles are based on the assumption that subcutaneous fat mass represents about 20% of total body fat
ANSWER: B   p. 256

42. Which of the following is an advantage of using the fatfold measurement over the body mass index measurement?

AP
A. It is easier to perform
B. It is less expensive to perform
C. It is better at predicting the level of risks for diseases
D. It can also predict the success of standard weight-loss programs
ANSWER: C p. 256

43. What is the range of body fat content of normal weight women?

K
A. 9-17%
B. 18-32%
C. 33-37%
D. 38-44%
ANSWER: B p. 257

44. What is the range of body fat content of normal weight men?

K
A. 5-9%
B. 10-14%
C. 15-22%
D. 23-28%
ANSWER: C p. 257

45. What is the chief advantage of measuring fatfold thickness of only the triceps area rather than at multiple body sites for the estimation of whole body fat stores?

K
A. It is least painful
B. It is easily accessible
C. There are no reliable tables of normal fatfold data for the other parts of the body
D. Since it is no different than the other body sites, it is representative of the entire body
ANSWER: B p. 257

46. All of the following are among techniques used to assess body fat content or distribution EXCEPT

K
A. waist-to-hip ratio.
B. underwater weighing.
C. bioelectric impedance.
D. radioactive fat count.
ANSWER: D p. 257

10   Chapter 8   Energy Balance and Weight Control

47. Which of the following is NOT a known side effect of a body fat level well below average in an otherwise normal individual?

AP A. Infertility
    B. Clinical depression
    C. Elevated body temperature
    D. Abnormal hunger regulation
    ANSWER: C   p. 257

48. What is the recommended minimum amount of body fat for women and for men?

K   A. 2-6% for each
    B. 18-22% for each
    C. 4-8% and 6-9%, respectively
    D. 12-16% and 5-10%, respectively
    ANSWER: D   p. 257

49. What is the weight classification assigned both to young women with 32% body fat and young men with 22% body fat?

K   A. Obese
    B. Normal
    C. Mildly overweight
    D. Slightly underweight
    ANSWER: A   p. 257

50. What is the rationale for the fat cell theory of obesity?

K   A. Fat cell number in an adult can decrease only by fasting
    B. Fat cell number continues to increase throughout adulthood
    C. Early overfeeding stimulates fat cells to increase abnormally in number
    D. Weight gain in adults can take place only by increasing the number of fat cells
    ANSWER: C   p. 258

51. Since obesity apparently has many causes, even in a single individual, the best attack on the problem seems to be

AP A. fasting.
    B. medicines.
    C. prevention.
    D. genetic counseling.
    ANSWER: C   p. 258

Chapter 8 Energy Balance and Weight Control 11

52. According to body mass index values, what fraction of the U.S. adult population is considered overweight?

K A. 1/20
  B. 1/10
  C. 1/8
  D. 1/4
  ANSWER: D p. 258

53. All of the following describe the behavior of fat cells EXCEPT

K A. the number decreases when fat is lost from the body.
  B. the storage capacity for fat depends on both cell number and cell size.
  C. the number increases at a faster rate in obese children than in lean children.
  D. the number increases several-fold during the growth years and tapers off when reaching adult status.
  ANSWER: A p. 258

54. What type of body lipid is especially known for its production of heat?

K A. Yellow fat
  B. White adipose tissue
  C. Brown adipose tissue
  D. Erythrocyte crimson fat
  ANSWER: C p. 258

55. What serves as the body's chief storage site for lipid?

K A. Yellow fat
  B. Brown adipose tissue
  C. White adipose tissue
  D. High-density lipoproteins
  ANSWER: C p. 258

56. What is the chief factor that determines a person's risk for obesity?

AP A. Genetics
  B. Environment
  C. Metabolic rate
  D. Fat content of diet
  ANSWER: A p. 259

57. What is the incidence of obesity in a person whose parents are both obese?

AP A. 10%
  B. 30%
  C. 60%
  D. 80%
  ANSWER: D p. 259

Chapter 8 Energy Balance and Weight Control

58. What is the incidence of obesity in a person whose parents are not obese?

AP
- A. 10%
- B. 30%
- C. 60%
- D. 80%

ANSWER: A   p. 259

59. Which of the following defines the body's set point?

K
- A. Minimum weight of a person
- B. Maximum weight of a person
- C. Point which a dieter plateaus and then drops weight quickly
- D. Point above which the body tends to lose weight and below which it tends to gain weight

ANSWER: D   p. 260

60. Which of the following promotes fat storage in adipocytes?

K
- A. Glucagon
- B. Lipoprotein lipase
- C. Cellulite synthetase
- D. Lipoprotein synthetase

ANSWER: B   p. 260

61. What is the most likely explanation for why women readily store fat around the hips whereas men readily store fat around the abdomen?

AP
- A. Differences in blood insulin levels
- B. Differences in the activity of lipoprotein lipase
- C. Differences in circulating lipid transport proteins
- D. Differences in the activity of lipoprotein synthetase

ANSWER: B   p. 260

62. Which of the following describes the condition whereby chronic dieters continue to increase body fat but cannot decrease it below a minimum level?

K
- A. Secondary obesity
- B. Primary hypertrophy
- C. Dieting-induced obesity
- D. Law of diminishing returns

ANSWER: C   p. 260

Chapter 8   Energy Balance and Weight Control   13

63. When making adjustments in the diet for reducing body weight, which of the following is most likely to remain at the same dietary level?

AP
    A.   Fat intake
    B.   Fiber intake
    C.   Protein intake
    D.   Carbohydrate intake
ANSWER: C   p. 261

64. What were the results from research studies on the adaptation response of normal-weight adults who were placed on either high-fat or low-fat diets?

K
    A.   Those on the high-fat diet adjusted their intake to match energy expenditure after 3 days
    B.   Those on the high-fat diet did not decrease total food intake enough to prevent a gain in weight
    C.   Those on the low-fat diet increased the quantity of food consumed in order to maintain body weight
    D.   Those on the low-fat diet showed a rapid fall in metabolic rate which increased slowly to normal by the end of 1 week, resulting in a slight gain in body weight
ANSWER: B   p. 262

65. What unexpected findings were obtained from studies in nonobese men who were allowed to eat at will from a high-fat (energy dense) diet?

K
    A.   The subjects overate, seeming to ingest the extra food in order to achieve some threshold of carbohydrate intake
    B.   The subjects gradually decreased the volume of food consumed so that energy intake became almost identical to that of the pre-study period
    C.   The subjects showed very large variations in their energy intakes, resulting in equal numbers whose body weights rose, fell, or remained the same
    D.   The subjects showed alternating periods of high food intake and low food intake, resulting in very little weight change and demonstrating the body's unusual ability to normalize energy intake when faced with an energy-dense diet
ANSWER: A   p. 262

66. Researchers have shown that in adults wanting to gain weight, the most rapid increase occurs when they consume a high level of dietary

K
    A.   fat.
    B.   fiber.
    C.   protein.
    D.   carbohydrate.
ANSWER: A   p. 263

14   Chapter 8   Energy Balance and Weight Control

67. All of the following represent findings from research studies on dietary fat intake in human beings EXCEPT

K
A. the intake of fat correlates directly with the amount of body fat.
B. the total energy intake of obese men correlates directly with body fat measurements.
C. the gain in body weight from overeating requires fewer kcal from a high-fat diet compared with a mixed diet.
D. the intake of fat as a percentage of total energy intake is similar to nonobese men eating the typical U.S. diet.
ANSWER: B   p. 263

68. What is the relationship between the amounts of energy required to convert dietary fat and dietary carbohydrate into stored fat?

K
A. Converting the carbohydrate to stored fat uses about 6 times more energy
B. Converting the dietary fat to stored fat uses about twice as much energy
C. Converting the carbohydrate to stored fat use about twice as much energy
D. Converting both of them to stored fat requires about the same amount of energy
ANSWER: A   p. 263

69. Which of the following is the most likely explanation for the body's higher metabolic efficiency of converting a molecule of corn oil into stored fat compared with a molecule of sucrose?

AP
A. The enzymes specific for metabolizing absorbed fat have been found to have higher activities than those metabolizing sucrose
B. The absorbed corn oil is transported to adipocytes at a faster rate than the absorbed sucrose, thereby favoring the uptake of corn oil fat
C. There are fewer metabolic reactions for disassembling the corn oil and re-assembling the parts into a triglyceride for uptake by the adipocytes
D. Since the energy content is higher in a molecule of corn oil than sucrose, conversion of these nutrients into stored fat requires a smaller percentage of the energy from the corn oil
ANSWER: C   p. 263

70. What is considered to be the most important single contributor to the obesity problem in the United States?

K
A. Overeating
B. Physical inactivity
C. Environmental factors
D. Overabundance of foods
ANSWER: B   p. 264

Chapter 8 Energy Balance and Weight Control   15

71. Television watching contributes to obesity for all of the following reasons EXCEPT

K
- A. it promotes inactivity.
- B. it promotes between-meal snacking.
- C. it replaces time that could be spent eating.
- D. it gives high exposure to energy-dense foods in the commercial advertisements.

ANSWER: C   p. 264

72. Approximately what percentage of people who lose weight by dieting fail to maintain the weight loss?

K
- A. 5
- B. 25
- C. 75
- D. 95

ANSWER: D   p. 265

73. Which of the following defines weight cycling?

K
- A. A series of weight loss and regain episodes that affects body composition and metabolism
- B. An ergonometric device designed to force the user to achieve higher levels of energy expenditure and thus weight loss
- C. A safe weight loss program consisting of a 2-week period of dieting and then 1 week off the diet, and repeating this cycle until the desired amount of body weight is lost
- D. A technique designed by the American Medical Association involving use of a combination of aerobic activities and light-weight strength conditioning weights as a safe method of weight loss

ANSWER: A   p. 266

74. Which of the following terms is NOT commonly used to describe the typical situation of an overweight individual who experiences repeated bouts of weight loss and re-gain, with the gain frequently to a greater body weight than before?

K
- A. Yo-yo effect
- B. Weight cycling
- C. Ratchet effect
- D. Elevator effect

ANSWER: D   p. 266

75. In the quest for achieving desirable body weight, adults have control over all of the following EXCEPT

AP
- A. diet.
- B. behavior.
- C. adipocyte number.
- D. physical activity.

ANSWER: C   p. 267

Chapter 8 Energy Balance and Weight Control

76. Which of the following is lost from the body when a person takes a diuretic for weight reduction?

AP
A. Water
B. Glycogen
C. Abdominal fat
D. Subcutaneous fat
ANSWER: A   p. 267

77. All of the following are characteristics of amphetamine use for weight reduction EXCEPT

K
A. they lead to dependency.
B. the weight lost is regained.
C. they reduce the appetite for prolonged periods.
D. they are considered to have little use in treating obesity.
ANSWER: C   p. 268

78. What range of energy intake per day would fall into the classification of a very-low-kcalorie diet?

K
A. 50-300 kcal.
B. 400-800 kcal.
C. 900-1200 kcal.
D. 1300-1400 kcal.
ANSWER: B   p. 269

79. Which of the following types of diets is the most likely to promote constipation?

K
A. Low-fat
B. High-fluid
C. Low-carbohydrate
D. High-carbohydrate
ANSWER: C   p. 269-270

80. Methods to induce weight loss by interfering with the amount of food consumed include all of the following EXCEPT

AP
A. liposuction.
B. wiring the jaw shut.
C. stapling the stomach.
D. inserting a balloon in the stomach.
ANSWER: A   p. 269

Chapter 8 Energy Balance and Weight Control   17

81. Which of the following does NOT describe very-low-energy diet formulas?

K
    A. They provide little or no fat
    B. They are designed to be adequate in nutrients
    C. They provide most of the energy as carbohydrate
    D. They provide about twice the RDA level of protein
ANSWER: C   p. 269-270

82. Which of the following is a feature of very-low-kcalorie diets?

K
    A. They lead to rapid weight loss
    B. They provide insufficient protein
    C. They promote conservation of lean body tissues
    D. They prolong the time to regain the lost weight
ANSWER: A   p. 269-270

83. Which of the following is a side effect of very-low-kcalorie diets?

K
    A. Blood pressure rises
    B. Cold intolerance develops
    C. Blood cholesterol levels fall
    D. Basal metabolism rises slightly
ANSWER: B   p. 270

84. What is considered to be a healthy rate of weight loss for most overweight people on a long term basis?

K
    A. 0.5-1 lb/week
    B. 2 to 3 lbs/week
    C. 4 to 5 lbs/week
    D. 7 to 8 lbs/week
ANSWER: A   p. 271

85. All of the following are sensible guidelines for diet plans EXCEPT

K
    A. consume low-fat foods regularly.
    B. eat rapidly to avoid prolonged contact with food.
    C. adjust energy intake downward as weight loss progresses.
    D. include vegetables, fruits, and grains as the mainstay of the diet.
ANSWER: B   p. 272

86. What is the best approach to weight loss?

AP
    A. Avoid foods containing carbohydrates
    B. Reduce daily energy intake and increase energy expenditure
    C. Eliminate all fats from the diet and decrease water intake
    D. Greatly increase protein intake to prevent body protein loss
ANSWER: B   p. 273

18   Chapter 8   Energy Balance and Weight Control

87. Which of the following would NOT be a recommendation of weight-reduction counseling?

AP
A. Reorganize some established behavior patterns
B. Use the exchange system to keep track of energy intake
C. Perform physical exercise to increase energy expenditure
D. Reduce daily energy intake to less than 1000 kcal to overcome the decrease in metabolic rate

ANSWER: D   p. 273

88. A desirable aid in a person's weight-loss diet program is to

AP
A. decrease water intake.
B. increase physical activity.
C. speed up thyroid activity with metabolic enhancers.
D. develop ketosis by maintaining carbohydrate intake as low as possible.

ANSWER: B   p. 273

89. The only way to avoid lean body losses while losing fat on a kilocalorie-restricted diet is to

AP
A. minimize water intake.
B. ingest additional protein.
C. include vigorous exercise.
D. decrease the amount of fat in the diet.

ANSWER: C   p. 273

90. In studies of weight loss in obese women, which of the following was a result of combining physical exercise with a weight reduction diet as compared with dieting without exercise?

AP
A. Stress level increased
B. More of the weight lost was fat
C. Appetite was more difficult to control
D. Basal metabolism slowed for several hours after exercise

ANSWER: B   p. 273

91. In people trying to change their eating habits, which of the following describes an essential part of behavior modification?

AP
A. Changes in behavior are more likely to occur when the antecedents are more intense
B. Feeling remorseful when behavior is inappropriate fosters more disciplined adherence to the diet later on
C. The consequences of behavior modification frequently result in changes of the cues or stimuli associated with food intake
D. One of the 4 parts of behavior modification includes some form of punishment only when eating behavior is uncontrollable

ANSWER: A   p. 274-276

Chapter 8 Energy Balance and Weight Control   19

92. An example of a behavior modification technique for weight control is to

AP
    A. feel guilty after you overeat.
    B. keep a record of your eating habits.
    C. always clean your plate when you eat.
    D. have someone watch you to prevent overeating.
    ANSWER: B   p. 275

93. All of the following are behavior modifications for losing weight EXCEPT

AP
    A. shopping only when not hungry.
    B. eating only in one place and in one room.
    C. participating in activities such as television viewing only when not eating.
    D. taking smaller portions of food but always eating everything on the plate quickly.
    ANSWER: D   p. 277

94. To help maximize the long-term success of a person's weight-loss program, which of the following personal attitudes should be encouraged in the individual?

AP
    A. Strongly believing that weight can be lost
    B. Viewing the body realistically as being fat rather than thin
    C. Refraining from expressing overconfidence in ability to lose weight
    D. Accepting that underexercising is a part of the lifestyle of most overweight people
    ANSWER: A   p. 278

95. Underweight is known to increase the risks for the all of the following EXCEPT

K
    A. diabetes.
    B. tuberculosis.
    C. digestive diseases.
    D. infertility in women.
    ANSWER: A   p. 279

96. Which is NOT a recommended strategy for weight gain in an underweight person?

AP
    A. Increase in activity
    B. Behavior modification training
    C. Forced awakening during the night for supplemental meals and snacks
    D. Consumption of regular meals and snacks that provide high-kcalorie foods in small volumes
    ANSWER: C   p. 280

20   Chapter 8 Energy Balance and Weight Control

97. Which of the following would NOT be part of a successful program of weight gain in an underweight individual?

AP
A. Physical exercise
B. Energy-dense foods
C. Energy-dense beverages
D. Large number of small meals
ANSWER: D   p. 280

98. Which of the following does NOT typically describe the person with anorexia nervosa?

K
A. Female
B. Teenaged
C. Uneducated
D. Middle-class
ANSWER: C   p. 286

99. In reality, a person with anorexia nervosa is

K
A. starving to death.
B. losing water weight only.
C. losing weight by fad dieting.
D. damaging herself psychologically only.
ANSWER: A   p. 286

100. Which of the following is in characteristic of anorexia norvosa?

A. It is easily self-diagnosed
B. Males account for about 5% of the cases
C. It damage the body less than starvation does
D. Treatment involving dietary intervention
ANSWER: B   p. 286-287

101. The adaptation response to anorexia nervosa includes all of the following EXCEPT

A. a fall in basal metabolic rate.
B. a rise in blood pressure.
C. a fall in blood proteins concentration.
D. a rise in blood vitamin A & E concentrations.
ANSWER: B   p. 287

102. Typical foods chosen by a person with bulimia during a binge include all of the following EXCEPT

AP
A. bread.
B. cookies.
C. ice cream.
D. vegetables.
ANSWER: D   p. 288

Chapter 8 Energy Balance and Weight Control

103. All of the following are common side effects of bulimia EXCEPT

    A. rectal bleeding.
    B. mineral imbalance.
    C. severe weight loss.
    D. ulceration of the esophagus.
    ANSWER: C   p. 288

104. The death rate of people with anorexia nervosa is about

    A. 1%
    B. 3%
    C. 6%
    D. 10%
    ANSWER: C   p. 288

105. Diet recommendation for bulimic include all of the following EXCEPT

    A. avoid "finger" foods to minimize overeating.
    B. eat cold foods to stimulate satiety.
    C. include fiber-rich foods.
    D. eat sitting down.
    ANSWER: B   p. 290

Essay Questions

247   106.   Define basal metabolic rate and discuss factors that increase and decrease it.

247   107.   List the major components that contribute to the body's daily expenditure of energy. Compare the relative contributions of a sedentary person with a marathon runner of the same body weight.

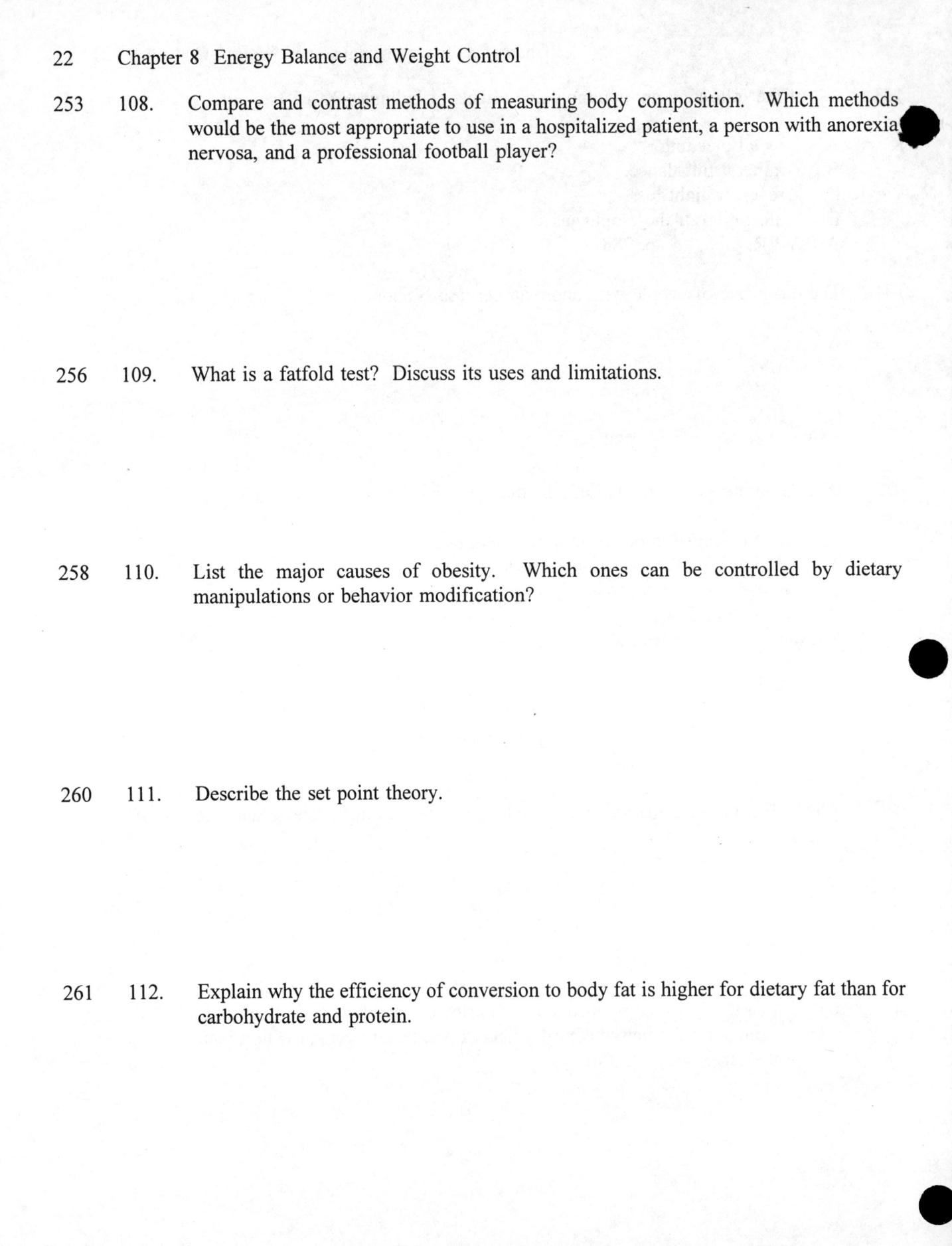

Chapter 8 Energy Balance and Weight Control

253 108. Compare and contrast methods of measuring body composition. Which methods would be the most appropriate to use in a hospitalized patient, a person with anorexia nervosa, and a professional football player?

256 109. What is a fatfold test? Discuss its uses and limitations.

258 110. List the major causes of obesity. Which ones can be controlled by dietary manipulations or behavior modification?

260 111. Describe the set point theory.

261 112. Explain why the efficiency of conversion to body fat is higher for dietary fat than for carbohydrate and protein.

266 113. List several factors that help identify inappropriate, unsound, and possibly dangerous commercial weight-loss programs.

267 114. Explain the attraction of unsound weight-loss procedures and plans to obese people.

268 115. List the approaches for reducing body weight that involve surgery or placement of devices that diminish food intake. What are the adverse side effects of these procedures?

271 116. Describe a good weight-reduction diet in relation to energy, protein, fat and carbohydrate content.

273 117. Explain the changes in metabolism consequent to a decrease in energy intake. How are these changes modified by regular physical exercise?

Chapter 8 Energy Balance and Weight Control

286   118.   List the adverse side effects of anorexia nervosa and bulimia. Describe the typical personality traits of individuals with these eating disorders.

289   119.   Discuss the characteristics of obese binge eating. What is known about its treatment?

CHAPTER 9
THE WATER-SOLUBLE VITAMINS: B VITAMINS AND VITAMIN C

MULTIPLE CHOICE

1. Which of the following vitamins would be removed in the production of skim milk?

AP
- A. Thiamin
- B. Vitamin A
- C. Riboflavin
- D. Vitamin B_{12}

ANSWER: B   p. 294

2. Expressions of vitamin levels in foods and in the body include all of the following EXCEPT

K
- A. grams.
- B. micrograms.
- C. milligrams.
- D. equivalents.

ANSWER: A   p. 294,303

3. General characteristics of the water-soluble vitamins include all of the following EXCEPT

K
- A. they must be consumed daily.
- B. excesses are eliminated from the kidneys.
- C. they are absorbed directly into the blood.
- D. toxic levels in the body are rarely found.

ANSWER: A   p. 294

Chapter 9 The Water-Soluble Vitamins: B Vitamins and Vitamin C

4. Which of the following is NOT a general characteristic of the fat-soluble vitamins?

K
A. Excesses are eliminated from the kidneys
B. Absorption is via the lymphatic circulation
C. Several of them require protein carriers for transport
D. They can be stored in relatively large amounts in certain body tissues
ANSWER: A   p. 294

5. Cooking a food in liberal amounts of water is LEAST likely to affect the vitamin content of

AP
A. folate.
B. vitamin A.
C. thiamin.
D. riboflavin.
ANSWER: B   p. 294

6. When vitamin B_1 is consumed in excess of needs, how does the body treat the excess?

AP
A. Not absorbed
B. Excreted in the urine
C. Excreted in the feces
D. Stored in liver, bone, and adipose tissue
ANSWER: B   p. 295

7. What is the primary excretory route for the water-soluble vitamins?

K
A. Bile
B. Kidney
C. Intestine
D. Perspiration
ANSWER: B   p. 295

8. What is the primary function of the B vitamins?

K
A. Energy source
B. Anticoagulation
C. Coenzyme participation
D. Antibody stabilization
ANSWER: C   p. 296

9. Which of the following explains why B vitamin deficiencies lead to lack of energy?

AP
A. B vitamins are a source of kilocalories
B. Absorption of carbohydrates and fats is decreased
C. Oxygen for energy metabolism cannot be transported to the cells
D. Coenzymes needed for energy metabolism are produced in insufficient amounts
ANSWER: D   p. 296

10. Which of the following functions has a requirement for thiamin?

AP A. Blood coagulation
    B. Formation of red blood cells
    C. Energy release from macronutrients
    D. Formation of epithelial cell mucopolysaccharides
    ANSWER: C   p. 296

11. Which of the following describes the basic function of a coenzyme?

K   A. Attaches to RNA to assist in the synthesis of an enzyme
    B. Attaches to cell membranes to assist in uptake of an enzyme
    C. Attaches to an enzyme and allows a chemical reaction to take place
    D. Attaches to an enzyme which allows for transport of the enzyme through the circulation
    ANSWER: C   p. 296

12. What is the primary chemical reaction in which thiamin participates as its coenzyme?

K   A. Transfers amine groups in the synthesis of amino acids
    B. Transfers hydrogen atoms in the synthesis of erythrocytes
    C. Assists in addition of methyl groups to compounds involved in energy metabolism
    D. Assists in removal of one carbon units from compounds involved in energy metabolism
    ANSWER: D   p. 296

13. Which of the following is the coenzyme form of thiamin?

K   A. Thiaminacide
    B. Thiamin pyrophosphate
    C. Thiamin adenine dinucleotide
    D. Thiamin flavin mononucleotide
    ANSWER: B   p. 296

14. Beriberi results from a deficiency of what vitamin?

K   A. Niacin
    B. Thiamin
    C. Vitamin C
    D. Vitamin B_{12}
    ANSWER: B   p. 297

15. The need for which of the following vitamins is related directly to the amount of energy expended?

K   A. Folate
    B. Thiamin
    C. Vitamin C
    D. Vitamin B_6
    ANSWER: B   p. 297

4   Chapter 9   The Water-Soluble Vitamins: B Vitamins and Vitamin C

16. What vitamin was discovered first?

K   A. Niacin
     B. Thiamin
     C. Vitamin A
     D. Ascorbic acid
     ANSWER: B   p. 297

17. Which of the following is a property of thiamin nutrition?

K   A. Participates in activation of prothrombin
     B. Significant amounts are found in leafy vegetables
     C. Requirements are proportional to energy expenditure
     D. Deficiency results in cheilosis and marked dermatitis
     ANSWER: C   p. 297

18. Which of the following diets is most likely to lead to beriberi?

AP   A. Low intakes of whole grains
     B. High intakes of polished rice
     C. High intakes of unrefined rice
     D. Low intakes of enriched grains
     ANSWER: B   p. 297

19. What type of yeast is commonly used as a nutrient supplement in the diets of vegetarians?

K   A. Flour yeast
     B. Baker's yeast
     C. Brewer's yeast
     D. Fortified yeast
     ANSWER: C   p. 298

20. Which of the following food groups ordinarily contains the highest amount of vitamins when expressed per kcalorie?

K   A. Dairy
     B. Meats
     C. Fruits
     D. Vegetables
     ANSWER: D   p. 298

21. Which of the following provides the most thiamin per serving size?

K   A. Ham
     B. Squash
     C. Whole milk
     D. Whole-grain breads
     ANSWER: A   p. 299-300

22. Of the following, which is the richest food source of thiamin?

AP   A. Milk
B. Pork
C. Lettuce
D. Refined rice
ANSWER: B   p. 300

23. Which of the following provides muscle tissue with the highest concentration of thiamin?

AP   A. Pig
B. Fish
C. Steer
D. Chicken
ANSWER: A   p. 300

24. Which of the following is a characteristic of thiamin stability in relation to cooking method?

K   A. Microwaving the food conserves much of the thiamin
B. Prolonged heating of the food has little, if any, affect on the thiamin
C. Boiling the food tends to conserve thiamin by forming a stable, hydrated complex
D. Steaming the food can lead to substantial thiamin loss due to the high heat needed to form the steam
ANSWER: A   p. 300

25. Riboflavin in its coenzyme form functions in the transfer of

K   A. methyl groups.
B. hydrogen atoms.
C. 1-carbon units.
D. 2-carbon units.
ANSWER: B   p. 300

26. Which of the following vitamins is involved substantially in energy transformation reactions?

K   A. Biotin
B. Cobalamin
C. Riboflavin
D. Pyridoxine
ANSWER: C   p. 300

27. Which of the following is indicative of a dietary deficiency of riboflavin?

K   A. Beriberi
B. Diarrhea
C. Keratomalacia
D. Inflamed eyelids
ANSWER: D   p. 301

6   Chapter 9 The Water-Soluble Vitamins: B Vitamins and Vitamin C

28.   What vitamin in milk provides about half of the amount available to the U.S. population?

AP   A.   Folate
       B.   Biotin
       C.   Riboflavin
       D.   Pantothenic acid
       ANSWER: C   p. 301

29.   If one identical twin who leads a sedentary lifestyle has an RDA of 1.3 mg for riboflavin, what would be the approximate allowance for the other twin who engages in regular physical activity?

AP   A.   1.3 mg
       B.   1.6 mg
       C.   1.9 mg
       D.   2.6 mg
       ANSWER: A   p. 301

30.   Riboflavin needs are more difficult to meet when the diet is low in

AP   A.   meats.
       B.   grains.
       C.   vegetables.
       D.   dairy foods.
       ANSWER: D   p. 301

31.   The signs and symptoms of riboflavin deficiency are known collectively as

K   A.   pellagra.
       B.   antiflavonosis.
       C.   ariboflavinosis.
       D.   flavin adenine dinucleosis.
       ANSWER: C   p. 301

32.   A deficiency of what vitamin produces a characteristic cracking and redness at the corners of the mouth?

K   A.   Biotin
       B.   Niacin
       C.   Riboflavin
       D.   Ascorbic acid
       ANSWER: C   p. 301

33.   Riboflavin is destroyed when exposed to which of the following?

K   A.   Heat
       B.   Acid
       C.   Alkali
       D.   Ultraviolet light
       ANSWER: D   p. 303

Chapter 9 The Water Soluble Vitamins: B Vitamins and Vitamin C   7

34. What type of container is best for protecting the riboflavin content of milk?

AP A. Airtight
    B. Cardboard
    C. Transparent glass
    D. Translucent plastic
    ANSWER: B   p. 303

35. When the diet contains an adequate amount of protein, what amino acid can be used by the body to synthesize niacin?

AP A. Lysine
    B. Valine
    C. Tryptophan
    D. Phenylalanine
    ANSWER: C   p. 303

36. Which of the following is a property of riboflavin in nutrition?

K   A. Stability to heat is good
    B. Deficiency leads to beriberi
    C. Requirements are proportional to body weight
    D. Significant amounts are found in citrus products
    ANSWER: A   p. 303

37. Which of the following is a property of niacin in nutrition?

K   A. It is susceptible to destruction in foods exposed to lights
    B. It participates primarily in reactions involving amino acids
    C. It can be soluble in water and lipids depending upon its chemical form
    D. It can be synthesized in the body from the essential amino acid tryptophan
    ANSWER: D   p. 303

38. Which of the following properties is shared by niacin and riboflavin coenzymes?

AP A. Unstable to irradiation
    B. Transfers hydrogen atoms
    C. Transfers carboxyl groups
    D. Unstable to metal cooking utensils
    ANSWER: B   p. 303

39. Which of the following is NOT among the common signs of pellagra?

K   A. Dementia
    B. Diarrhea
    C. Dermatitis
    D. Demineralization
    ANSWER: D   p. 304

8   Chapter 9   The Water-Soluble Vitamins: B Vitamins and Vitamin C

40. A diet low in protein and in which corn is a principal food has been found to cause a deficiency of what vitamin?

AP
A. Niacin
B. Thiamin
C. Vitamin C
D. Vitamin B_{12}
ANSWER: A   p. 304

41. A general niacin deficiency is manifested in abnormalities of all of the following organs/systems EXCEPT

K
A. skin.
B. skeletal.
C. nervous system.
D. gastrointestinal tract.
ANSWER: B   p. 304

42. Which of the following nutrients functions to prevent the appearance of a bilateral, symmetrical dermatitis, especially on areas exposed to the sun?

AP
A. Niacin
B. Choline
C. Inositol
D. Riboflavin
ANSWER: A   p. 304

43. What vitamin deficiency disease appeared in people who had subsisted on a diet that was high in corn and low in protein?

K
A. Scurvy
B. Pellagra
C. Wet beriberi
D. Pernicious anemia
ANSWER: B   p. 304

44. What is the term that identifies the characteristic cutaneous tingling sensations and reddening of the skin after ingesting a pharmacologic dose of nicotinic acid?

AP
A. Niacin flush
B. NAD dermatitis
C. Niacin erythremia
D. Bilateral symmetrical dermatitis
ANSWER: A   p. 304

Chapter 9   The Water Soluble Vitamins: B Vitamins and Vitamin C   9

45. Which of the following overt side effect(s) is likely to appear after a person ingests a high quantity of nicotinic acid?

AP
    A.   Constipation
    B.   Mental confusion
    C.   Painful, tingling, itching sensation
    D.   Hair loss, bloating, and photophobia
ANSWER: C   p. 304

46. Which of the following is a feature of niacin nutrition?

K
    A.   Low doses may lead to kidney stones
    B.   High doses may lower blood cholesterol
    C.   Low doses may lead to heartburn and low blood pressure
    D.   High doses may elevate red blood cell count in mildly anemic individuals
ANSWER: B   p. 304

47. Which of the following represents the minimum amount of vitamin C that would be considered a pharmacologic level for normal adults?

AP
    A.   25 mg
    B.   50 mg
    C.   100 mg
    D.   200 mg
ANSWER: D   p. 304

48. When taken in large doses, which of the following vitamins is associated with liver injury and peptic ulcers?

AP
    A.   Niacin
    B.   Thiamin
    C.   Vitamin B_6
    D.   Vitamin B_{12}
ANSWER: A   p. 305

49. Large doses of nicotinic acid are known to result in all of the following EXCEPT

K
    A.   liver injury.
    B.   peptic ulcer disease.
    C.   laboratory evidence of diabetes.
    D.   disappearance of learning disorders in children.
ANSWER: D   p. 305

Chapter 9 The Water-Soluble Vitamins: B Vitamins and Vitamin C

50. A typical diet of a 50 kg woman provides the RDA level of protein. The protein contains an average of 1% tryptophan and 2% tyrosine. Approximately how many niacin equivalents are contributed by the diet?

AP
    A. 2
    B. 5
    C. 7
    D. 10
    ANSWER: C   p. 305

51. All of the following are features of biotin in nutrition EXCEPT

K
    A. it functions in the breakdown of amino acids and fatty acids.
    B. it functions as a carrier of carbon dioxide in energy metabolism.
    C. a deficiency can be induced by ingesting large quantities of raw egg whites.
    D. a deficiency can be induced by ingesting large amounts of thiamin and folic acid which interfere with its absorption.
    ANSWER: D   p. 305

52. Among the following compounds that serve as coenzymes in metabolism, which is considered a vitamin for human beings?

K
    A. Biotin
    B. Choline
    C. Inositol
    D. Lipoic acid
    ANSWER: A   p. 305,318

53. Which of the following statements confirms our knowledge of water-soluble vitamin toxicity?

K
    A. Toxicity symptoms for vitamin B_6 can be severe and irreversible
    B. Toxicity symptoms for vitamin C include constipation and hyperactivity
    C. Toxicities of the B-vitamins occur almost as often from foods as from supplements
    D. Toxicity of niacin has been reported in body builders taking large amounts of amino acid supplements
    ANSWER: A   p. 305,309,322,327

54. Which of the following foods contains a protein that decreases bioavailability of biotin?

K
    A. raw egg
    B. aged wine
    C. aged cheese
    D. raw cauliflower
    ANSWER: A   p. 306

Chapter 9 The Water Soluble Vitamins: B Vitamins and Vitamin C   11

55.   What vitamin forms a part of coenzyme A?

K   A.   Biotin
      B.   Folate
      C.   Riboflavin
      D.   Pantothenic acid
      ANSWER: D   p. 307

56.   A protein that binds with biotin (thus inhibiting absorption) is found in which food?

K   A.   Aged cheese
      B.   Raw egg whites
      C.   Whole wheat bread
      D.   Unhomogenized milk
      ANSWER: B   p. 307

57.   Biotin can be synthesized by

K   A.   avidin.
      B.   the skin.
      C.   the liver.
      D.   intestinal bacteria.
      ANSWER: D   p. 307

58.   Which of the following vitamins is synthesized by intestinal bacteria?

K   A.   folate
      B.   biotin
      C.   cyanocobalamin
      D.   pantothenic acid
      ANSWER: B   p. 307

59.   Which of the following is required in the diet of human beings?

K   A.   Biotin
      B.   Choline
      C.   Inositol
      D.   Lipoic acid
      ANSWER: A   p. 307

60.   What vitamin is involved intensively in amino acid metabolism?

K   A.   Biotin
      B.   Vitamin A
      C.   Vitamin B_6
      D.   Riboflavin
      ANSWER: C   p. 308

12   Chapter 9   The Water-Soluble Vitamins: B Vitamins and Vitamin C

61. Which of the following is NOT a characteristic of vitamin B_6 in nutrition?

AP
- A. It is stored in muscle tissue
- B. It is required in amounts proportional to energy expenditure
- C. It can lead to irreversible nerve damage when taken in large doses
- D. It functions, in part, in the synthesis of glycine and glutamic acid

ANSWER: B   p. 309

62. All of the following are features of vitamin B_6 metabolism EXCEPT

K
- A. alcohol intake promotes its destruction and excretion.
- B. it functions primarily as the coenzyme pyridoxal phosphate.
- C. deficiency may result in people being treated for tuberculosis.
- D. it enhances physical performance when supplied at a level of 1 mg/g of dietary protein.

ANSWER: D   p. 309

63. What vitamin was taken in large amounts by many women in the early 1980's in hopes of combatting the symptoms of pre-menstrual syndrome?

K
- A. Thiamin
- B. Inositol
- C. Cobalamin
- D. Vitamin B_6

ANSWER: D   p. 309

64. On a per-kcalories basis, which of the following foods is richest in vitamin B_6?

AP
- A. Meats
- B. Fruits
- C. Legumes
- D. Vegetables

ANSWER: D   p. 311

65. Which of the following is an essential nutrient for human beings?

K
- A. Folate
- B. Choline
- C. Inositol
- D. Lipoic acid

ANSWER: A   p. 311

66. Which of the following vitamins is generally found in a form that is bound to one or more glutamic acid molecules in food?

K
- A. Folate
- B. Thiamin
- C. Vitamin B_6
- D. Ascorbic acid

ANSWER: A   p. 311

67. All of the following are properties of folate in nutrition EXCEPT

K A. it requires vitamin B_{12} to function properly.
   B. it is needed for proper functioning of vitamin B_{12}.
   C. it functions primarily in the transfer of carbon dioxide units.
   D. it requires enzymes on the intestinal mucosa to enhance its absorption from most foods.
   ANSWER: C   p. 311

68. What vitamin is involved mainly with the replacement of red blood cells and digestive tract cells?

AP A. Folate
    B. Niacin
    C. Thiamin
    D. Riboflavin
    ANSWER: A   p. 313

69. Which of the following is NOT known to affect the body's folate status?

K A. Smoking
   B. Aspirin
   C. Some anticancer drugs
   D. Some antituberculosis drugs
   ANSWER: D   p. 313

70. A person with a disorder that limits production of bile is at increased risk for deficiency of

AP A. folate.
    B. niacin.
    C. riboflavin.
    D. ascorbic acid.
    ANSWER: A   p. 313

71. What is the most likely explanation for the impaired functioning of the GI tract resulting from folate deficiency?

AP A. Since folate is required for bile synthesis, folate deficiency results in insufficient bile production thereby promoting fat malabsorption and diarrhea
    B. Since folate functions, in large part, in the process of cell renewal, a deficiency slows mucosal cell replacement thereby resulting in decreased GI functioning
    C. The anemia of folate deficiency results in decreased oxygen supply to body tissues, with the intestines being particularly affected because of its high metabolic activity
    D. Since folate functions, in part, in the synthesis of pancreatic digestive enzymes, a deficiency leads to decreased enzymatic capacity in the intestines thereby resulting in malabsorption
    ANSWER: B   p. 313

14   Chapter 9   The Water-Soluble Vitamins: B Vitamins and Vitamin C

72. Physiological stresses such as blood loss, burns, measles, and cancer are known to increase the risk of deficiency particularly for

AP
A. biotin.
B. folate.
C. riboflavin.
D. pantothenic acid
ANSWER: B   p. 313

73. What is the RDA for folate for a woman weighing 132 pounds?

AP
A. 180 µg
B. 220 µg
C. 242 µg
D. 400 µg
ANSWER: A   p. 313

74. Which of the following activities is shared by vitamin B_{12} and folate?

AP
A. Both are required for nucleic acid synthesis
B. Both are considered problem nutrients for strict vegetarians
C. Both are found in significant amounts in green leafy vegetables
D. Both require intrinsic factor for their release from food proteins
ANSWER: A   p. 313,318

75. Which of the following is associated with a deficiency of folate?

K
A. Hemolysis
B. Hypoxemia
C. Hemolytic anemia
D. Large-cell type anemia
ANSWER: D   p. 314

76. Which of the following foods is highest in folate?

K
A. Meats
B. Starches
C. Dairy products
D. Green leafy vegetables
ANSWER: D   p. 314

77. Which of the following is representative of folate availability in foods?

K
A. Good sources are dairy products and meats
B. Poor sources are fruit juices and vegetable juices
C. Only about 10% of the amount in foods is bioavailable
D. Much of the vitamin is unstable to ordinary cooking temperatures
ANSWER: D   p. 314

78. Which of the following is required for the absorption of dietary vitamin B$_{12}$?

K
    A. Bile
    B. Lipase
    C. Intrinsic factor
    D. Carboxypeptidase
    ANSWER: C   p. 316

79. A similar type of anemia is produced when there is a deficiency of either

AP
    A. riboflavin or niacin.
    B. vitamin B$_{12}$ or folate.
    C. thiamin or riboflavin.
    D. vitamin B$_6$ or vitamin B$_{12}$.
    ANSWER: B   p. 316

80. What is the function of intrinsic factor in vitamin B$_{12}$ absorption?

K
    A. It catalyzes release of the vitamin from its protein-bound form
    B. It attaches to the vitamin thereby allowing absorption from the intestines
    C. It acts as a storage protein for the vitamin within the intestinal epithelial cells
    D. It acts as a cofactor for mucosal enzymes involved in absorption of the vitamin
    ANSWER: B   p. 316

81. What is the most common treatment for pernicious anemia?

AP
    A. Injection of cobalamin
    B. Topical administration of liver extract
    C. Oral supplements of B-vitamin complex
    D. A diet high in liver and green leafy vegetables
    ANSWER: A   p. 316

82. Which of the following vitamins has an RDA?

K
    A. Biotin
    B. Choline
    C. Cobalamin
    D. Pantothenic acid
    ANSWER: C   p. 316

83. Which of the following is a property of vitamin B$_{12}$?

K
    A. It is efficiently recycled by the body
    B. It is necessary for protection from pinpoint hemorrhages
    C. It requires attachment to fatty acids for transport in the circulation
    D. It is absorbed from the stomach with the aid of a special binding protein
    ANSWER: A   p. 316-317

16   Chapter 9   The Water-Soluble Vitamins: B Vitamins and Vitamin C

84. What is the most likely reason for the development of a vitamin B_{12} deficiency?

AP A. Inadequate intake
    B. Increased excretion
    C. Inadequate absorption
    D. Increased losses in food preparation
    ANSWER: C   p. 316

85. Among the following water-soluble vitamins, a secondary deficiency would most likely be seen for

AP A. biotin.
    B. thiamin.
    C. vitamin C.
    D. vitamin B_{12}.
    ANSWER: D   p. 316

86. Why are vegetarians at risk of developing vitamin B_{12} deficiency?

AP A. Vegetarian diets inhibit absorption of the vitamin
    B. Vegetarian diets provide insufficient amounts of the vitamin
    C. High fiber content of vegetarian diets causes decreased storage by the liver
    D. High fiber content of vegetarian diets causes increased excretion of the vitamin
    ANSWER: B   p. 318

87. Which of the following is NOT a vitamin for human beings?

K   A. Cobalamin
    B. Ubiquinone
    C. Pyridoxine
    D. Pantothenic acid
    ANSWER: B   p. 318

88. Which of the following acids is NOT required in the diet of human beings?

K   A. Folic acid
    B. Lipoic acid
    C. Ascorbic acid
    D. Pantothenic acid
    ANSWER: B   p. 318

89. Of the following foods, which would be the only source of vitamin B_{12}?

AP A. Hot dog
    B. Pecan pie
    C. Cauliflower
    D. Blueberry muffin
    ANSWER: A   p. 318

Chapter 9   The Water Soluble Vitamins: B Vitamins and Vitamin C   17

90. If a person refrained from ingesting any of the water-soluble vitamins, deficiency symptoms would appear last for

AP
A. folate.
B. vitamin C.
C. vitamin B$_1$.
D. vitamin B$_{12}$.
ANSWER: D   p. 318

91. Normally, the body's storage and re-utilization of vitamin B$_{12}$ prevents a primary or secondary deficiency from occurring until after about

AP
A. 3 weeks.
B. 3 years.
C. 3 months.
D. several days.
ANSWER: B   p. 318

92. Which of the following is known to perform an essential function in the human body?

K
A. Inositol
B. Ubiquinone
C. Pangamic acid
D. Para-aminobenzoic acid
ANSWER: A   p. 318

93. Which of the following characteristics is shared by vitamins B$_6$, B$_{12}$, C and folate?

AP
A. Prevention of anemia
B. Required in glycolysis
C. Required in microgram quantities
D. Found in citrus products and legumes
ANSWER: A   p. 319

94. Which of the following is frequently affected by deficiencies of the B vitamins?

K
A. Bones
B. Tongue
C. Eyesight
D. Hair and nails
ANSWER: B   p. 322

95. Which of the following is an overt sign of a possible B vitamin deficiency?

AP
A. Anemia
B. Smooth tongue
C. Abnormal liver function
D. Abnormal heart function
ANSWER: B   p. 322

Chapter 9 The Water-Soluble Vitamins: B Vitamins and Vitamin C

96. In what capacity does vitamin C function?

K   A. Energy release from nutrients
     B. Cofactor in collagen formation
     C. Cofactor with calcium in blood coagulation
     D. Coenzyme in the formation of red blood cells
     ANSWER: B   p. 324

97. Which of the following is a general function of vitamin C?

K   A. Antiviral agent
     B. Antifungal agent
     C. Anticancer agent
     D. Antioxidant agent
     ANSWER: D   p. 324

98. The protein that requires ascorbic acid for its formation is

K   A. keratin.
     B. albumin.
     C. collagen.
     D. hydroxyproline.
     ANSWER: C   p. 324

99. What is the minimum amount of ascorbic acid that will prevent the appearance of scorbutic symptoms in human beings?

K   A. 10 mg
     B. 30 mg
     C. 50 mg
     D. 60 mg
     ANSWER: A   p. 325

100. If you have been consuming adequate amounts of vitamin C followed by no vitamin C in the diet for two days, which of the following will happen?

AP A. Signs of vitamin C deficiency will appear almost immediately
     B. You will probably notice that you bruise very easily on the second day
     C. The body's pool of vitamin C will be diminished but no deficiency symptoms are likely to appear
     D. Nothing: since vitamin C is stored in the liver, well-nourished people can go for several months with no dietary vitamin C before they develop deficiency symptoms
     ANSWER: C   p. 326

Chapter 9 The Water Soluble Vitamins: B Vitamins and Vitamin C   19

101. Which of the following is an early sign of vitamin C deficiency?

K   A. Bleeding gums
    B. Pernicious anemia
    C. Appearance of a cold
    D. Hysteria and depression
    ANSWER: A   p. 326

102. Which of the following circumstances has NOT been shown to benefit from intakes of vitamin C above the RDA?

AP A. Infections
    B. Major surgery
    C. Psychological stress
    D. Oral contraceptive use
    ANSWER: C   p. 326

103. Which of the following symptoms is indicative of a deficiency of vitamin C?

K   A. Hair loss
    B. Muscle spasms
    C. Bilateral symmetrical dermatitis
    D. Subcutaneous pinpoint hemorrhages
    ANSWER: D   p. 326

104. What term is used to describe the outcome of a diagnostic test that apparently shows that you have mononucleosis when in reality you do not?

AP A. True positive
    B. True negative
    C. False positive
    D. False negative
    ANSWER: C   p. 326

105. In the United States, what is the adult RDA for vitamin C?

K   A. 10 mg
    B. 30 mg
    C. 60 mg
    D. 75 mg
    ANSWER: C   p. 327

106. Which of the following is a possible withdrawal symptom from chronic vitamin C megadoses?

AP A. Diarrhea
    B. Bleeding gums
    C. GI discomfort
    D. Metallic taste
    ANSWER: B   p. 328

20   Chapter 9   The Water-Soluble Vitamins: B Vitamins and Vitamin C

107. What is the only food group that provides ample amounts of vitamin C?

K   A.   Milk group
      B.   Meat group
      C.   Bread-cereal group
      D.   Vegetable-fruit group
      ANSWER: D   p. 328

108. Which of these meals is lacking in vitamin C?

AP   A.   Roast beef, carrots, noodles, and tea
       B.   Hot dog, cabbage, french fries, and milk
       C.   Roast beef, broccoli, noodles, and coffee
       D.   Spaghetti with tomato sauce, meatball, garlic bread, and red wine
       ANSWER: A   p. 328-330

109. What food group is a rich source of vitamin C?

K   A.   Milk group
      B.   Meat group
      C.   Bread-cereal group
      D.   Vegetable-fruit group
      ANSWER: D   p. 328

110. Which of the following would be a very good source of vitamin C for the lacto-ovo-vegetarian?

AP   A.   Eggs
       B.   Milk
       C.   Broccoli
       D.   Whole-grain bread
       ANSWER: C   p. 328

111. All of the following are consequences of ingesting excess vitamin C supplements EXCEPT

AP   A.   they frequently cause diarrhea.
       B.   they appear safe at levels up to 300 mg/day.
       C.   they enhance the action of anticlotting medications.
       D.   they interfere with laboratory urine tests for the diagnosis of diabetes.
       ANSWER: C   p. 328

112. Which of the following would be the poorest dietary source of vitamin C?

AP   A.   Liver
       B.   Potatoes
       C.   Whole grains
       D.   Cruciferous vegetables
       ANSWER: C   p. 328-330

Chapter 9 The Water Soluble Vitamins: B Vitamins and Vitamin C   21

113. What is the benefit of using controls in an experiment?

AP
A. The size of the groups is very large
B. The subjects do not know anything about the experiment
C. The subjects who are treated are balanced against the placebos
D. The subjects are similar in all respects except for the treatment being tested
ANSWER: D   p. 332

114. What is the benefit of using placebos in an experiment?

AP
A. All subjects are similar
B. All subjects receive a treatment
C. Neither subject nor researcher know who is receiving treatment
D. One group of subjects receives a treatment and the other group receives nothing
ANSWER: B   p. 332

115. What is the meaning of a double-blind experiment?

K
A. Both subject groups take turns getting each treatment
B. Neither group of subjects knows whether they are in the control or experiment group
C. Neither subjects nor researchers know which subjects are in the control or experiment group
D. Both subject groups know whether they are in the control or experiment group but the researchers do not
ANSWER: C   p. 332

116. What is the benefit of using a large sample size in an experiment?

AP
A. Chance variation is ruled out
B. There will be no placebo effect
C. The experiment will be double-blind
D. The control group will be similar to the experimental group
ANSWER: A   p. 332

117. Which of the following represents the results of well-controlled studies of vitamin C supplementation on the resistance to, and recovery from, colds?

AP
A. There was a reduction in the duration of colds by 50% on the average
B. There was only a minor effect on reducing the number and severity of colds
C. There was a significant reduction in the number of colds only in people who consumed more than one gram a day
D. There was a significant reduction in the number of colds only in people who consumed more than three grams per day
ANSWER: B   p. 333

Chapter 9 The Water-Soluble Vitamins: B Vitamins and Vitamin C

Essay Questions

304,309,322,326   118. Under what circumstances can water-soluble vitamins be toxic? Give several examples.

316-318   119. Define intrinsic factor and discuss its relationship to vitamin B_{12} absorption. What other factors are associated with vitamin B_{12} absorption? What is the most common cause of vitamin B_{12} deficiency? How is vitamin B_{12} deficiency treated under these conditions?

316-318   120. Discuss the interrelationships of folate and vitamin B_{12} in the diagnosis and treatment of large-cell type anemia.

318   121. Why might vegans have a normal vitamin B_{12} status?

319-321   122. Discuss the roles of the B vitamins in energy metabolism.

321-322   123.   Discuss similarities in the deficiency symptoms of the B vitamins.

325-326   124.   Under what conditions and for what reasons would intakes of vitamin C above the RDA be desirable?

328   125.   Discuss how megadoses of vitamin C could possibly lead to symptoms of scurvy.

CHAPTER 10
THE FAT-SOLUBLE VITAMINS: A, D, E, AND K

MULTIPLE CHOICE

1. Which of the following is NOT a feature of the fat-soluble vitamins?

   AP
   A. Irregularly excreted from the body
   B. Found in the fat and oily parts of foods
   C. Transported permanently to the liver and adipose tissue
   D. Pose a greater risk for developing a toxicity than water-soluble vitamins
   ANSWER: C   p. 337

2. What is the major carrier of the fat-soluble vitamins from the intestinal epithelial cell to the circulation?

   K
   A. Albumin
   B. Cholesterol
   C. Chylomicrons
   D. Liposoluble binding proteins
   ANSWER: C   p. 337

3. Which of the following is NOT a fat-soluble vitamin?

   K
   A. Retinol
   B. Tocopherol
   C. Phylloquinone
   D. Cyanocobalamin
   ANSWER: D   p. 337,355,359

1

Chapter 10   The Fat-Soluble Vitamins: A, D, E, and K

4. As far as is known, vitamin A does NOT play an important role in which of the following processes?

AP
    A. Blood clotting
    B. Growth of bones and teeth
    C. Synthesis of visual pigment
    D. Maintaining mucous membranes

ANSWER: A   p. 337

5. Which of the following is a property of the fat soluble vitamins?

K
    A. Most of them are synthesized by intestinal bacteria
    B. Intestinal transport occurs by way of the portal circulation
    C. Toxicity risk is higher for vitamins E and K than other fat soluble vitamins
    D. Deficiencies result in a slower onset of symptoms than from the water-soluble vitamins
ANSWER: D   p. 337

6. Which of the following is responsible for transporting vitamin A from the liver to other tissues?

K
    A. Albumin
    B. Rhodopsin
    C. Transcarotenoid protein
    D. Retinol-binding protein
ANSWER: D   p. 337

7. What form of vitamin A is active in the visual response?

K
    A. Opsin
    B. Keratin
    C. Retinal
    D. Carotene
ANSWER: C   p. 338

8. How many different forms of vitamin A are active in the body?

K
    A. 1
    B. 2
    C. 3
    D. 5
ANSWER: C   p. 338

9. Which of the following describes an event in the visual response process?

K A. Light energy strikes the retina and excites pigments to release retinol
   B. Light energy strikes the cornea and excites pigments to release retinoic acid
   C. Visual pigments deep in the brain are excited by light transmitted through the retina
   D. Epithelial cells on the surface of the eye respond to light energy by transmitting opsin molecules along nerve pathways to the brain
   ANSWER: A   p. 338

10. All of the following are forms of vitamin A EXCEPT

K A. retinol.
   B. retinal.
   C. retinoic acid.
   D. retinoquinone.
   ANSWER: D   p. 338

11. Which of the following functions of vitamin A accounts for most of the body's need for the vitamin?

AP A. Promoting good night vision
   B. Assisting in immune reactions
   C. Promoting the growth of bones
   D. Maintaining mucous membranes
   ANSWER: D   p. 340

12. The adult RDA for vitamin A is approximately

K A. 400 mg.
   B. 1,000 mg.
   C. 1,000 retinol equivalents.
   D. 5,000 retinol equivalents.
   ANSWER: C   p. 341

13. Approximately what percent of the body's vitamin A stores are found in the liver?

K A. 20
   B. 50
   C. 70
   D. 90
   ANSWER: D   p. 342

14. The effects of vitamin A deficiency are most severe in what population group?

AP A. Adults
   B. Elderly
   C. Newborns
   D. Adolescents
   ANSWER: C   p. 342

4   Chapter 10   The Fat-Soluble Vitamins: A, D, E, and K

15. What is the most probable reason for widespread vitamin A deficits in children?

AP
- A. Low intake of vegetables
- B. High requirements for the nutrient
- C. Increased utilization due to vaccinations
- D. Inadequate intakes by mother during pregnancy

ANSWER: A   p. 342

16. Vitamin A supplements are helpful in treating which of the following conditions?

AP
- A. Acne
- B. Rickets
- C. Osteomalacia
- D. Night blindness

ANSWER: D   p. 342, 346

17. What tissue contains the majority of the body's store of vitamin A?

K
- A. Liver
- B. Adipose
- C. Retinal cells
- D. Intestinal mucosal cells

ANSWER: A   p. 342

18. If a normal, healthy adult were to begin consuming a vitamin A poor diet, approximately how much time would pass before the first deficiency symptoms would appear?

K
- A. 2 weeks
- B. 1 to 2 months
- C. 6 months
- D. 1 to 2 years

ANSWER: D   p. 342

19. Studies in developing countries have demonstrated that the mortality rate of children with measles can be significantly reduced by providing large supplements of

K
- A. iron.
- B. vitamin A.
- C. folic acid.
- D. phylloquinone.

ANSWER: B   p. 342

20. Which of the following is most likely to occur from a dietary deficiency of vitamin A?

AP
- A. Osteomalacia
- B. Osteoporosis
- C. Xerophthalmia
- D. Prolonged blood-clotting time

ANSWER: C   p. 343

Chapter 10 The Fat-Soluble Vitamins: A, D, E, and K   5

21. Which of the following is likely to induce vitamin A toxicity?

AP
A. Eating liver more than once a week
B. Consuming high-dosage vitamin A supplements
C. Drinking 2 quarts of vitamin A-fortified milk daily
D. Consuming too many dark green and deep orange vegetables
ANSWER: B   p. 344

22. Which of the following disorders is shared by a deficiency of vitamin A or folic acid?

AP
A. Anemia
B. Nyctalopia
C. Hemorrhaging
D. Osteomalacia
ANSWER: A   p. 344

23. Which of the following poses the greatest health risk when consumed in large amounts?

AP
A. Wheat germ
B. Desiccated liver
C. Nutritional yeast
D. Vitamin A and D supplements
ANSWER: D   p. 345, 341

24. Which of the following is the most likely side effect for a person who regularly consumes large quantities of carrots or carrot juice?

AP
A. Bone pain
B. Dermatitis
C. Skin yellowing
D. Vitamin A toxicity
ANSWER: C   p. 345

25. In which of the following individuals would vitamin A toxicity be most likely to occur?

AP
A. Adolescent women
B. Overweight adults
C. Those taking vitamin A supplements
D. Those consuming more than 100 g of carrots daily
ANSWER: C   p. 346

26. Which of the following substances is converted to vitamin A in the body?

K
A. Carotene
B. Xanthophyll
C. Chlorophyll
D. Cholesterol
ANSWER: A   p. 347

6   Chapter 10   The Fat-Soluble Vitamins: A, D, E, and K

27. On the average, one retinol equivalent is equal to about how many international units?

K   A.   3
       B.   5
       C.   8
       D.   10
       ANSWER: B   p. 347

28. All of the following are good sources of vitamin A EXCEPT

AP   A.   liver.
       B.   pears.
       C.   apricots.
       D.   sweet potatoes.
       ANSWER: B   p. 347-349

29. Which of the following foods is a very good source of vitamin A?

K   A.   Corn
       B.   Pumpkin pie
       C.   Baked potato
       D.   Whole-grain bread
       ANSWER: B   p. 347-349

30. Which of the following functions is shared by carotene and vitamin E?

AP   A.   Inhibition of oxidation
       B.   Prevention of keratinization
       C.   Prevention of hemolytic anemia
       D.   Inhibition of bone calcium loss
       ANSWER: A   p. 347,354

31. If the diet contains precursor vitamin A, which of the following tissues can use it to form vitamin A?

AP   A.   Eyes
       B.   Kidneys
       C.   Adipose cells
       D.   Intestinal cells
       ANSWER: D   p. 347

32. Which of the following food substances can be converted to vitamin A in the body?

K   A.   Tryptophan
       B.   Chlorophyll
       C.   Xanthophyll
       D.   Beta-carotene
       ANSWER: D   p. 347

Chapter 10   The Fat-Soluble Vitamins: A, D, E, and K   7

33. Which of the following can be used by the body to synthesize vitamin D?

AP
A. Bone
B. Carotene
C. Tryptophan
D. Exposure to sunlight
ANSWER: D   p. 349

34. Which of the following is a feature of vitamin D?

AP
A. Toxicity from vitamin D may result from overexposure to the sun
B. Requirements are much higher in the elderly due to degenerative bone diseases
C. Fortification of milk with the vitamin is common in order to provide children with a reliable source
D. Absorption from most food sources is very poor, necessitating addition of liberal quantities to grain products
ANSWER: C   p. 349-351

35. All of the following are characteristics of vitamin D nutrition EXCEPT

K
A. deficient intake may lead to altered bone composition.
B. excessive intake may lead to mineral deposits in the kidneys.
C. fortified milk is the major dietary source in the U.S. population.
D. the requirement is increased in most people who are exposed to the sun.
ANSWER: D   p. 349-353

36. To avoid vitamin A toxicity, young children should not consume diets which exceed the RDA by more than

AP
A. 3 times.
B. 6 times.
C. 10 times.
D. 20 times.
ANSWER: A   p. 349

37. In what tissues must a molecule of vitamin D be chemically altered to yield a compound that is fully active?

AP
A. Liver only
B. Kidney only
C. Liver and kidney
D. Liver and intestines
ANSWER: C   p. 349

8   Chapter 10   The Fat-Soluble Vitamins: A, D, E, and K

38. What is the main function(s) of vitamin D?

K   A.   Promote secretion of calcitonin
    B.   Promote synthesis of 7-dehydrocholesterol
    C.   Promote synthesis of carotenoids and control absorption of fat soluble vitamins
    D.   Promote calcium and phosphorus absorption and promote calcium mobilization from bone
    ANSWER: D   p. 350

39. In what system would the effects of a vitamin D deficiency be most readily observed?

AP A.   Nervous
    B.   Skeletal
    C.   Muscular
    D.   Circulatory
    ANSWER: B   p. 350

40. Which of the following symptoms would indicate a vitamin D deficiency?

K   A.   Bowed legs
    B.   Rupture of red blood cells
    C.   Frequent respiratory infections
    D.   Abnormally high blood calcium level
    ANSWER: A   p. 350

41. Which of the following conditions or diseases are known to be caused by a deficiency of the same nutrient?

AP A.   Osteomalacia and rickets
    B.   Xerophthalmia and breath pentane release
    C.   Kwashiorkor and fibrocystic breast disease
    D.   Hemolytic anemia and large-cell type anemia
    ANSWER: A   p. 350

42. Which of the following compounds is known to function like a hormone?

K   A.   Vitamin D
    B.   Vitamin K
    C.   Phylloquinone
    D.   Alpha-tocopherol
    ANSWER: A   p. 350

43. What is the name of the vitamin D-deficiency disease in adults?

K   A.   Rickets
    B.   Osteomalacia
    C.   Keratomalacia
    D.   Hyperkeratosis
    ANSWER: B   p. 351

Chapter 10   The Fat-Soluble Vitamins: A, D, E, and K   9

44. Which of the following may result from excessive intakes of vitamin D by adults?

AP   A. Increased bone density
     B. Increased bone calcification
     C. Deformity of leg bones, ribs, and skull
     D. Mineral deposits in soft tissues such as the kidney
     ANSWER: D   p. 351

45. What is the RDA for vitamin D in individuals over 25 years of age?

K   A. 5 µg
     B. 8 µg
     C. 10 µg
     D. 14 µg
     ANSWER: A   p. 351

46. All of the following are other names for vitamin D EXCEPT

K   A. calciferol.
     B. calcitonin.
     C. ergocalciferol.
     D. cholecalciferol.
     ANSWER: B   p. 351

47. Which of the following conditions is known to lead to formation of mineral deposits in the blood vessels and kidney?

AP   A. Excessive intake of vitamin D
     B. Inadequate intake of vitamin D
     C. Excessive intake of tocopherols
     D. Inadequate intake of tocopherols
     ANSWER: A   p. 351

48. Which of the following is the most reliable source of vitamin D in the diet?

AP   A. Meat
     B. Fortified milk
     C. Fruits and vegetables
     D. Enriched breads and cereals
     ANSWER: B   p. 353

49. Which of the following enables most of the world's population to maintain adequate vitamin D status?

AP   A. Outdoor exposure of the body to sunlight
     B. Wide availability of low-cost fish products
     C. Wide availability of food assistance programs
     D. World Health Organization distribution of vitamin D capsules
     ANSWER: A   p. 353

10   Chapter 10   The Fat-Soluble Vitamins: A, D, E, and K

50.   The main function of vitamin E in the body is to act as a(n)

K   A.   coenzyme.
    B.   peroxide.
    C.   antioxidant.
    D.   free radical.
    ANSWER: C   p. 354

51.   In what capacity does vitamin E participate in the metabolism of free radicals?

K   A.   Carrier
    B.   Promoter
    C.   Scavenger
    D.   Synthesizer
    ANSWER: C   p. 354

52.   Which of the following can be used as indirect evidence of vitamin E deficiency?

AP A.   Skin peroxidation index
    B.   Fecal free radical activity
    C.   Blood ergocalciferol level
    D.   Breath pentane concentration
    ANSWER: D   p. 354

53.   Which of the following is a feature of vitamin E?

AP A.   Functions as a hormone-like substance
    B.   Toxicity symptoms include bone abnormalities
    C.   Important food sources include enriched breads and pasta
    D.   Deficiencies occur from inability to absorb dietary lipids
    ANSWER: D   p. 354

54.   Which of the following features are shared by vitamins C and E?

AP A.   Both function as antioxidants
    B.   Both require bile for absorption
    C.   Neither participates in protein synthesis
    D.   Neither is affected by the processing of foods
    ANSWER: A   p. 354

55.   All of the following show benefits from vitamin E supplements EXCEPT

AP A.   premature infants.
    B.   people exposed to air pollution.
    C.   women with fibrocystic breast disease.
    D.   people with problems of sexual impotence.
    ANSWER: D   p. 355-356

Chapter 10 The Fat-Soluble Vitamins: A, D, E, and K

56. Nutritional muscular dystrophy in animals can be produced by feeding a diet deficient in

AP
    A. vitamin A.
    B. vitamin D.
    C. vitamin E.
    D. vitamin K.
    ANSWER: C   p. 355

57. Which of the following may result from vitamin E deficiency?

K
    A. Rickets
    B. Peroxidation
    C. Xerophthalmia
    D. Erythrocyte hemolysis
    ANSWER: D   p. 356

58. What is the reason that vitamin E deficiencies are rarely observed in human beings?

AP
    A. The vitamin is not essential
    B. The vitamin is so widespread in foods
    C. Most people take vitamin E supplements
    D. The vitamin can be synthesized by the body
    ANSWER: B   p. 356

59. Which of the following are major sources of vitamin E in the diet?

K
    A. Meats
    B. Citrus fruits
    C. Vegetable oils
    D. Milk and dairy products
    ANSWER: C   p. 356

60. Increasing the amount of polyunsaturated fats in the diet increases the need for

AP
    A. vitamin A.
    B. vitamin D.
    C. vitamin E.
    D. vitamin K.
    ANSWER: C   p. 356

61. Which of the following contains the highest concentration of vitamin E?

AP
    A. Butter
    B. Carrots
    C. Milk fat
    D. Corn oil
    ANSWER: D   p. 356-358

12 Chapter 10 The Fat-Soluble Vitamins: A, D, E, and K

62. Which of the following conditions may benefit from vitamin E therapy?

AP A. Diabetes
    B. Pernicious anemia
    C. Muscular dystrophy
    D. Intermittent claudication
    ANSWER: D   p. 356

63. In what chief capacity does vitamin K function?

K   A. Blood clotting
    B. Energy metabolism
    C. Calcium utilization
    D. Epithelial tissue renewal
    ANSWER: A   p. 358

64. Which of the following vitamins is synthesized in the intestines by bacteria?

K   A. Vitamin A
    B. Vitamin D
    C. Vitamin E
    D. Vitamin K
    ANSWER: D   p. 358

65. Which of the following substances requires vitamin K for its synthesis in the liver?

AP A. Opsin
    B. Albumin
    C. Calcitonin
    D. Prothrombin
    ANSWER: D   p. 358

66. Which of the following is a feature of vitamin K?

K   A. It participates in synthesis of bone proteins
    B. Large amounts can be stored in adipose tissue
    C. Good food sources are legumes and raw fruits
    D. Intestinal bacterial synthesis provides over 90% of the body's need for most people
    ANSWER: A   p. 358

67. Knowing the role of vitamin K in the body, in what organ would you expect to find it in large quantities?

AP A. Liver
    B. Pancreas
    C. Gallbladder
    D. Small intestine
    ANSWER: A   p. 358

Chapter 10 The Fat-Soluble Vitamins: A, D, E, and K   13

68. Which of the following is a property of the tocopherols?

K
A. Easily destroyed by air and heat
B. Act as precursors for the menaquinones
C. May dissolve from foods into cooking water
D. Absorbed from the intestines into the portal circulation
ANSWER: A   p. 358

69. The synthesis of which of the following is known to require vitamin K?

K
A. Albumin
B. GI mucosa
C. Prothrombin
D. Mucopolysaccharides
ANSWER: C   p. 358

70. Of the following, which would most likely induce a vitamin K deficiency?

AP
A. Achlorhydria
B. Antibiotic therapy
C. Presence of oxalic acid in food
D. Insufficient intake of green leafy vegetables
ANSWER: B   p. 359

71. In what population group is vitamin K deficiency most often observed?

K
A. Adults
B. Elderly
C. Newborns
D. Teenagers
ANSWER: C   p. 359

72. What type of foods should be limited in individuals taking anticoagulant medicines?

AP
A. Cold water fish
B. Processed soups
C. Enriched breads
D. Green leafy vegetables
ANSWER: D   p. 359

73. All of the following are features of vitamin K in nutrition EXCEPT

AP
A. infants frequently require a supplement at birth.
B. good food sources are plants of the cabbage family.
C. risk of deficiency is increased in people taking antibiotics for prolonged periods.
D. gut microflora synthesis supplies sufficient amounts to meet the needs of all healthy adults.
ANSWER: D   p. 359

14   Chapter 10   The Fat-Soluble Vitamins: A, D, E, and K

74. The process of bone remodeling is known to be dependent on all of the fat-soluble vitamins EXCEPT

K
A. vitamin A.
B. vitamin K.
C. vitamin E.
D. vitamin D.
ANSWER: C   p. 360

75. Which of the following statements is representative of vitamin supplementation practices?

AP
A. Most people who take supplements consume a poor diet
B. Most people should take supplements daily because of the great difficulty in obtaining the needed amounts from food
C. People who have low energy intakes or are pregnant are at risk for developing deficiencies and may benefit from supplementation
D. People should take supplements daily because nutrition surveys in the U.S. and Canada have detected deficiencies in some population groups
ANSWER: C   p. 363

76. Groups of people who are at risk for developing marginal deficiencies and may benefit from taking vitamin supplements include all of the following EXCEPT

AP
A. athletes.
B. food faddists.
C. pregnant or lactating women.
D. people with low energy intakes, such as habitual dieters and the elderly.
ANSWER: A   p. 363

77. All of the following are known to occur from a mild iron overdose EXCEPT

AP
A. nausea.
B. GI distress.
C. black tongue.
D. black diarrhea.
ANSWER: C   p. 364

78. The known dangers of taking vitamin supplements include all of the following EXCEPT

K
A. vitamin toxicity.
B. the taker may ignore warning signs of a disease.
C. the taker may feel a false sense of security and consume a poor diet.
D. pathogenic bacterial overgrowth of the large intestines leading to increased risk of infection.
ANSWER: D   p. 364

79. If a person needs a supplement, what kind should be taken?

AP
    A. High dose vitamin supplement
    B. High dose mineral supplement
    C. Vitamin-mineral supplement at or below the RDA
    D. Vitamin-mineral supplement at up to 5 times the RDA
    ANSWER: C   p. 365

Essay Questions

341,350   80. Explain why vitamin A and vitamin D may function as hormones rather than as vitamins.

346   81. Why are children more likely than others to be affected by vitamin A toxicity?

349   82. Describe how the body can synthesize vitamin D with the help of sunlight.

350   83. Compare and contrast the characteristics of the two deficiency diseases osteomalacia and rickets.

16   Chapter 10   The Fat-Soluble Vitamins: A, D, E, and K

355   84.   Describe false claims of vitamin E supplementation.

358   85.   Discuss the conditions under which deficiencies of vitamin K are most likely to occur.

363   86.   Discuss the use and abuse of nutrient supplements.

CHAPTER 11
THE BODY FLUIDS AND THE MAJOR MINERALS

MULTIPLE CHOICE

1. Which of the following is NOT a function of water in the body?

K   A. Lubricant
      B. Source of energy
      C. Component of compounds
      D. Participant in chemical reactions
      ANSWER: B   p. 369

2. Which of the following contributes most to the weight of the human body?

K   A. Iron
      B. Water
      C. Calcium
      D. Protein
      ANSWER: B   p. 370

3. Which of the following helps to regulate thirst?

K   A. Brain stem
      B. Cerebellum
      C. Optic nerve
      D. Hypothalamus
      ANSWER: D   p. 370

Chapter 11 The Body Fluids and the Major Minerals

4. What pituitary hormone regulates kidney retention of water?

K
A. Thyroxine
B. Cortisone
C. Epinephrine
D. Antidiuretic hormone
ANSWER: D   p. 370

5. What organ provides the major control for homeostasis of body fluids?

AP
A. Liver
B. Heart
C. Kidneys
D. Skeletal muscle
ANSWER: C   p. 370

6. Factors that are effective in regulating the body's water balance include all of the following EXCEPT

K
A. adrenaline.
B. aldosterone.
C. angiotensin.
D. antidiuretic hormone.
ANSWER: A   p. 370

7. What is the function of renin?

K
A. Activates angiotensin
B. Activates antidiuretic hormone
C. Stimulates the thirst mechanism
D. Stimulates water absorption from the GI tract
ANSWER: A   p. 370

8. What is the minimum amount of water excreted each day as urine that is needed to carry away the body's waste products?

K
A. 100 ml
B. 250 ml
C. 500 ml
D. 1,000 ml
ANSWER: C   p. 371

Chapter 11 The Body Fluids and the Major Minerals

9. What is the recommended water intake of a 65 kg adult with an energy expenditure of 2,500 kcal?

AP
- A. 250 to 500 ml
- B. 650 to 1300 ml
- C. 1,000 ml
- D. 2,500 to 3,250 ml

ANSWER: D   p. 371

10. Ions that carry a positive charge are called

K
- A. anions.
- B. cations.
- C. mineralytes.
- D valence ions.

ANSWER: B   p. 372

11. Which of the following is a feature of water?

K
- A. Not a vital nutrient
- B. Not found in beverages
- C. Oxidized to yield energy
- D. Generated from oxidation of energy nutrients

ANSWER: D   p. 372

12. The daily loss of water via the kidneys, lungs, feces, and skin approximates

K
- A. 0 to 0.5 liter.
- B. 0.5 to 1.5 liters.
- C. 1.5 to 2.5 liters.
- D. 3.0 to 4.0 liters.

ANSWER: C   p. 372

13. All of the following are properties of electrolytes EXCEPT

K
- A. they attract water.
- B. they are charged particles.
- C. they carry electrical current.
- D. they include fat soluble as well as water soluble particles.

ANSWER: D   p. 372-373

14. What is the term for the pressure that develops when two solutions of varying concentrations are separated by a membrane?

K
- A. Hypotension
- B. Hypertension
- C. Osmotic pressure
- D. Hypertonic pressure

ANSWER: C   p. 372

4   Chapter 11 The Body Fluids and the Major Minerals

15. Which of the following describes a way to make an electrolyte solution?

AP
- A. Dissolve a teaspoon of salt in a glass of water
- B. Vigorously shake a mixture of corn oil and water
- C. Dissolve a pinch of corn starch in a glass of water
- D. Vigorously shake a pinch of table sugar in warm water

ANSWER: A   p. 372

16. What is the force that moves water into a space where a solute is more concentrated?

K
- A. Buffer action
- B. Osmotic pressure
- C. Permeable selectivity
- D. Electrolyte imbalance

ANSWER: B   p. 373

17. What is the major extracellular cation?

K
- A. Sodium
- B. Sulfate
- C. Protein
- D. Potassium

ANSWER: A   p. 373,377

18. What is the major intracellular cation?

K
- A. Sodium
- B. Calcium
- C. Phosphate
- D. Potassium

ANSWER: D   p. 373,382

19. What is the major extracellular anion?

K
- A. Sodium
- B. Lactate
- C. Sulfate
- D. Chloride

ANSWER: D   p. 373,381

20. What is the major intracellular anion?

K
- A. Protein
- B. Sodium
- C. Phosphate
- D. Bicarbonate

ANSWER: C   p. 373

Chapter 11 The Body Fluids and the Major Minerals   5

21. What is the sodium pump?

K   A. A cell membrane enzyme that pumps sodium into the cell
    B. A cell membrane enzyme that pumps sodium out of the cell
    C. A mechanism present throughout interstitial fluid for draining sodium from the circulation
    D. A mechanism present in the kidneys for exchanging sodium with lactic acid for regulating organic acid concentration
    ANSWER: B   p. 374

22. Normally, what is the relationship of the amount of sodium excreted to the amount ingested that day?

AP A. Sodium intake is higher
    B. Sodium excretion is higher
    C. Sodium intake and excretion are equal
    D. Sodium excretion is unrelated to intake
    ANSWER: C   p. 375

23. In a normal individual with a daily requirement of 500 mg sodium, what would be the sodium balance after consuming 10 g of common salt?

AP A. Equilibrium
    B. Slight positive balance
    C. Strong positive balance
    D. Moderate positive balance
    ANSWER: A   p. 375

24. When a person looses fluid by sweating or bleeding, what minerals are lost in greatest quantity?

AP A. Sodium and chloride
    B. Bicarbonate and sulfate
    C. Calcium and magnesium
    D. Potassium and phosphate
    ANSWER: A   p. 376

25. What organ is the chief regulator of the body's acid-base balance?

K   A. Skin
    B. Liver
    C. Kidneys
    D. Stomach
    ANSWER: C   p. 377

Chapter 11 The Body Fluids and the Major Minerals

26. Which of the following is a feature of sodium nutrition?

K
- A. It has no RDA because diets rarely lack sodium
- B. It has no RDA because the kidneys are highly efficient at regulating sodium balance
- C. The RDA is 3 g, an amount which has been shown to have little or no effect on blood pressure
- D. The RDA is only 500 mg because the body possesses an unusually efficient retention mechanism

ANSWER: A   p. 377

27. What is another term for hypertension?

K
- A. High blood sodium
- B. High blood pressure
- C. Excessive mental stress
- D. Excessive muscular contraction

ANSWER: B   p. 378

28. How much sodium is contained in a fast-food deluxe hamburger that lists a salt content of 2.5 g?

AP
- A. 100 mg
- B. 125 mg
- C. 1,000 mg
- D. 2,500 mg

ANSWER: C   p. 378

29. What is the greatest single source of sodium in the diet?

AP
- A. Processed foods
- B. Unprocessed foods
- C. Natural salt content of foods
- D. Salt added during cooking and at the table

ANSWER: A   p. 379

30. Which of the following does NOT supply high amounts of sodium?

AP
- A. Sausage and frankfurters
- B. Canned and instant soups
- C. Onions and onion powder
- D. American cheese and catsup

ANSWER: C   p. 380

Chapter 11 The Body Fluids and the Major Minerals   7

31.   Which of the following is a major function of chloride?

K   A.   Participates in wound healing
     B.   Helps maintain gastric acidity
     C.   Acts as principal intracellular electrolyte
     D.   Protects bone structures against degeneration
     ANSWER: B   p. 381

32.   All of the following are characteristics of chloride in nutrition EXCEPT

K   A.   deficiencies are extremely rare.
     B.   intake is related, in large part, to sodium intake.
     C.   the RDA has recently been set at 10 mg/kg body weight.
     D.   it is necessary for maintaining electrolyte balance of body fluids.
     ANSWER: C   p. 381

33.   Which of the following is the primary function of potassium?

K   A.   Participates in wound healing
     B.   Helps maintain gastric acidity
     C.   Acts as principal intracellular electrolyte
     D.   Protects bone structures against degeneration
     ANSWER: C   p. 382

34.   Which of the following is an early symptom of potassium deficiency?

K   A.   Extreme thirst
     B.   Muscle weakness
     C.   Profound sweating
     D.   Lowered blood pressure
     ANSWER: B   p. 382

35.   Which of the following is NOT a common food source of potassium?

AP   A.   Cheese
     B.   Potatoes
     C.   Dried fruits
     D.   Orange juice
     ANSWER: A   p. 382

36.   Which of the following groups of healthy people risk potassium depletion?

AP   A.   Athletes who are body-builders
     B.   Construction workers in cold climates
     C.   People who ingest fewer than 800 kcalories/day
     D.   People who consume insufficient amounts of salted foods
     ANSWER: C   p. 382

Chapter 11 The Body Fluids and the Major Minerals

37. All of the following are features of potassium in nutrition EXCEPT

AP A. intakes in the U.S. show wide variation.
    B. per serving size, legumes are a rich source.
    C. foods lose large amounts during processing.
    D. per serving size, bananas are a rich source.
    ANSWER: D   p. 382

38. Which of the following is NOT a feature of potassium deficiency?

K   A. Prolonged vomiting and dehydration are known to lead to deficiencies
    B. Deficiencies occur due to excessive losses rather than to insufficient intakes
    C. Chronic use of certain diuretics and laxatives are known to lead to deficiencies
    D. Dietary deficiencies are common due to availability of only a few good food sources
    ANSWER: D   p. 382

39. Almost all (99%) of the calcium in the body is used to

AP A. provide energy for cells.
    B. provide rigidity for the bones and teeth.
    C. regulate the transmission of nerve impulses.
    D. maintain the blood level of calcium within very narrow limits.
    ANSWER: B   p. 384

40. Which of the following regulates the level of calcium in the blood?

K   A. Glucagon and epinephrine
    B. Dietary intake of calcium
    C. Parathormone and calcitonin
    D. Dietary intake of phosphorus
    ANSWER: C   p. 384

41. Which of the following is a feature of potassium supplements?

AP A. Can cause toxicity
    B. Should always be taken with diuretics
    C. Necessary in treatment of low blood pressure
    D. Absorption of the mineral decreases markedly as intake increases
    ANSWER: A   p. 384

42. Calcium absorption is facilitated by the presence of

K   A. fiber.
    B. lactose.
    C. phytic acid.
    D. oxalic acid.
    ANSWER: B   p. 385

Chapter 11 The Body Fluids and the Major Minerals   9

43. Which of the following represents the LEAST likely cause for an abnormal blood calcium level?

AP A. Diseases of the liver
    B. Diseases of the kidney
    C. Insufficient dietary intake
    D. Altered secretion of parathormone
    ANSWER: C   p. 385

44. How much calcium would be typically absorbed by a normal adult with a calcium intake of 1,000 mg?

AP A. 100 mg
    B. 300 mg
    C. 600 mg
    D. 950 mg
    ANSWER: B   p. 385

45. All of the following are known to enhance calcium absorption from the GI tract EXCEPT

K   A. lactose.
    B. pregnancy.
    C. oxalic acid.
    D. stomach acid.
    ANSWER: C   p. 385

46. All of the following dietary substances are known to adversely affect calcium balance EXCEPT

K   A. high fiber diet.
    B. lactose in the diet.
    C. phytic acid in the diet.
    D. phosphorus in the diet at a level 3 times that of calcium.
    ANSWER: B   p. 385

47. All of the following characteristics are shared by calcium and magnesium EXCEPT

AP A. both are involved in bone formation.
    B. both are involved in blood clotting.
    C. both are found in abundance in dairy products.
    D. either may result in tetany when blood levels become abnormally low.
    ANSWER: C   p. 385,392

10   Chapter 11   The Body Fluids and the Major Minerals

48.   As far as is known, which of the following is NOT a process that involves calcium?

K   A.   pH regulation
      B.   Blood clotting
      C.   Nerve transmission
      D.   Maintenance of heart beat
      ANSWER: A   p. 387

49.   What is the RDA for calcium for adults beyond 25 years of age?

K   A.   500 mg
      B.   800 mg
      C.   1000 mg
      D.   1200 mg
      ANSWER: B   p. 387

50.   Which of the following is a good source of dietary calcium?

K   A.   Fruits
      B.   Breads
      C.   Enriched grains
      D.   Green vegetables
      ANSWER: D   p. 388

51.   Which of the following vegetable greens shows the lowest bioavailability of calcium?

K   A.   Kale
      B.   Spinach
      C.   Broccoli
      D.   Mustard greens
      ANSWER: B   p. 389

52.   Which of the following is a feature of osteoporosis?

K   A.   It is most common in men over 45 years of age
      B.   It has virtually no effect on blood calcium levels
      C.   It results from short-term deprivation of dietary calcium
      D.   It causes significant alterations in the blood levels of parathormone and calcitonin
      ANSWER: B   p. 390

53.   Which of the following is a feature of phosphorus?

K   A.   Involved in energy exchange
      B.   Absorption efficiency is about 95%
      C.   Ranks lowest among the minerals in amount present in the body
      D.   Ranks highest among the minerals in amount present in the body
      ANSWER: A   p. 391

Chapter 11 The Body Fluids and the Major Minerals 11

54. Which of the following minerals is involved in the transportation of lipids through the body's lymph and blood systems?

K
    A. Iron
    B. Sodium
    C. Calcium
    D. Phosphorus
    ANSWER: D   p. 391

55. Which of the following minerals is LEAST likely to be deficient in anyone's diet?

AP
    A. Iron
    B. Calcium
    C. Chromium
    D. Phosphorus
    ANSWER: D   p. 391

56. What is hydroxyapatite?

K
    A. Abnormal cellular structures seen in osteoporosis
    B. The calcium-rich crystalline structure of teeth and bones
    C. A calcium regulatory hormone secreted from the trabeculae region of bone
    D. A compound in plant foods that binds to calcium and phosphorus and inhibits absorption
    ANSWER: B   p. 391

57. Which of the following is a function of magnesium?

K
    A. Transport of oxygen
    B. Prevention of anemia
    C. Production of thyroid hormone
    D. Catalyst in energy metabolism
    ANSWER: D   p. 392

58. Where is the majority of the body's magnesium found?

K
    A. Bones
    B. Teeth
    C. Fatty tissue
    D. Cells of soft tissue
    ANSWER: A   p. 392

59. On a per kcalorie basis, which of the following are the best sources of magnesium?

AP
    A. Meats
    B. Fruits
    C. Breads
    D. Vegetables
    ANSWER: D   p. 392

Chapter 11 The Body Fluids and the Major Minerals

60. Sulfur is present in practically all

K   A. vitamins.
      B. proteins.
      C. fatty acids.
      D. carbohydrates.
      ANSWER: B   p. 394

61. Some amino acids can link to each other by bridges made of

K   A. sulfur.
      B. calcium.
      C. chloride.
      D. magnesium.
      ANSWER: A   p. 394

62. Which of the following does NOT have a high sulfur content?

AP   A. Skin
      B. Hair
      C. Teeth
      D. Nails
      ANSWER: C   p. 394

63. What is the major source of dietary sulfur?

K   A. Fats
      B. Protein
      C. Mineral salts
      D. Carbohydrates
      ANSWER: B   p. 394

64. Which of the following is a function of bone trabeculae?

K   A. Storage site for calcium
      B. Storage site for vitamin D
      C. Involved in synthesis of vitamin D
      D. Involved in synthesis of calcitonin
      ANSWER: A   p. 396

Essay Questions

369   65. Identify some of the common substances found in foods that combine with minerals to form complexes the body cannot absorb. In what foods are they found and what minerals are affected?

Chapter 11 The Body Fluids and the Major Minerals   13

369   66. Compare and contrast the major functions of minerals and vitamins.

370,374   67. Describe the role of the kidneys in regulating acid-base balance.

379   68. What are the major sources of sodium in the diet of the U.S. population?

384   69. What are the functions of parathormone, calcitonin, and vitamin D in the regulation of calcium metabolism?

387   70. What is calmodulin and how does it function to deliver messages?

388   71. List 5 milk substitutes that are relatively low in lactose.

400-403   72. Discuss major risk factors in the development of osteoporosis. What population groups are most at risk? What dietary measures are advocated for high risk groups?

CHAPTER 12
THE TRACE MINERALS

MULTIPLE CHOICE

1. Which of the following is a feature of iron nutrition?

   K   A. Most people absorb about 50-60% of dietary iron
       B. Many people do not eat enough iron-containing foods
       C. Iron plays an important role in the synthesis of thyroxine
       D. Iron deficiency represents the second most common mineral deficiency in the U.S.
   ANSWER: B   p. 406-410

2. Which of the following is a characteristic of the trace minerals?

   K   A. Transported primarily by red blood cells
       B. Found in very small quantities in the body
       C. Absorbed from the intestines to the lymph circulation
       D. Absorbed from the intestine with greater efficiencies than the macro minerals
   ANSWER: B   p. 406

3. What iron-containing compound carries oxygen in the bloodstream?

   K   A. Ferritin
       B. Myoglobin
       C. Hemoglobin
       D. Transferrin
   ANSWER: C   p. 406

1

2   Chapter 12   The Trace Minerals

4. What is the oxygen carrying protein of muscle cells?

K   A.   Myoglobin
     B.   Hemoglobin
     C.   Cytochrome
     D.   Transferrin
     ANSWER: A   p. 406

5. Which of the following is a characteristic of iron transport?

K   A.   Albumin is the major iron transport protein in the blood
     B.   Transferrin in the blood carries iron to the bone marrow
     C.   Hemochromatosis results from inability to absorb and transport iron
     D.   Ferritin functions by transporting iron from the spleen to the bone marrow
     ANSWER: B   p. 407-408

6. Which of the following is a protein that carries iron through the circulation to the tissues?

K   A.   Albumin
     B.   Hemosiderin
     C.   Transferrin
     D.   Metallothionein
     ANSWER: C   p. 407-408

7. Which of the following compounds provides a major storage reservoir for iron?

K   A.   Ferritin
     B.   Myoglobin
     C.   Hemoglobin
     D.   Transferrin
     ANSWER: A   p. 408

8. What is the average lifespan of red blood cells?

K   A.   Two weeks
     B.   One month
     C.   Four months
     D.   Six months
     ANSWER: C   p. 408

9. Under normal circumstances, what is the average percentage of dietary iron that is absorbed?

K   A.   2 to 5
     B.   10 to 15
     C.   50 to 60
     D.   90 to 95
     ANSWER: B   p. 408

10. Which of the following is a characteristic of iron utilization?

K
   A. Most of the body's iron is recycled
   B. The chief storage site for iron is the intestinal epithelium
   C. Iron from supplements is better absorbed than iron from foods
   D. Iron from non-heme food sources is absorbed better than from heme food sources
ANSWER: A   p. 408

11. How would the body respond typically to loss of blood from hemorrhage?

AP
   A. More transferrin is produced to allow absorption and transport of more iron
   B. The average life of the red blood cell is increased in order to allow better tissue oxygenation
   C. Less iron storage proteins are produced which increases the amount of iron available for synthesis of new red blood cells
   D. The liver and muscles release their supply of stored red blood cells which compensates, in part, for the decrease in red blood cell concentration of the circulation
ANSWER: A   p. 408

12. Low levels of blood hemoglobin usually indicate a deficiency of

AP
   A. zinc.
   B. iron.
   C. copper.
   D. manganese.
ANSWER: B   p. 409

13. The most common tests to diagnose iron deficiency include all of the following measures EXCEPT

AP
   A. size of red blood cells.
   B. number of red blood cells.
   C. DNA content of red blood cells.
   D. hemoglobin content of red blood cells.
ANSWER: C   p. 409

14. Which of the following symptoms would ordinarily NOT be found in individuals with iron-deficiency anemia?

AP
   A. Fatigue
   B. Headaches
   C. Concave nails
   D. Diminished sense of smell
ANSWER: D   p. 409-419

4   Chapter 12   The Trace Minerals

15. Which of the following population groups is LEAST susceptible to iron deficiency anemia?

AP A. Older infants
    B. Children 2-10 years of age
    C. Men 20-45 years of age
    D. Women of childbearing age
    ANSWER: C   p. 410

16. What type of anemia results from iron deficiency?

K   A. Hemolytic
    B. Megaloblastic
    C. Hypochromic microcytic
    D. Hyperchromic macrocytic
    ANSWER: C   p. 410

17. What percent of the world's population is thought to be affected by iron-deficiency anemia?

K   A. 2
    B. 4
    C. 10
    D. 15
    ANSWER: D   p. 410

18. What is the name given to the ingestion of nonnutritive substances?

K   A. Pica
    B. Tetany
    C. Goiter
    D. Hemosiderosis
    ANSWER: A   p. 411

19. What is the major cause of iron deficiency?

K   A. Blood loss
    B. Poor nutrition
    C. Hereditary defect
    D. Parasitic infections of the GI tract
    ANSWER: B   411

20. Poor tolerance to cold is a recently recognized symptom of which of the following?

K   A. Iron toxicity
    B. Zinc toxicity
    C. Iron deficiency
    D. Zinc deficiency
    ANSWER: C   p. 411

21. Approximately how much iron would be provided by a balanced diet supplying 2000 kcalories?

AP
   A.   3 mg
   B.   6 mg
   C.   12 mg
   D.   30 mg
ANSWER: C   p. 412

22. What is the RDA for iron for females 11-50 years old?

K
   A.   8 mg
   B.   10 mg
   C.   15 mg
   D.   22 mg
ANSWER: C   p. 412

23. Which of the following describes one aspect of iron toxicity?

K
   A.   Among men in the United States, it is more common than iron-deficiency anemia
   B.   In adults, the consumption of alcohol is somewhat protective against absorption of excess iron
   C.   In most people with this disorder, infections are rare because bacteria are killed by excess iron in the blood
   D.   It is usually caused by a virus that attacks the intestinal mucosal cells leading to unregulated and excessive iron absorption
ANSWER: A   p. 412

24. Which of the following foods should be particularly limited in the diet of individuals with hemochromatosis?

AP
   A.   Dairy products
   B.   Fluoridated water
   C.   Carbonated beverages
   D.   Iron-fortified cereals
ANSWER: D   p. 412

25. Iron deficiency in children is likely to result from a diet that overemphasizes

AP
   A.   milk.
   B.   cereals.
   C.   vegetables.
   D.   dried beans.
ANSWER: A   p. 413

Chapter 12 The Trace Minerals

26. In the United States, iron is currently added to which of the following foods?

K
   A. Milk and cheese
   B. Breads and cereals
   C. Peanut butter and jellies
   D. Orange juice and tomato juice
   ANSWER: B   p. 413

27. A child diagnosed with iron-deficiency anemia would most likely benefit from increasing the consumption of which of the following foods?

AP
   A. Milk
   B. Red meat
   C. Fresh fruits
   D. Yellow vegetables
   ANSWER: B   p. 413

28. Which of the following is a feature of iron absorption?

K
   A. It is lower in people with iron toxicity
   B. It is higher in people with severe iron deficiency
   C. It is lower when iron is in the form of heme rather than non-heme
   D. It is higher in adults than children due to more mature intestinal function
   ANSWER: B   p. 413-415

29. If a normal, healthy young adult woman loses an average of 2 mg/day of iron from the body, approximately how much should she consume from the diet to remain in iron balance?

AP
   A. 2 mg/day
   B. 4 mg/day
   C. 10 mg/day
   D. 20 mg/day
   ANSWER: D   p. 413

30. Which of the following characteristics is shared by zinc and iron?

AP
   A. Good food sources include dairy products
   B. Proteins in the blood are needed for their transport
   C. Severe deficiencies lead to delay in the onset of puberty
   D. Doses of 10 times the RDA are known to cause death in children
   ANSWER: B   413,421

31. Which of the following foods provides iron in the most absorbable form?

AP
   A. Rice
   B. Spinach
   C. Hamburger
   D. Iron-fortified baby cereal
   ANSWER: C   p. 415

Chapter 12   The Trace Minerals   7

32. Which of the following nutrients enhances iron absorption from the intestinal tract?

K
   A. Biotin
   B. Calcium
   C. Vitamin D
   D. Vitamin C
   ANSWER: D   p. 415

33. All of the following are known to reduce the absorption of iron EXCEPT

K
   A. tea.
   B. coffee.
   C. sugars.
   D. phytates.
   ANSWER: C   p. 415

34. Absorption of iron from supplements is improved by taking them with

AP
   A. tea.
   B. meat.
   C. milk.
   D. whole grain bread.
   ANSWER: B   p. 415

35. Which of the following is known to enhance iron absorption?

K
   A. Tea
   B. Coffee
   C. Foods containing vitamin C
   D. Foods containing vitamin E
   ANSWER: C   p. 415

36. All of the following factors are known to reduce the absorption of iron EXCEPT

K
   A. phytates.
   B. MPF factor.
   C. tannic acid in tea.
   D. EDTA in food additives.
   ANSWER: B   p. 415

37. All of the following factors are known to enhance the absorption of iron EXCEPT

K
   A. MPF factor.
   B. stomach acid.
   C. ascorbic acid.
   D. calcium from milk.
   ANSWER: D   p. 415

8   Chapter 12   The Trace Minerals

38. When eaten in the same meal, which of the following foods enhances the absorption of iron in legumes?

AP
A. Nuts
B. Fiber
C. Oranges
D. Whole-grain breads
ANSWER: C   p. 415

39. Which of the following is NOT a source of iron in the diet?

K
A. Red meat
B. Iron cookware
C. Iron-fortified bread
D. EDTA food additives
ANSWER: D   p. 415-416

40. All of the following characteristics are shared by iron and zinc EXCEPT

K
A. absorption is inhibited by fiber.
B. absorption is inhibited by cow's milk.
C. transport in the blood is primarily by albumin.
D. absorption rises with increased needs of the body.
ANSWER: C   p. 415,421

41. If cow's milk is found to contain unusually high levels of iodine, what is the most likely explanation?

AP
A. Storage of milk in galvanized tanks
B. Grazing of cows on high iodine soils
C. Addition of fortified salt at the milk processing plant
D. Exposure of cows to iodide-containing medications and disinfectants
ANSWER: D   p. 415

42. When calculating the amount of iron that can be absorbed from a meal, all of the following factors are considered EXCEPT

K
A. fiber content.
B. heme iron content.
C. vitamin C content.
D. nonheme iron content.
ANSWER: A   p. 416

Chapter 12   The Trace Minerals   9

43. Which of the following individuals would most likely need an iron supplement?

AP
A. One-year old
B. Elderly female
C. Pregnant female
D. Adolescent female
ANSWER: C   p. 416

44. Which of the following is the most effective strategy and least costly for preventing an iron deficiency?

AP
A. Consume iron supplements at a level 2-3 times the RDA
B. Switch to iron cooking utensils and eat 4 servings of red meat daily
C. Eat small amounts of citrus products and increase intake of low fat milk
D. Eat small quantities of meat, fish and poultry frequently together with liberal amounts of vegetables and legumes
ANSWER: D   p. 417

45. What is the name of the binding protein for zinc?

K
A. Ligand
B. Ferritin
C. Hemosiderin
D. Metallothionein
ANSWER: D   p. 418

46. What tissue contains the greatest quantity of the body's zinc?

K
A. Bone
B. Liver
C. Muscle
D. Prostate gland
ANSWER: C   p. 418

47. In a healthy individual who suddenly fails to obtain adequate dietary zinc, which of the following signs is observed first?

AP
A. Decrease in body weight
B. Decrease in prostate gland zinc
C. Decrease in blood level of zinc
D. Decrease in ability to taste salt
ANSWER: C   p. 418

10   Chapter 12   The Trace Minerals

48. Zinc is known to play an important role in all of the following functions EXCEPT

AP
   A. wound healing.
   B. production of sperm.
   C. synthesis of retinal.
   D. oxidation of polyunsaturated fatty acids.
   ANSWER: D   p. 418

49. Which of the following minerals undergoes enteropancreatic circulation during normal metabolism?

K
   A. Iron
   B. Zinc
   C. Copper
   D. Fluoride
   ANSWER: B   p. 418

50. Which of the following characteristics are shared by iron and zinc?

AP
   A. Neither functions in the maintenance of blood glucose
   B. Neither is circulated from the pancreas to the intestines and back to the pancreas
   C. Both are absorbed into intestinal epithelial cells but may then be lost by normal villus cell renewal processes
   D. Both are absorbed into intestinal mucosal cells and bound to metallothionein for transport first to the liver
   ANSWER: C   p. 418

51. Which of the following is thought to regulate the absorption of zinc?

K
   A. Metallothionein in the intestinal cells
   B. Iron releasing enzymes in the intestinal mucosa
   C. Pancreatic juice containing iron-absorption enhancers
   D. Bile acids which complex with iron and promote its absorption
   ANSWER: A   p. 419

52. Which of the following is a known side effect of prolonged ingestion of excessive amounts of zinc supplements?

AP
   A. Iron toxicity due to increased ferritin synthesis
   B. Zinc salt deposits in soft tissues such as the heart and kidneys
   C. Copper deficiency due to interference with copper absorption
   D. Mineral binding protein deficiency due to a decrease in metallothionein production
   ANSWER: C   p. 419,421

Chapter 12   The Trace Minerals   11

53. Which of the following is a binder found in whole-grain cereals that hinders the absorption of zinc?

K   A.   Iron
      B.   EDTA
      C.   Calcium
      D.   Phytic acid
      ANSWER: D   p. 420

54. What dietary ratio of iron to zinc inhibits zinc absorption?

K   A.   0.5 to 1
      B.   1 to 1
      C.   Less than 2 to 1
      D.   Greater than 2 to 1
      ANSWER: D   p. 420

55. What is the chief transport substance for zinc in the circulation?

K   A.   Albumin
      B.   Metallothionein
      C.   Carbonic anhydrase
      D.   High-density lipoproteins
      ANSWER: A   p. 420

56. Which of the following would be the minimum amount of dietary iron known to impair zinc absorption in an individual with a zinc intake of 15 mg?

AP   A.   5 mg
       B.   15 mg
       C.   32 mg
       D.   60 mg
       ANSWER: C   p. 420

57. All of the following are known to result from excessive zinc intake EXCEPT

K   A.   galvanized liver and kidneys.
      B.   inhibition of iron absorption.
      C.   inhibition of copper absorption.
      D.   decreases in high-density lipoproteins.
      ANSWER: A   p. 420-421

12 Chapter 12 The Trace Minerals

58. According to the Committee on Dietary Allowances, what is the bioavailability of dietary zinc?

K   A. 20%
      B. 35%
      C. 50%
      D. 70%
      ANSWER: A   p. 421

59. Deficiency of which of the following minerals is associated with retarded growth and sexual development in children?

K   A. Zinc
      B. Iron
      C. Iodine
      D. Chromium
      ANSWER: A   p. 421

60. Conditions associated with zinc deficiency include all of the following EXCEPT

K   A. altered taste.
      B. kidney failure.
      C. abnormal dark vision.
      D. poor healing of wounds.
      ANSWER: B   p. 421-422

61. Which of the following represents the most reliable dietary source of zinc?

K   A. Milk
      B. Fiber
      C. Fruits
      D. Meat and whole-grain cereals
      ANSWER: D   p. 421

62. Zinc is highest in foods that also contain a high amount of

AP   A. fat.
      B. fiber.
      C. protein.
      D. carbohydrate.
      ANSWER: C   p. 421

63. All of the following are symptoms of zinc deficiency EXCEPT

K   A. anemia.
      B. altered taste acuity.
      C. impaired dark vision.
      D. increased susceptibility to infection.
      ANSWER: A   p. 421

64. What mineral may be found in toxic amounts in orange juice that is stored in a galvanized container?

AP   A. Iron
B. Zinc
C. Copper
D. Iodine
ANSWER: B   p. 421

65. Which of the following may result from iodine deficiency?

K   A. Gout
B. Goiter
C. Anemia
D. Hypertension
ANSWER: B   p. 424

66. What mineral is critical to the synthesis of thyroxin?

K   A. Iron
B. Copper
C. Iodine
D. Magnesium
ANSWER: C   p. 424

67. A woman with a severe iodine deficiency during pregnancy may have a child who develops

AP   A. anemia.
B. rickets.
C. cretinism.
D. allergies.
ANSWER: C   p. 424

68. What is the response of the pituitary gland of a person who is deficient in iodine?

AP   A. Increase in its size to trap more iodine
B. Increase in its size to trap more thyroxine
C. Increased release of thyroid-stimulating hormone
D. Decreased release of thyroid-stimulating hormone
ANSWER: C   p. 424

69. What nutrient deficiency during pregnancy may give rise to a child with cretinism?

AP   A. Iodine
B. Copper
C. Chromium
D. Molybdenum
ANSWER: A   p. 424

14   Chapter 12   The Trace Minerals

70. Under which of the following conditions are supplements of zinc known to be beneficial?

AP A. In the treatment of colds
    B. In the treatment of Menkes' syndrome
    C. In the treatment of toxicity from certain other metals
    D. In the treatment of slow growth syndrome in U.S. children
    ANSWER: C   p. 424

71. Which of the following is a feature of iodide utilization?

K   A. It is an integral part of pituitary thyroid stimulating hormone
    B. Ingestion of plants of the cabbage family stimulates iodide uptake
    C. A deficiency or a toxicity leads to enlargement of the thyroid gland
    D. The amount in foods is unrelated to the amount of iodine present in the soil
    ANSWER: C   p. 424-425

72. A person ingesting large amounts of thyroid antagonist substances is at high risk of developing

AP A. toxic goiter.
    B. simple goiter.
    C. high blood T_3 levels.
    D. high blood thyroxin levels.
    ANSWER: A   p. 424

73. Which of the following foods are known to contain goitrogens?

AP A. Shellfish
    B. Whole grains
    C. Cauliflower and broccoli
    D. Strawberries and raspberries
    ANSWER: C   p. 424

74. Which of the following is the richest source of iodine?

AP A. Corn
    B. Salmon
    C. Lake trout
    D. Orange juice
    ANSWER: B   p. 425

75. Which of the following could result from an excessive intake of iodine?

AP A. Goiter
    B. Skin rashes
    C. Dehydration
    D. Thyroid gland enlargement
    ANSWER: D   p. 425

76. Which of the following would be the most appropriate food source of iodide for a person who lives around the Great Lakes area?

AP A. Fresh water fish
    B. Iodized table salt
    C. Locally grown produce
    D. Plants of the cabbage family
    ANSWER: B   p. 425

77. Which of the following minerals is a cofactor in the formation of hemoglobin?

K   A. Iodine
    B. Copper
    C. Sodium
    D. Calcium
    ANSWER: B   p. 426

78. All of the following conditions are known to lead to copper deficiency EXCEPT

K   A. zinc excess.
    B. iodide deficiency.
    C. protein deficiency.
    D. iron-deficiency anemia.
    ANSWER: B   p. 426

79. Which of the following minerals functions primarily in reactions that consume oxygen?

K   A. Zinc
    B. Copper
    C. Chromium
    D. Molybdenum
    ANSWER: B   p. 426

80. Which of the following characteristics are shared by copper and fluoride?

AP A. Both serve as cofactors for a number of enzymes
    B. Neither is involved in the integrity of bones and teeth
    C. Both are obtained from drinking water in significant amounts
    D. Neither is known to be toxic at intakes of 10 times the estimated safe and adequate dietary intake
    ANSWER: C   p. 426

81. Which of the following does NOT have an RDA?

K   A. Iron
    B. Zinc
    C. Iodine
    D. Copper
    ANSWER: D   p. 427

Chapter 12 The Trace Minerals

82. Which of the following represents a significant source of copper in the U.S. diet?

K
- A. Tomatoes
- B. Dairy products
- C. Drinking water
- D. Vegetables of the cabbage family

ANSWER: C   p. 427

83. Characteristics of manganese in nutrition include all of the following EXCEPT

K
- A. good sources are plant foods.
- B. deficiencies are seen primarily in the elderly.
- C. absorption is inhibited by calcium supplements.
- D. toxicity is more common from environmental contamination than from the diet.

ANSWER: B   p. 427

84. Which of the following mechanisms explains why fluoride is effective in controlling tooth decay?

AP
- A. Helps form decay-resistant enamel
- B. Helps regulate calcium levels in saliva
- C. Inhibits growth of decay-producing bacteria
- D. Changes the pH of the mouth, inhibiting bacterial growth

ANSWER: A   p. 428

85. What is the most reliable source of dietary fluoride?

K
- A. Public water
- B. Dark green vegetables
- C. Milk and milk products
- D. Meats and whole-grain cereals

ANSWER: A   p. 428

86. Which of the following is known to cause discolored enamel of the teeth?

K
- A. Excessive fluoride in the water
- B. Excessive intake of simple sugars
- C. Insufficient fluoride in the water
- D. Inability of the body to absorb fluoride

ANSWER: A   p. 428

87. Fluoride deficiency is best known to lead to

K
- A. dental decay.
- B. osteoporosis.
- C. discoloration of teeth.
- D. nutritional muscular dystrophy.

ANSWER: A   p. 428

Chapter 12 The Trace Minerals   17

88. How much drinking water must be consumed to meet the recommended intake of fluoride if the water is fluoridated at 1 ppm?

AP
- A. 1 liter
- B. 2 liters
- C. 3 liters
- D. 4 liters

ANSWER: A   p. 428

89. What is the primary mechanism associated with the role of fluoride in prevention of dental caries?

K
- A. Fluoride increases calcium absorption which increases crystal formation of teeth
- B. Decay is inhibited due to neutralization of organic acids produced by bacteria on the teeth
- C. Decay is reduced due to the inhibitory effects of fluoride on growth of bacteria on the teeth
- D. Fluoride becomes incorporated into the crystalline structure of teeth which inhibits tooth decay

ANSWER: D   p. 428

90. A biologically important chromium compound is

K
- A. insulin tolerance factor.
- B. glucose tolerance factor.
- C. chromium insulin factor.
- D. glucose chromium factor.

ANSWER: B   p. 429

91. One of the chief functions of chromium is in the metabolism of

K
- A. iron.
- B. proteins.
- C. carbohydrates.
- D. metallothionein.

ANSWER: C   p. 429

92. Which of the following is known to accelerate excretion of chromium from the body?

AP
- A. High intake of liver
- B. High intakes of cheeses
- C. High intake of refined simple sugars
- D. High intake of whole-grain products containing fiber

ANSWER: C   p. 429

18   Chapter 12   The Trace Minerals

93. Which of the following is an important function of selenium?

K   A. Helps blood to clot
     B. Stabilizes the alcohol content of beer
     C. Acts as a cross-linking agent in collagen
     D. Inhibits the oxidation of polyunsaturated fatty acids
     ANSWER: D   p. 430

94. Which of the following population groups has been shown to benefit from chromium supplementation?

AP   A. Infants with hemolytic anemia
      B. Elderly with mild osteoporosis
      C. Children with moderate lead poisoning
      D. People with blood glucose abnormalities
      ANSWER: D   p. 430

95. All of the following are characteristics of chromium in nutrition EXCEPT

K   A. good food sources include whole grains, nuts, and cheeses.
     B. marginal intakes are most likely to be found in the elderly.
     C. only about 10% of U.S. adults ingest the suggested minimum intake.
     D. supplements are without benefit in people with abnormalities of blood glucose.
     ANSWER: D   p. 430

96. Which of the following nutrients has functions similar to those of vitamin E?

AP   A. Iron
      B. Selenium
      C. Chromium
      D. Molybdenum
      ANSWER: B   p. 430

97. Which of the following is a property of selenium in nutrition?

K   A. It participates in the functioning of insulin
     B. Significant food sources include dairy and unprocessed vegetables
     C. Severe deficiency is associated with heart disease in children in China
     D. It has no RDA but the estimated safe and adequate dietary intake is only 2-3 µg/day
     ANSWER: C   p. 430-431

98. Which of the following has been found to result from excessive intakes of molybdenum?

AP   A. Goiter
      B. Diabetes
      C. Goutlike symptoms
      D. Atherosclerotic lesions
      ANSWER: C   p. 431

Chapter 12   The Trace Minerals   19

99.   Which of the following is a characteristic of the mineral molybdenum?

K
A.   Deficiency symptoms in animals and people are unknown
B.   Participates as a coenzyme in the synthesis of nucleic acids
C.   Unusually poor food sources are milk and leafy green vegetables
D.   Toxicity symptoms in human beings include damage to red blood cells
ANSWER: B   p. 431

100.   What mineral is part of vitamin B_{12}?

K
A.   Copper
B.   Cobalt
C.   Nickel
D.   Vanadium
ANSWER: B   p. 432

101.   Which of the following trace minerals is known to be involved in bone calcification?

K
A.   Tin
B.   Cobalt
C.   Silicon
D.   Vanadium
ANSWER: C   p. 432

102.   Evidence to date in animals and/or human beings indicates that normal bone metabolism requires all of the following trace minerals EXCEPT

AP
A.   boron.
B.   silver.
C.   silicon.
D.   vanadium.
ANSWER: B   p. 432

103.   Which of the following elements is known to be essential for animals but not for human beings?

K
A.   Silicon
B.   Selenium
C.   Chromium
D.   Molybdenum
ANSWER: A   p. 432

104.   All of the following are common signs of lead toxicity EXCEPT

K
A.   diarrhea.
B.   lethargy.
C.   dermatitis.
D.   irritability.
ANSWER: C   p. 439

Chapter 12 The Trace Minerals

105. What is the most common cause of lead poisoning in infants?

K
- A. Maternal passage of lead to fetus
- B. Ingestion of flakes of lead-based wall paint
- C. Contaminated water used to make infant formula
- D. Preparation of infant formula in galvanized containers

ANSWER: C   p. 439

106. What is the most realistic advice for reducing lead exposure of a person whose home has lead-soldered plumbing?

AP
- A. Whenever possible boil the water to vaporize the lead and thus decrease the amount remaining in the water
- B. Since upon sitting overnight the lead in hot water pipes settles out, draw the drinking water from this source first
- C. Since the first water drawn from the tap each day is highest in lead, let the water run a few minutes before using it
- D. Add a small amount of citrus juice to the water to provide citric acid to complex with the lead and inhibit its absorption

ANSWER: C   p. 439

Essay Questions

406-434   107. Choose any 3 trace elements and discuss their major functions, deficiency symptoms, toxicity symptoms, and food sources.

412   108. Discuss the pros and cons of increasing the iron level of enriched bread in the United States.

413   109. Discuss factors that influence the bioavailability of dietary iron. What are good sources of bioavailable iron? What factors interfere with iron absorption?

Chapter 12   The Trace Minerals   21

413   110.   Explain the difference between heme and nonheme iron. How can the efficiency of absorption be increased for both types of iron?

415   111.   What factors are known to reduce or enhance iron absorption?

420   112.   What are the signs and symptoms of zinc deficiency? Which ones have similarities to other nutrient deficiencies?

425   113.   What factors account for the dramatic increase and subsequent decrease in iodine intakes observed in the United States since 1960?

426   114.   Explain how a deficiency of copper can lead to "iron deficiency" anemia.

428   115.   Discuss the essential nature of fluoride. What level in the diet is considered optimal? What are the effects of excess fluoride intake and how does toxicity usually occur?

Chapter 12 The Trace Minerals

429   116. Discuss the essential nature of chromium. What population groups are most likely to be deficient in chromium? List good food sources of chromium.

432   117. Make several general statements about trace elements in nutrition, including general food sources, deficiencies, toxicities, interactions, and the need for supplements.

438   118. Discuss the effects of lead exposure on health and human performance. What strategies are most effective at minimizing exposure to lead in the environment?

CHAPTER 13
FITNESS: PHYSICAL ACTIVITY, NUTRIENTS, AND BODY ADAPTATIONS

MULTIPLE CHOICE

1. All of the following are acceptable definitions of the term fitness EXCEPT

K   A.   the ability of the body to resist stress.
     B.   the ability of the body to perform physical activity without undue stress.
     C.   the ability to maintain a normal body composition and remain free of injury while performing strenuous physical tasks.
     D.   the ability to meet normal physical demands while maintaining an energy reserve sufficient to overcome an immediate challenge.
ANSWER: C   p. 443

2. Which of the following is generally NOT associated with a regular program of physical fitness?

K   A.   Lowering of bone density
     B.   Lowering of blood pressure
     C.   Lowering of blood cholesterol
     D.   Lowering of resting pulse rate
ANSWER: A   p. 443

2   Chapter 13   Fitness: Physical Activity, Nutrients, and Body Adaptations

3. Leading a sedentary life may lead to development of all of the following EXCEPT

AP
- A. obesity.
- B. cardiovascular disease.
- C. accelerated bone losses.
- D. increased aerobic capacity.

ANSWER: D   p. 443

4. The components of fitness include all of the following EXCEPT

K
- A. strength.
- B. flexibility.
- C. bone fragility.
- D. cardiovascular endurance.

ANSWER: C   p. 444

5. The belief that fitness develops in response to demand and diminishes in response to lack of demand is called the

K
- A. fitness principle.
- B. exercise principle.
- C. use-disuse principle.
- D. cardiovascular principle.

ANSWER: C   p. 444

6. Which of the following is a characteristic of the body's muscle fibers?

K
- A. Slow-twitch fibers are best suited to carry out aerobic work
- B. Fast-twitch fibers are best suited to carry out prolonged endurance exercise
- C. There are four major groups which work in pairs to initiate contraction and relaxation
- D. One fiber type has an unlimited potential to adapt in size whereas others are restricted in their development

ANSWER: A   p. 445

7. A muscle that increases size in response to use is an example of

AP
- A. atrophy.
- B. hypertrophy.
- C. muscular endurance.
- D. muscle engorgement.

ANSWER: B   p. 445

8. The effect of regular exercise on heart and lung function is known as

K
- A. muscle fitness.
- B. muscle endurance.
- C. cardiovascular endurance.
- D. cardiovascular conditioning.

ANSWER: D   p. 446

Chapter 13 Fitness: Physical Activity, Nutrients, and Body Adaptations

9. Which of the following is NOT derived directly from cardiovascular conditioning?

K   A. Slowed resting pulse
     B. Increased flexibility
     C. Increased breathing efficiency
     D. Increased blood volume and oxygen delivery
ANSWER: B   p. 446

10. With aerobic training, muscle cells show all of the following changes EXCEPT

AP   A. they hold more myoglobin.
      B. they become stronger in the lungs.
      C. they hold more fat oxidizing enzymes.
      D. they draw less oxygen due to increased efficiency of aerobic metabolism.
ANSWER: D   p. 446

11. According to the American College of Sports Medicine, which of the following would meet the exercise schedule to maintain an appropriate level of fitness?

K   A. 2 hours of aerobic exercise daily
     B. 1 hour of aerobic exercise 4 times a week
     C. 5 minutes of aerobic exercise 2 times a week
     D. 20 minutes of aerobic exercise 3 times a week
ANSWER: D   p. 447-448

12. An appropriate program for a person to achieve a well-rounded level of fitness includes all of the following EXCEPT

AP   A. aerobic work.
      B. daily workouts.
      C. nutritious diet.
      D. resistance work for muscle strength.
ANSWER: B   p. 448

13. What substance contains the chemical energy that drives muscle contraction?

K   A. ATP
     B. Glucose
     C. Fatty acids
     D. Phosphocreatine
ANSWER: A   p. 448

4   Chapter 13   Fitness: Physical Activity, Nutrients, and Body Adaptations

14. What high-energy compound acts as a reservoir of energy for the maintenance of a steady supply of ATP?

K A. Glycerol
  B. Glycogen
  C. Fatty acids
  D. Phosphocreatine
  ANSWER: D p. 449

15. During physical performance, what is the role of phosphocreatine?

K A. Removal of lactic acid
  B. Transfer of energy to make ATP
  C. Removal of nitrogen waste products
  D. Transfer of phosphate to muscle fiber
  ANSWER: B p. 449

16. What is the usual fate of muscle glycogen during exercise?

AP A. Utilized as a fuel within the muscle cell only
  B. Released into the bloodstream to provide fuel for brain cells
  C. Released into the bloodstream to replenish liver glycogen as needed
  D. Utilized to support lung and heart function under conditions of intense physical performance
  ANSWER: A p. 449

17. If muscle work is anaerobic, which of the following can NOT serve as fuel?

AP A. Fat
  B. Protein
  C. Carbohydrate
  ANSWER: A p. 450-451

18. During the first 20 minutes of moderate exercise, the body uses about

K A. 50% of the available fat.
  B. 10% of the available water.
  C. 90% of the available protein.
  D. 20% of the available glycogen.
  ANSWER: D p. 450-451

19. Which of the following is LEAST likely to affect the size of the body's glycogen stores?

AP A. Exercise regimen
  B. Fat content of the diet
  C. Type of supplements taken
  D. Carbohydrate content of the diet
  ANSWER: C p. 450

Chapter 13 Fitness: Physical Activity, Nutrients, and Body Adaptations

20. Which of the following diets has consistently allowed superior performance regarding physical endurance in athletes?

AP A. High fat diet
    B. High protein diet
    C. High carbohydrate diet
    D. Normal mixed diet with vitamin supplements
    ANSWER: C   p. 450

21. Which of the following activities depletes glycogen most quickly?

AP A. Jogging
    B. Walking
    C. Swimming
    D. Sprinting
    ANSWER: D   p. 450

22. How much time is usually needed in vigorous activity to cause depletion of glycogen reserves?

K   A. 1 hour
    B. 2 hours
    C. 3 hours
    D. 4 hours
    ANSWER: B   p. 450

23. What dietary nutrients are most effective at raising muscle glycogen concentrations?

AP A. Fats
    B. Proteins
    C. Carbohydrates
    D. Chromium and iron
    ANSWER: C   p. 450

24. What is the predominant fuel used by muscle cells during low or moderate intensity activity?

K   A. Fat
    B. Protein
    C. Glycogen
    D. Blood glucose
    ANSWER: A   p. 451

6   Chapter 13 Fitness: Physical Activity, Nutrients, and Body Adaptations

25. A tissue deprived of an oxygen supply during exercise would have an accumulation of

AP A. ATP.
    B. lactic acid.
    C. glucose-1-phosphate.
    D. TCA cycle intermediates.
    ANSWER: B   p. 451

26. Which of the following is a common product of anaerobic metabolism?

AP A. Lactic acid
    B. Phytic acid
    C. Phosphoric acid
    D. Hydrochloric acid
    ANSWER: A   p. 451

27. A deficit of oxygen built up by the body performing an exercise so demanding that the cardiovascular system could not deliver oxygen fast enough to support aerobic metabolism is called

AP A. oxygen debt.
    B. exercise fatigue.
    C. cardiovascular debt.
    D. lactic acid overload.
    ANSWER: A   p. 451

28. Which of the following substances increases in muscles during increasing exercise intensity?

AP A. ATP
    B. Glycogen
    C. Lactic acid
    D. Phosphocreatine
    ANSWER: C   p. 451

29. What is the Cori cycle?

K   A. The coordinated muscle contraction sequence of slow-twitch and fast-twitch fibers
    B. A process in the liver that regenerates glucose from lactic acid released by muscles
    C. An exercise machine that allows development of both aerobic and anaerobic capacities
    D. A group of enzymatic reactions to accelerate muscle glycogen repletion in the trained athlete
    ANSWER: B   p. 452

Chapter 13   Fitness: Physical Activity, Nutrients, and Body Adaptations

30. When a marathon runner experiences the phenomenon known as "hitting the wall," what nutrient is most likely depleted?

AP
   A.   Water
   B.   Protein
   C.   Glucose
   D.   Fatty acids
ANSWER: C   p. 452

31. What cellular organelles are responsible for producing ATP aerobically?

K
   A.   Ribosomes
   B.   Golgi bodies
   C.   Mitochondria
   D.   Cell membranes
ANSWER: C   p. 453

32. Which of the following is a property of conditioned muscles?

K
   A.   They can store more glycogen
   B.   They are more efficient at converting fat to glucose
   C.   They contain less mitochondria due to increased glucose utilization
   D.   They rely less on fat breakdown and more on glucose oxidation for energy
ANSWER: A   p. 453

33. Which of the following describes fat utilization during physical activity?

AP
   A.   Fat that is stored closest to the exercising muscle is oxidized first
   B.   Fat oxidization makes more of a contribution as the intensity of the exercise increases
   C.   Fat oxidation may continue at an above normal rate for some time after cessation of physical activity
   D.   Fat is burned in higher quantities during short high-intensity exercises than prolonged low-intensity exercises
ANSWER: C   p. 453

34. Which of the following is an effect of physical fitness on fat metabolism?

AP
   A.   Fatty acid release from adipose cells into muscle cells becomes more efficient
   B.   Fat oxidation by the whole body is higher throughout the day rather than only during exercise
   C.   Fatty acid energy release requires less oxygen on a per-kcal basis than does the use of glucose
   D.   Fat utilization slows down and liver glucose release rises in response to adaptation of the body's hormonal profile
ANSWER: B   p. 454

Chapter 13 Fitness: Physical Activity, Nutrients, and Body Adaptations

35. Athletes can safely add muscle tissue by

AP
   A. tripling protein intake.
   B. taking hormones duplicating those of puberty.
   C. putting a demand on muscles making them work harder.
   D. relying on protein for muscle fuel and decreasing intake of carbohydrates.
   ANSWER: C   p. 455

36. Which of the following is NOT known to modify the body's use of protein?

AP
   A. Diet
   B. The degree of training
   C. Exercise intensity and duration
   D. Vitamin supplements above the RDA
   ANSWER: D   p. 455-460

37. Which of the following is an effect of exercise on protein metabolism?

AP
   A. Protein use as a fuel is lowest in endurance athletes
   B. Protein synthesis is inhibited during exercise and for some time thereafter
   C. Protein use during physical performance is generally not related to carbohydrate content of the diet
   D. Protein synthesis is increased slightly during exercise but diminishes by a like amount to remain in balance
   ANSWER: B   p. 455

38. Which of the following is a role of diet in physical activity?

AP
   A. Diets high in fat lead to a fall in amino acid utilization for fuel
   B. Diets lacking in carbohydrates lead to increased amino acid utilization for fuel
   C. Deficiencies of vitamins have no effect on performance provided that all other nutrients are adequate
   D. Deficiencies of minerals have no effect on performance provided that all other nutrients are adequate
   ANSWER: B   p. 456-457

39. How do the protein needs for athletes compare with those for non-athletes?

AP
   A. Same
   B. Slightly lower
   C. Slightly higher
   D. Markedly higher
   ANSWER: C   p. 457

Chapter 13 Fitness: Physical Activity, Nutrients, and Body Adaptations

40. According to the American Dietetic Association, how many grams of protein per day does a 70 kg athlete need to consume?

AP
    A. 56
    B. 70
    C. 105
    D. 140
    ANSWER: B   p. 457

41. Which of the following describes the role of protein in the diet of athletes?

K
    A. The need for protein is highest in weight lifters and body builders
    B. The need for protein is higher in marathon runners than body builders
    C. The need for protein is best met by increasing the level to 20-25% of total energy content of the diet
    D. The need for protein in most athletes generally would NOT be sufficient from diets meeting energy requirements but containing only 10% of the energy as protein
    ANSWER: B   p. 457

42. Which of the following represents current knowledge of the role of vitamin and mineral supplements in physical performance?

K
    A. When taken right before an event, they have been shown to benefit performance
    B. Moderate amounts have been shown to improve the performance of most elite athletes
    C. They are needed in high amounts to meet the needs of athletes exposed to hot and humid weather conditions
    D. Supplements are not recommended since there is no difference in the RDA of physically active people compared with sedentary people
    ANSWER: D   p. 457-459

43. What nutrient is important in transport of oxygen in blood and in muscle tissue and energy transformation reactions?

AP
    A. Iron
    B. Calcium
    C. Thiamin
    D. Vitamin C
    ANSWER: A   p. 458

44. Which of the following nutrients is important for both collagen formation and hormone synthesis?

K
    A. Iron
    B. Zinc
    C. Calcium
    D. Vitamin C
    ANSWER: D   p. 458

10   Chapter 13 Fitness: Physical Activity, Nutrients, and Body Adaptations

45. What is the minimum amount of fluid that an athlete should drink for each pound of body weight lost during an activity?

AP
    A. One-half pound
    B. One pound
    C. Two pounds
    D. Three pounds
    ANSWER: B   p. 459

46. All of the following are characteristics of heat stroke EXCEPT

K
    A. it is rarely fatal.
    B. it is due, in part, to dehydration.
    C. it is caused by heat buildup in the body.
    D. its symptoms include headache, nausea, and mental changes.
    ANSWER: A   p. 459

47. A person engaged in physically active work in hot humid weather and who wears a rubber suit to promote weight loss is at high risk of experiencing

AP
    A. ketosis.
    B. hypothermia.
    C. heat stroke.
    D. overhydration.
    ANSWER: C   p. 459

48. What would be the minimum amount of body water loss necessary to bring about a reduction in work capacity of an average 165 pound individual?

AP
    A. 1½ liters
    B. 3½ liters
    C. 6 liters
    D. 10 liters
    ANSWER: A   p. 459

49. A person engaged in an endurance event has lost two liters of body water by sweating. What would be the approximate energy loss associated with the evaporation of the sweat?

AP
    A. 100 kcal
    B. 500 kcal
    C. 850 kcal
    D. 1200 kcal
    ANSWER: D   p. 459

Chapter 13 Fitness: Physical Activity, Nutrients, and Body Adaptations

50. Which of the following is a feature of water metabolism during exercise?

K   A. The maximum loss of fluid per hour of exercise is about 0.5 liters
     B. In cold weather, the need for water falls dramatically because the body does not sweat
     C. Sweat losses can exceed the capacity of the GI tract to absorb water resulting in some degree of dehydration
     D. Heavy sweating leads to a marked rise in the thirst sensation to stimulate water intake which delays the onset of dehydration

ANSWER: C   p. 459

51. All of the following are valid reasons for consuming sports drinks by athletes EXCEPT

K   A. they may provide a psychological advantage.
     B. they are better than water at preventing sodium depletion.
     C. they contain a source of fuel which may enhance performance in endurance events.
     D. they have a good taste which encourages their consumption and ensures adequate hydration.

ANSWER: B   p. 460

52. Which of the following would be the best choice for an athlete who needs to rehydrate?

AP A. "Sweat" replacers
     B. Salt tablets and tap water
     C. Diluted juice or cool water
     D. Water warmed to body temperature

ANSWER: C   p. 460

53. Which of the following is a benefit of glucose polymer sports drinks as compared with sugar containing drinks?

K   A. They supply more energy per gram of carbohydrate
     B. They require less digestion and therefore are absorbed faster into the circulation
     C. They attract less water in the GI tract and thus allow more water to remain in the circulation
     D. They are absorbed much more slowly and therefore provide a more even carbohydrate load to the body

ANSWER: C   p. 460

54. What is the recommended amount of water to meet the needs of athletes?

K   A. 1-1½ ml per kcal expended
     B. 5-7 ml per kcal expended
     C. 1,000 ml per hour of activity
     D. 1,500 ml per hour of activity

ANSWER: A   p. 460

12   Chapter 13 Fitness: Physical Activity, Nutrients, and Body Adaptations

55. All of the following are characteristics of electrolyte metabolism in sports <u>EXCEPT</u>

K   A. the trained athlete actually loses less electrolytes than the untrained person.
      B. replenishment of lost electrolytes in most athletes can be accomplished by ingesting a regular diet.
      C. sweating leads to significant losses of calcium, sulfur, and chromium which can be replaced by including skim milk in the diet.
      D. salt tablet supplements to replace electrolyte losses of sweat are known to cause fluid retention in the GI tract, irritation of the stomach, and vomiting.
ANSWER: C   p. 461

56. Which of the following is a known feature of iron nutrition in athletes?

K   A. Iron in sweat represents the major route of iron loss from the body
      B. Iron deficiency affects a higher percentage of male athletes than female athletes
      C. Sports anemia is successfully treated by increasing dietary iron to levels 2-3 times the RDA
      D. Iron losses in runners occur when blood cells are squashed by the impact of the foot on a hard surface
ANSWER: D   p. 462

57. Which of the following is a characteristic of athletic amenorrhea?

K   A. It increases the risk of bone loss
      B. It is defined, in part, by high estrogen concentration and fertility
      C. It develops more often in females who began training in their early thirties
      D. It has been shown to bear no association with body fat levels in all studies to date
ANSWER: A   p. 463

58. Weight standards for the general female population may not be appropriate for women athletes because

K   A. the bodies of some women athletes are denser than nonathletes and therefore contribute more weight.
      B. the bodies of some women athletes have less bone and muscle tissue and thus contribute less weight.
      C. the bodies of some women athletes can store very high levels of glycogen which can significantly alter body weight.
      D. the bodies of women athletes who practice fluid restriction to achieve a certain weight show erroneous body weight measurements.
ANSWER: A   p. 464

59. What nutrient is depleted most rapidly during physical exercise?

K   A. Iron
      B. Water
      C. Glucose
      D. Glycogen
ANSWER: B   p. 464

Chapter 13 Fitness: Physical Activity, Nutrients, and Body Adaptations

13

60. What type of meal is best for the most rapid repletion of glycogen stores after physical activity?

AP
    A. Mixed meal taken within 4 hours
    B. Mixed meal taken within 30 minutes
    C. High-carbohydrate meal taken within 2½ hours
    D. High-carbohydrate meal taken within 15 minutes
    ANSWER: D   p. 466

61. Which of the following should be a component of a healthy diet for athletes?

AP
    A. Salt tablets
    B. Protein powders
    C. Nutrient dense foods
    D. Vitamin and mineral supplements
    ANSWER: C   p. 467

62. What should be the composition of the last meal before an athletic event?

AP
    A. High-protein, providing 30 kcal per kg body weight
    B. Vegetable and fruit juices providing 100 to 200 kcal
    C. High-carbohydrate, low-fiber, providing 300 to 800 kcal
    D. High-fiber providing 200 to 300 kcal and liberal amounts of fluid which is beneficially retained by the fiber in the GI tract
    ANSWER: C   p. 468

63. Which of the following describes the usefulness of branched-chain amino acid supplements in physical performance?

K
    A. They may improve performance in events lasting under 1 hour
    B. They may improve performance in events lasting more than 3 hours
    C. They increase the rate of lactic acid production by muscle and therefore speed up the Cori cycle
    D. They significantly lower the rate of glucose utilization and thus delay the onset of carbohydrate depletion
    ANSWER: B   p. 471

64. An athlete who believes in soda loading as a means of improving performance would, right before the event, consume

AP
    A. caffeine tablets.
    B. sodium bicarbonate.
    C. a carbonated beverage.
    D. a lactose containing beverage.
    ANSWER: B   p. 472

14   Chapter 13 Fitness: Physical Activity, Nutrients, and Body Adaptations

65. Which of the following substances, when taken in moderation within two hours of the event, may improve athletic performance?

AP A. Niacin
    B. Protein
    C. Caffeine
    D. Vitamin C
    ANSWER: C   p. 472-473

Essay Questions

444   66.   List the diseases associated with a sedentary lifestyle.

449-457   67.   Discuss the use of protein, fat, and carbohydrate as fuels during low, moderate, and intense exercise.

459-462   68.   Discuss the need for water in maintaining physical performance. What are the symptoms of dehydration? What are the recommendations for ensuring that the body is well-hydrated prior to an athletic event?

462-463   69.   Compare and contrast the characteristics of sports anemia with the anemia that would be found in marathon runners.

Chapter 13 Fitness: Physical Activity, Nutrients, and Body Adaptations

464-467   70.   Describe an appropriate diet for athletic performance.

462-463   71.   Discuss the effects of athletic training on iron nutrition.

466   72.   Explain the training technique of glycogen loading. What are its advantages and disadvantages?

472   73.   Discuss factors that should be used to identify nutrition quackery in the physical fitness area.

472-473   74.   Discuss the use of baking soda and caffeine in athletic performance.

473-475   75.   Discuss the hazards of using anabolic steroids, human growth hormone, and blood doping as means of improving physical performance.

CHAPTER 14
CONSUMER CONCERNS ABOUT FOODS

MULTIPLE CHOICE

1. Which of the following appears first on the Food and Drug Administration's priority concerns for food safety?

   K   A.   Food additives
         B.   Pesticide residues
         C.   Food-borne illnesses
         D.   Environmental contaminants
   ANSWER: C   p. 478

2. Which of the following is NOT among the major food safety concerns of the FDA?

   K   A.   Pesticide residues
         B.   Proper food disposal
         C.   Environmental contaminants
         D.   Nutritional adequacy of foods
   ANSWER: B   p. 478

3. What is the leading cause of food contamination in the U.S.?

   K   A.   Naturally occurring toxicants
         B.   Food poisoning from microbes
         C.   Pesticide residues from farmers
         D.   Food additives from the food industry
   ANSWER: B   p. 478

Chapter 14 Consumer Concerns About Foods

4. What is the most common pathogenic microorganism in U.S. foods?

K
   A. Salmonella
   B. Campylobacter jejuni
   C. Staphylococcus aureas
   D. Clostridium perfringens
ANSWER: B   p. 478

5. Which of the following is the major food source for transmission of Campylobacter jejuni?

K
   A. Raw poultry
   B. Uncooked seafood
   C. Contaminated water
   D. Imported soft cheeses
ANSWER: A   p. 478

6. Which of the following is an example of food intoxication?

AP
   A. Addition of alkaline and acidic agents to foods
   B. Illness produced by acute overconsumption of high-fat foods
   C. Addition of alcohol containing beverages in the cooking of foods
   D. Illness produced from ingestion of food contaminated with natural toxins
ANSWER: D   p. 478

7. How often is a food-borne illness experienced by the average person?

K
   A. Once per week
   B. Once per month
   C. Once per year
   D. Once per 5 years
ANSWER: C   p. 478

8. What branch of the Department of Health and Human Services is responsible for monitoring food-borne illness?

K
   A. EPA
   B. FAO
   C. CDC
   D. WHO
ANSWER: C   p. 479

9. What is the largest single group of food additives?

K
   A. Flavoring agents
   B. Antimicrobial agents
   C. Artificial sweeteners
   D. Artificial coloring agents
ANSWER: A   p. 497

Chapter 14 Consumer Concerns About Foods 3

10. What is the international agency that has adopted standards to regulate the use of pesticides?

K
A. WHO
B. FDA
C. CDC
D. USDA
ANSWER: A   p. 479

11. Which of the following is a characteristic of botulism illness?

K
A. It is rarely fatal and victims usually recover completely
B. It is caused by a toxic compound rather than by invasion of pathogenic bacteria
C. It most often occurs from eating foods that were stored under aerobic conditions of high pH
D. It is caused by ingestion of food contaminated with a combination of aflatoxin and mold
ANSWER: B   p. 479

12. When milk held in the refrigerator for an extended period of time is found to be spoiled, it is

AP
A. a normal occurrence.
B. an indication the sterilization process was inadequate.
C. an indication the pasteurization process was inadequate.
D. usually the result of accidental contamination by the retailer.
ANSWER: A   p. 479

13. What organism is the most deadly cause of food-borne illness in the United States?

K
A. Salmonella
B. Clostridium botulinum
C. Staphylococcus aureus
D. Listeria monocytogenes
ANSWER: B   p. 479

14. Clostridium botulinum poisoning is a hazard associated with

K
A. nitrosamines.
B. rotting vegetables.
C. undercooked poultry.
D. improperly canned vegetables.
ANSWER: D   p. 479

4   Chapter 14 Consumer Concerns About Foods

15. Which of the following foods are associated with illness from Salmonella?

AP
- A. Raw vegetables
- B. Pickled vegetables
- C. Home-canned vegetables
- D. Raw meats, poultry, and eggs

ANSWER: D   p. 480

16. What organism is primarily responsible for causing "traveler's" diarrhea?

K
- A. Salmonella
- B. Escherichia coli
- C. Clostridium botulinum
- D. Staphylococcus aureus

ANSWER: B   p. 480

17. A patient reports that since returning from overseas travel to a developing country, she has been experiencing stomach cramps and diarrhea. Which of the following food-borne organisms is most likely responsible for these symptoms?

AP
- A. E. coli
- B. Clostridium botulinum
- C. Clostridium perfringens
- D. Listeria monocytogenes

ANSWER: A   p. 480

18. A patient with a high temperature complains of headache, stomach ache, fever, and vomiting. Upon questioning, he admits to eating several raw eggs the day before. The most likely organism causing these symptoms is

AP
- A. E. coli.
- B. Salmonella.
- C. Perfringens.
- D. Campylobacter jejuni.

ANSWER: B   p. 480

19. A child is brought in to the emergency room with breathing difficulties. He also has difficulty swallowing and speaking. The mother mentions that he ate some home-canned beans yesterday. You suspect microbiological food poisoning. The most likely toxin is

K
- A. botulium.
- B. giardiasis exotoxin.
- C. campylobacteria toxin.
- D. salmonella enterotoxin.

ANSWER: A   p. 480

Chapter 14 Consumer Concerns About Foods 5

20. Approximately what fraction of all food-borne illnesses occurs from preparing foods in the home kitchen?

K A. 1/10
  B. 1/4
  C. 1/3
  D. 1/2
  ANSWER: C p. 481

21. Which of the following would most likely result from the practice in which cooked hamburger patties are removed from the grill and placed immediately on the same plate that held the uncooked patties?

AP A. Flavor declination
  B. Meat juice retention
  C. Fat drippings exudation
  D. Microbial cross-contamination
  ANSWER: D p. 481

22. Which of the following methods of thawing meats or poultry increases health risk?

K A. In the refrigerator
  B. At room temperature
  C. In a microwave oven
  D. Under cool running water
  ANSWER: B p. 481-482

23. All of the following are rules to prevent illness from <u>Salmonella</u> EXCEPT

AP A. use hands to mix foods.
  B. thaw meats in the refrigerator.
  C. use a meat thermometer to avoid undercooking.
  D. use hot, soapy water to wash hands, utensils, and countertops.
  ANSWER: A p. 481-484

24. Which of the following foods is best known to transmit hepatitis?

K A. Poultry
  B. Seafood
  C. Legumes
  D. Raw vegetables
  ANSWER: B p. 481

Chapter 14   Consumer Concerns About Foods

25. Which of the following is a characteristic of meat contamination?

K
- A. A USDA seal of inspection does not insure the absence of harmful bacteria
- B. The presence of naturally occurring antibodies in meats slows down the growth of harmful organisms
- C. Ground meat is more resistant to contamination because of the high heat released by the grinding machines
- D. When properly informed, consumers should be able to detect the presence of harmful bacteria by odor or taste

ANSWER: A   p. 481

26. What type of seafood is responsible for between 80% and 90% of all sickness caused by eating seafood?

K
- A. Tuna
- B. Raw shellfish
- C. Raw fatty fish
- D. Cooked shellfish

ANSWER: B   p. 481

27. What is the risk of getting sick from eating seafood in the U.S.?

K
- A. 1 in 250
- B. 1 in 2,500
- C. 1 in 25,000
- D. 1 in 250,000

ANSWER: D   p. 481

28. What is the risk of getting sick from eating chicken in the U.S.?

K
- A. 1 in 250
- B. 1 in 2,500
- C. 1 in 25,000
- D. 1 in 250,000

ANSWER: C   p. 481

29. What is the "2-40-140" rule?

K
- A. A guide to minimize microbial growth on foods by restricting the food's exposure at 40°-140°F to a maximum of 2 hours
- B. A guide to minimize microbial growth on meats and poultry by cooking for a minimum of 40 minutes at 140°F for each two pounds of food
- C. A treatment regimen for suspected food poisoning that involves drinking 40 ounces of fluid every two hours for an average 140-pound person
- D. A safety regimen for people who work at eating establishments which involves washing the hands twice every 40 minutes in water with a temperature of at least 140°F

ANSWER: A   p. 481

30. What is the risk of getting sick from eating raw or undercooked seafood?

K A. 1 in 1,000-2,000
  B. 1 in 5,000-10,000
  C. 1 in 20,000-25,000
  D. 1 in 50,000-75,000
  ANSWER: A p. 482

31. What is the primary cause of foodborne illness in seafood?

K A. Poor worker hygiene
  B. Environmental contamination
  C. Inadequate storage conditions
  D. Toxins produced by certain marine fish
  ANSWER: B p. 482

32. Which of the following is the most appropriate method to thaw turkey?

AP A. In the refrigerator
  B. At room temperature
  C. On top of a warm oven
  D. Under very low heat in the oven
  ANSWER: A p. 482

33. Which of the following is known to serve as a food source of botulism poisoning in infants?

K A. Milk
  B. Eggs
  C. Honey
  D. Cheese
  ANSWER: C p. 483

34. If you suspect that you are suffering from a food-borne illness, appropriate actions to take include all of the following EXCEPT

AP A. notify the Health Hazard Evaluation Board of the FDA.
  B. drink clear liquids to help combat diarrhea and vomiting, and call a physician.
  C. find a portion of the remaining suspected food and taste it to detect any off flavors.
  D. find the remainder of the suspected food and store it in the refrigerator for possible inspection by health authorities.
  ANSWER: C p. 484

35. What are the chances of contracting diarrhea from travel to other countries?

K A. 1 in 2
  B. 1 in 10
  C. 1 in 100
  D. 1 in 1,000
  ANSWER: A p. 484

8   Chapter 14   Consumer Concerns About Foods

36. Which of the following is inappropriate advice on sanitation for someone traveling to another country?

AP
   A. Drink all beverages without ice
   B. Boil the local water before use to kill microbes
   C. Drink carbonated beverages because they inhibit growth of bacteria in the drink
   D. Eat vegetables raw with the peel to decrease risk from wash-water contamination
ANSWER: D   p. 484

37. Which of the following are examples of heavy metals?

K
   A. Mercury and lead
   B. Iron and chromium
   C. Carbon and nitrogen
   D. Molybdenum and fluoride
ANSWER: A   p. 485

38. Which of the following is a feature of an organic halogen?

K
   A. Heavy metal
   B. Safe additive
   C. Toxic chemical
   D. Component of most proteins
ANSWER: C   p. 486

39. What was the toxic substance that accidentally found its way into the food chain in the early 1970's and to which almost all of Michigan's residents became exposed?

K
   A. Lead acetate
   B. Methylmercury
   C. <u>Listeria monocytogenes</u>
   D. Polybrominated biphenyl
ANSWER: D   p. 486

40. Which of the following is an example of heavy metal exposure from foods?

AP
   A. Cooking foods for prolonged periods in iron utensils
   B. Ingestion of food containing high amounts of mercury
   C. Ingestion of food supplements containing high levels of calcium and sodium salts
   D. Cooking foods over superheated charcoal containing high levels of copper and iron
ANSWER: B   p. 486-488

Chapter 14   Consumer Concerns About Foods   9

41. Which of the following is a feature of naturally occurring food toxicants?

K A. Lima beans contain deadly cyanide compounds
   B. The toxic solanine in potatoes is inactivated by cooking
   C. The toxic laetrile substance in certain fruit seeds is a moderately effective cancer cure
   D. Mustard greens and radishes contain compounds that are known to worsen a cholesterol problem
   ANSWER: A   p. 488

42. What organization is responsible for approving the use of a pesticide on food?

K A. EPA
   B. FDA
   C. WHO
   D. DDT
   ANSWER: A   p. 489

43. What organization is responsible for enforcing the tolerances that are set for a pesticide on food?

K A. EPA
   B. FDA
   C. WHO
   D. DDT
   ANSWER: B   p. 489

44. What term is used to describe the highest level of a pesticide that is allowed in a food when the pesticide is used according to label directions?

K A. Toxicity level
   B. Tolerance level
   C. Risk concentration
   D. Optimum concentration
   ANSWER: B   p. 489

45. All of the following are features of pesticide tolerance levels EXCEPT

K A. they have been set for over 300 chemicals.
   B. they represent the maximum safe residue in foods.
   C. they are equivalent to amounts that should kill pests but not harm laboratory animals.
   D. they are equivalent to a level of 0.1% to 1% of the amount that causes no effect in laboratory animals.
   ANSWER: C   p. 489

10   Chapter 14   Consumer Concerns About Foods

46. According to FDA's monitoring practices, what percentage of <u>domestic</u> food samples showed pesticide residue levels that exceeded the maximum permissible amount?

K   A. 2
     B. 5
     C. 50
     D. 75
     ANSWER: A   p. 490

47. According to FDA's monitoring practices, what percentage of <u>imported</u> food samples showed pesticide residue levels that exceeded the maximum permissible amount?

K   A. 4
     B. 12
     C. 67
     D. 99
     ANSWER: A   p. 490

48. What category is assigned to additives put in foods after a rational decision-making process?

K   A. Indirect
     B. Incidental
     C. Intentional
     D. Contaminants
     ANSWER: C   p. 492-493

49. All of the following practices are known to minimize exposure to food pesticide residues EXCEPT

K   A. throwing away the outer leaves of leafy vegetable.
     B. using a knife to peel citrus fruits rather than biting into the peel.
     C. throwing away the fats and oils in broths and pan drippings from cooked meats.
     D. washing waxed fruits and vegetables in water to remove the wax-impregnated pesticides.
     ANSWER: D   p. 492

50. What is the classification given to a substance put into food to give a certain color?

AP   A. Indirect additive
     B. Incidental additive
     C. Peripheral additive
     D. Intentional additive
     ANSWER: D   p. 492

Chapter 14 Consumer Concerns About Foods 11

51. What classification is given to a substance that leaches from the inside lining of a can of fruit to the food, resulting in an off-flavor?

AP   A.   Direct additive
      B.   Indirect additive
      C.   Migratory contamination
      D.   Peripheral contamination
      ANSWER: B   p. 492

52. What organization regulates and monitors the use of chemical additives?

K   A.   FDA
     B.   HRS
     C.   WHO
     D.   USDA
     ANSWER: A   p. 493

53. What list is composed of substances widely used for many years without apparent ill effects?

K   A.   FDA
     B.   GRAS
     C.   Delaney
     D.   Additive Safety
     ANSWER: B   p. 493

54. Which of the following dictates that an additive must not have been found to be a carcinogen in any test on animals or human beings?

K   A.   Additive Rules
     B.   Delaney Clause
     C.   FDA GRAS List
     D.   Contaminant Law
     ANSWER: B   p. 493

55. What is the origin of the quotation "No additive shall be deemed to be safe if it is found to induce cancer when ingested by man or animal?"

K   A.   GRAS list
     B.   Delaney Clause
     C.   WHO Mandate of 1985
     D.   USDA Bulletin of 1962
     ANSWER: B   p. 493

Chapter 14   Consumer Concerns About Foods

56. Caffeine is permitted as a food additive because it is part of the

AP
A. GRAS list.
B. Delaney Clause.
C. WHO Mandate of 1985.
D. USDA Bulletin of 1962.
ANSWER: A   p. 493

57. The law on additive safety puts the burden of proof on the

K
A. FDA.
B. manufacturer.
C. scientific community.
D. consumer advocacy groups.
ANSWER: B   p. 494

58. What is the term that describes the allowance of most additives in foods at levels 100 times below those at which the risks of adverse effects are known to be zero?

K
A. Toxicity range
B. Zone of hazard
C. Acceptable area
D. Margin of safety
ANSWER: D   p. 494

59. What level of cancer risk to human beings from a food additive is accepted by the FDA?

K
A. 0
B. 1 in 1,000
C. 1 in 1,000,000
D. 1 in 100,000,000
ANSWER: C   p. 494

60. Which of the following statements is used to help define the safety of additives?

K
A. The capacity of a substance to harm living organisms is a measure of its toxicity
B. The capacity of a substance to harm living organisms is a measure of its hazard level
C. The capacity of a substance to produce injury should be independent of its level of use
D. The capacity of a substance to produce injury under conditions of use is a measure of its toxicity
ANSWER: A   p. 494

Chapter 14 Consumer Concerns About Foods 13

61. Which of the following substances in the diet would typically have the lowest margin of safety?

AP   A. Table-salt
      B. Pesticides
      C. Preservatives
      D. Color additives
      ANSWER: A   p. 494

62. Which of the following activities would result in the LEAST exposure to nitrites?

AP   A. Eating bacon
      B. Drinking beer
      C. Driving a new car
      D. Smoking cigarettes
      ANSWER: A   p. 494-496

63. Of the following, which is the most widely used antimicrobial agent?

K   A. Sugar
      B. Saccharin
      C. Sodium nitrite
      D. Sodium propionate
      ANSWER: A   p. 495

64. Which of the following is NOT among the features of nitrites?

K   A. Preserves color
      B. Imparts off-flavors
      C. Present in natural foods
      D. Protects against bacterial growth
      ANSWER: B   p. 495

65. What is the "redeeming characteristic" of sodium nitrite which prompted the FDA to delay action on banning the substance?

K   A. Helps reduce oxidation of vitamin E
      B. Helps prevent botulism food poisoning
      C. Helps prevent rancidity of cured meats
      D. Helps retain the pink color in cured meats
      ANSWER: B   p. 495

66. All of the following are among the characteristics of antimicrobial food additives EXCEPT

K   A. nitrates also preserve the color of hot dogs.
      B. ordinary baking powder is one of the most common.
      C. sodium propionate is used in cheeses and margarine.
      D. nitrites can be converted to cancer-causing substances in the stomach.
      ANSWER: B   p. 495

14 Chapter 14 Consumer Concerns About Foods

67. Which of the following properties are shared by vitamins C and E, BHA and BHT, and sulfites?

AP
    A. Flavor enhancers
    B. Antimicrobial agents
    C. Antioxidant activities
    D. Incidental food additives
    ANSWER: C   p. 496

68. Which of the following is NOT one of the features of sulfites?

K
    A. Improves flavor
    B. Used to prevent oxidation
    C. Destroys appreciable amounts of thiamin
    D. Causes adverse reactions in some people with asthma
    ANSWER: A   p. 496

69. When a slice of fresh apple turns a brown color it is most likely the result of

AP
    A. oxidation.
    B. dehydration.
    C. microbial contamination.
    D. ethylene oxide treatment in the ripening process.
    ANSWER: A   p. 496

70. What vitamin undergoes the most destruction in foods preserved with sulfites?

K
    A. Folate
    B. Vitamin K
    C. Vitamin B_1
    D. Ascorbic acid
    ANSWER: C   p. 496

71. Which of the following is a feature of sulfite food additives?

K
    A. They are frequently used in wines
    B. They inhibit growth of certain microbes
    C. They interact with folate to inhibit its absorption
    D. They are one of the few substances to have virtually no side effects
    ANSWER: A   p. 496

72. What substance is added to foods by processors to inhibit the formation of nitrosamines in nitrite-preserved products?

K
    A. Sulfites
    B. Solanine
    C. Cyanogens
    D. Vitamin E
    ANSWER: D   p. 496

Chapter 14 Consumer Concerns About Foods 15

73. All of the following are among antioxidant agents used by food processors EXCEPT

K   A. BHA.
      B. BHT.
      C. solanine.
      D. vitamin E.
      ANSWER: C   p. 496

74. Approximately how many color additives are currently approved for use by the FDA?

K   A. 7
      B. 20
      C. 33
      D. 100
      ANSWER: A   p. 497

75. Which of the following is a flavor-enhancing food additive?

K   A. BHT
      B. Beta-carotene
      C. Sodium propionate
      D. Monosodium glutamate
      ANSWER: D   p. 497

76. What food additive is thought to be associated with Chinese restaurant syndrome?

K   A. Nitrites
      B. Carotenoids
      C. Monosodium glutamate
      D. Polybrominated biphenyl
      ANSWER: C   p. 497

77. What is the chief source of radiolytic products in foods?

AP   A. Irradiation
      B. PBB plus UV light
      C. Radium contamination
      D. Heavy metal contamination
      ANSWER: A   p. 498

78. Which of the following is a feature of food additives?

K   A. Irradiation is classified as a food additive
      B. Sulfites act to retard growth of pathogenic organisms
      C. Nitrites may form URP's when the food is overheated
      D. Carotenoids are used to retard formation of nitrosamines
      ANSWER: A   p. 498

16   Chapter 14   Consumer Concerns About Foods

79. Which of the following is an example of an indirect food additive?

K   A. Nitrites
    B. Vitamin E
    C. Irradiation
    D. Tin from the can
    ANSWER: D   p. 499

80. Which of the following toxic substances are formed from production of paper products used in food packaging?

K   A. PBB's
    B. URP's
    C. Dioxins
    D. BHT and BHA
    ANSWER: C   p. 500

81. Which of the following is a property of hormones used in food production?

K   A. Bovine growth hormone is used to stimulate growth of calves in the U.S.
    B. Most European countries began using these growth hormones 10 years before approval in the U.S.
    C. The cost of using these hormones usually results in higher-priced but better quality products
    D. They are naturally occurring substances and therefore require only minimal regulation by the FDA
    ANSWER: A   p. 500-501

82. All of the following are examples of currently utilized systems in food biotechnology EXCEPT

K   A. irradiation.
    B. antisense genes.
    C. recombinant DNA.
    D. transgenic bacteria.
    ANSWER: A   p. 501-502

83. Which of the following is a feature affecting the public water supply?

K   A. Surface water is derived primarily from underground aquifers
    B. Contaminants break down more slowly in groundwater than in surface water
    C. Groundwater sources are most susceptible to contamination by runoff of pesticides and wastes from highways
    D. Contaminants such as gasoline from leaking underground storage tanks are most likely to affect the quality of surface water
    ANSWER: B   p. 503-504

Chapter 14 Consumer Concerns About Foods   17

84. Which of the following is a characteristic of home water treatments?

K
- A. Boiling the water may actually increase the concentration of heavy metals
- B. Most home filtration systems are highly efficient at removing virtually all types of contaminants
- C. Boiling the water is effective at removing all organic chemicals as well as killing microorganisms
- D. Most home filtration systems combine the processes of heavy metal removal, killing of microorganisms, softening of the water, plus addition of enhancers

ANSWER: A   p. 505

85. Which of the following is a feature of bottled waters that are sold to consumers?

K
- A. Bottled water is classified as a food and is regulated by the FDA
- B. Cost and stability are the two main reasons for choosing to use bottled water
- C. Bottled water is classified as an indirect additive to the diet and is regulated by the EPA
- D. Government regulations mandate that labels on bottled water reveal sources and heavy metal content

ANSWER: A   p. 506

86. Which of the following types of drinking water contains the lowest amount of minerals?

AP
- A. Hard water
- B. Spring water
- C. Natural water
- D. Distilled water

ANSWER: D   p. 506

87. The amount of energy required to manufacture a six-pack of diet soda is about equivalent to the energy provided by

AP
- A. 2½ lbs of sugar.
- B. 6 grams of lipid.
- C. 60 grams of starch.
- D. 3½ lbs of corn oil.

ANSWER: A   p. 509

88. All of the following are examples of fossil fuels EXCEPT

K
- A. oil.
- B. coal.
- C. Geritol.
- D. natural gas.

ANSWER: C   p. 510

18   Chapter 14   Consumer Concerns About Foods

89. Worldwide trends that characterize the 1990's include all of the following EXCEPT

K   A.   shrinking of desert areas.
    B.   thinning of the ozone layer.
    C.   higher levels of carbon dioxide in the atmosphere.
    D.   increasing salt concentration of food-producing land.
    ANSWER: A   p. 510

90. What term applies to the practice of replacing cut trees with an equal number of new ones?

AP A.   Forest preservation
    B.   Forest equalization
    C.   Equilibrium harvesting
    D.   Sustainable management
    ANSWER: D   p. 510

91. Approximately how much carbon dioxide is formed for every gallon of gas consumed by an automobile?

K   A.   1 ounce
    B.   10 ounces
    C.   10 pounds
    D.   20 pounds
    ANSWER: D   p. 511

92. Approximately how much water is required each day to produce the average person's intake of meat, milk, and eggs?

AP A.   1 gallon
    B.   10 gallons
    C.   50 gallons
    D.   100 gallons
    ANSWER: D   p. 511

93. Which of the following is a characteristic of beef production practices?

K   A.   Regulations prohibit the production of beef for pet food
    B.   Beef production in the U.S. uses about 70% of the grain raised in the country
    C.   Beef that has been obtained from the rainforest is so identified on food labels
    D.   Range-fed beef causes slightly greater environmental pollution than feedlot beef
    ANSWER: B   p. 511

Chapter 14 Consumer Concerns About Foods   19

94. What is the chief reason why people living in poverty and hunger bear numerous children?

K
- A. Birth control expenses are prohibitive
- B. Only a small percentage of the children may survive
- C. The low educational level of adults limits their understanding of family planning
- D. The parents seek greater fulfillment through having more children since there are few other interests in their lives

ANSWER: B   p. 513

95. Which of the following meats typically contains the highest content of fat?

K
- A. Grain-fed beef
- B. Salt-water fish
- C. Range-fed buffalo
- D. Farm-raised chicken

ANSWER: A   p. 514

96. Which of the following packaging materials is LEAST biodegradable?

K
- A. Paper bag
- B. Foam carton
- C. Fiber carton
- D. Butcher paper

ANSWER: B   p. 515

97. All of the following are properties of dioxins in the environment EXCEPT

K
- A. they cause cancer in fish.
- B. they actually lead to closing of people's water wells when found in the water.
- C. they are more prevalent now due to increased forest fires releasing dioxin vapors.
- D. they are produced by reaction of naturally occurring ammonia with the chlorine bleach discharged by the paper pulp industry.

ANSWER: C   p. 515

98. Which of the following is a feature of plastic bags in the environment?

K
- A. Some contain mercury
- B. They are manufactured primarily from cellulose
- C. Most are now made to fully degrade in landfills
- D. Some now contain inactive microbes that are activated to degrade the bag when exposed to outdoor weather conditions

ANSWER: A   p. 515

20   Chapter 14   Consumer Concerns About Foods

99. Which of the following ethnic meals is most likely to be prepared in a style that preserves nutrient content yet minimizes energy use?

K   A.   Asian meals
      B.   Italian meals
      C.   French cuisine
      D.   Continental cuisine
ANSWER: A   p. 516

100. In general, which of the following uses the LEAST amount of energy to cook a food?

K   A.   Barbecuing
      B.   Microwaving
      C.   Oven baking
      D.   Boiling on a stove
ANSWER: B   p. 516

101. Which of the following is a characteristic of aluminum use in the U.S.?

K   A.   Foil is usually not recyclable
      B.   The mining of this metal is less destructive to the environment than of most other metals
      C.   The lifespan of aluminum cooking utensils is among the lowest of the metallic products
      D.   Release of CFC's into the atmosphere is one of the highest for aluminum utensil production
ANSWER: A   p. 516

102. What appliance uses the greatest amount of energy in most people's homes?

K   A.   Range
      B.   Dishwasher
      C.   Blow dryer
      D.   Refrigerator
ANSWER: D   p. 516

103. What is considered the best recommendation for dealing with an old and inefficient refrigerator?

K   A.   Replace it
      B.   Lower the thermostat setting
      C.   Install new insulating gaskets around the door
      D.   Install one of the new energy-regulating devices that attaches to the motor's components
ANSWER: A   p. 516

104. What are the two major types of solar homes?

K A. Neutron and photon
   B. Active and passive
   C. Direct and indirect
   D. Thermal and infrared
   ANSWER: B   p. 517

105. What is the chief factor that prevents most people from installing solar energy equipment and appliances?

K A. Short life-span
   B. High initial cost
   C. Unreliability of the technology
   D. Inability to run the home's major appliances efficiently
   ANSWER: B   p. 517

106. All of the following steps will reduce the amount of energy used to run a water heater EXCEPT

K A. place the water heater on a timer.
   B. wrap the water tank in an insulating blanket.
   C. install an electric unit rather than a natural gas unit.
   D. set the water heater thermostat no higher than 130°F.
   ANSWER: C   p. 517

107. Which of the following statements reflects a difference between compact fluorescent light bulbs and incandescent light bulbs?

K A. Fluorescent bulbs use about 75% less energy
   B. Fluorescent bulbs last about 1½ times longer
   C. Fluorescent bulbs give off more heat and can supply some of a room's heating needs
   D. Fluorescent bulbs rated at 75-watts give the identical light output to 100-watt incandescent bulbs
   ANSWER: A   p. 517

108. What is the average weight of trash produced weekly by a U.S. family of four?

K A. 10 lbs
   B. 40 lbs
   C. 100 lbs
   D. 150 lbs
   ANSWER: C   p. 517

Chapter 14 Consumer Concerns About Foods

109. What percentage of metals mined in the U.S. is recycled?

K
- A. 5
- B. 30
- C. 50
- D. 85

ANSWER: B   p. 518

Essay Questions

478-482   110. List three major pathogenic microbes that are transmitted by foods, their food sources, symptoms of sickness, and methods of prevention.

481-483   111. What precautions should consumers take when selecting and consuming seafood?

484   112. Explain the precautions that should be taken to minimize the risk of traveler's diarrhea.

487-488   113. Give several examples of naturally occurring toxicants in foods and appropriate methods to minimize exposure to them.

496	114.	What are sulfites? Explain current FDA regulations regarding their use.
496-500	115.	Discuss the concerns of the public regarding the use of pesticides. Describe methods to minimize intake of pesticide residues on foods.
496-497	116.	List the major antioxidant additives in the food supply and their side effects in human beings.
498	117.	What is irradiation? Explain the pros and cons of irradiation as a food-processing method.
499-501	118.	Give examples of different types of indirect food additives and explain how they become part of the food supply.

24   Chapter 14   Consumer Concerns About Foods

501-502   119.   a.   Describe the basic processes used in recombinant DNA technology for the production of foods.

            b.   What are the advantages and disadvantages of using recombinant DNA technology to improve the food supply?

505-506   120.   Explain the differences among spring water, natural water, mineral water, hard water, and distilled water.

CHAPTER 15
NUTRITION ASSESSMENT

MULTIPLE CHOICE

Objective 1 Describe the components of a nutritional assessment process.

1. The purposes of a nutritional assessment is to:

K   A.   detect malnutrition.
    B.   detect people at risk for malnutrition.
    C.   identify area for dietary improvement.
    D.   do all of the above
    ANSWER: D   p. 521

2. The purpose of obtaining a historical information is to assess for:

K   A.   low socioeconomic status.
    B.   food and drug interactions.
    C.   nutrient deficiencies.
    D.   health factors that affect nutritional status.
    ANSWER: D   p. 522

Chapter 15 Nutrition Assessment

3. Which of the following data is the least important component of a client's nutritional assessment?

K   A.   Weight
      B.   Medication
      C.   Serum albumin
      D.   Current address
      ANSWER: D   p. 525, 530, 532

4. The easiest method used by nurses to collect a food intake data is a:

K   A.   food diary.
      B.   24 hour recall or usual intake.
      C.   3 day diet history.
      D.   food frequency questionnaire.
      ANSWER: B   p. 526

5. Of the factors listed, the *most* objective measure of nutritional status is the:

K   A.   evaluation of biochemical tests.
      B.   self reported height and weight.
      C.   evaluation of a food frequency questionnaire.
      D.   observation of meal consumption by the client's friend.
      ANSWER: A   p. 540

Objective 2 Compare and contrast the four different methods of obtaining food intake data.

6. Assuming that each method is performed reliably, valuable food intake data can be obtained from the:

K   A.   Usual intake.
      B.   Food record.
      C.   24-hour recall.
      D.   Food frequency checklist.
      ANSWER: B   p. 527

7. Which of the following is a limitation to the value of the twenty-four hour recall?

K   A.   The process is time consuming
      B.   Clients often keep poor records
      C.   The method excludes recording of beverages
      D.   A twenty-four hour period may not be typical
      ANSWER: D   p. 526

Chapter 15 Nutrition Assessment

8. Which of the following statements describe advantages of food records?

K
- A. Food intake is recorded promptly after eating
- B. The individual assumes an active role in record keeping
- C. The individual becomes aware of personal food choices
- D. All of the above

ANSWER: D   p. 527

9. Which of the following statements is the *best* way to begin the interview for a 24-hour dietary history?

AP
- A. "What did you have for breakfast today?"
- B. "You do eat breakfast everyday, don't you?"
- C. "Do you begin the day with juice or coffee?"
- D. "What is the first thing you ate or drank when you woke up?"

ANSWER: D   p. 525

*10. According to the Daily Food Guide, the recommended minimum number of servings per day from the breads/cereal group is:

AP
- A. 2 to 4
- B. 3 to 5
- C. 4 to 6
- D. 6 to 11

ANSWER: D   refer to Food Pyramid p. 33

Objective 3 Describe the relationship between anthropometric data and body composition and development.

11. Anthropometric measurements compare an individual with:

K
- A. another individual.
- B. population standards specific for age.
- C. population standards specific for gender.
- D. population standards specific for gender and age.

ANSWER: D   p. 530

12. Head circumference in an infant can help predict all of the following *except*:

K
- A. age.
- B. brain size.
- C. growth rate.
- D. protein-energy malnutrition.

ANSWER: A   p. 532

4   Chapter 15 Nutrition Assessment

13. Which of the following measures are useful for estimating muscle mass in a client?

K   A.   Midarm circumference and waist-to-hip ratio
       B.   Triceps fatfold thickness and waist-to-hip ratio
       C.   Biceps fatfold thickness and midarm circumference
       D.   Triceps fatfold thickness and midarm circumference
       ANSWER: D   p. 536

14. A waist to hip ratio (WHR) of .95 or greater in men or 0.8 or greater in women is associated with:

K   A.   increased longevity.
       B.   less than adequate fat stores.
       C.   increased risk for obesity related diseases.
       D.   lower incidence of cardiovascular disease.
       ANSWER: C   p. 537

15. The best use of triceps skinfold and midarm muscle circumference in a hospital setting is to:

AP   A.   determine nutritional deficiency disease.
        B.   plan the most appropriate weight loss program.
        C.   determine percent body fat and percent protein lost.
        D.   measure changes in fat stores and somatic protein reserve over time.
        ANSWER: D   p. 530

For question 16:
Mrs. Falwell is 5'4" and weighs 110 lbs. During the interview, she mentions she has lost "a lot of weight" over the last five years. She reports her highest weight at 135 lbs.

16. What is her *ideal* body weight?

AN   A.   100 lbs.
        B.   110 lbs.
        C.   120 lbs.
        D.   135 lbs.
        ANSWER: C   p. 533

17. The desirable weights for a female 5'5" tall and a male 5'10" are:

AP   A.   120, 160.
        B.   125, 166.
        C.   130, 160.
        D.   135, 165.
        ANSWER: B   p. 533

Chapter 15 Nutrition Assessment 5

Objective 4 Analyze physical changes associated with nutrient deficiencies and toxicity.

18. A young adult with spoon-shaped ridged, brittle nails might be deficient in:

K   A.   iron.
      B.   calcium.
      C.   vitamin A.
      D.   vitamin B.
      ANSWER: A   p. 540

19. John Jones is a 56 year old male who has been in intensive care for three weeks. He has been fed with enteral solutions. At the time of admission he weighed 166 lbs. Today he weighs 160 lbs. On assessing him you note dry, brittle hair, scaly skin and enlarged cervical lymph nodes. These findings suggest a need to further assess:

AN   A.   iodine status.
       B.   vitamin B status.
       C.   vitamin A status.
       D.   protein-energy status.
       ANSWER: D   p. 540

*20. The vitamin deficiency most commonly associated with alcoholics is:

K   A.   thiamin.
      B.   vitamin D.
      C.   vitamin E.
      D.   ascorbic acid.
      ANSWER: A   Highlight 7

*21. Dorothy Wilson is a 75 year old black woman who is lactose intolerant and unable to consume dairy products. She lives alone and does not purchase fresh fruits and vegetables. She came to the clinic with a smooth, swollen, purple tongue. Which of the following nutrient deficiencies might be suspected?

AP/AN
       A.   Protein
       B.   Vitamin D
       C.   Vitamin B
       D.   Vitamin C
       ANSWER: C

*22. The overzealous use of sun block clues the assessor to further evaluate:

AP   A.   vitamin C status.
       B.   vitamin D status.
       C.   niacin status.
       D.   thiamin status.
       ANSWER: B

Chapter 15 Nutrition Assessment

For question 23:
Mr. Smith is a 42 year old man with a positive family history of coronary artery disease. His current diet is high in kcal, saturated fat and cholesterol.

*23. Which physical finding would *best* correlate with this assessment data?

AP   A.   glossitis
        B.   cheilosis
        C.   xanthomas
        D.   constipation
        ANSWER: C

Objective 5 Identify the laboratory tests that reflect nutritional status.

24. Which of the following nutrition assessment techniques is a measure of protein status?

K   A.   Serum albumin
    B.   Body Mass Index
    C.   Tricep skinfold thickness
    D.   Visual Assessment of the oral cavity
    ANSWER: A   p.542

*25. A serum albumin of 2.5 g/dl in a stable adult male with malnutrition suggests:

C   A.   iron deficiency.
    B.   a normal finding.
    C.   short-term protein malnutrition.
    D.   long-term protein malnutrition.
    ANSWER : D

26. Iron deficiency can best be detected early by which of the following tests?

K   A.   Hematocrit
    B.   Hemoglobin
    C.   Serum ferritin
    D.   Erythrocyte protoporphyrin
    ANSWER: C   p.545

27. One test for adequacy of vitamin B_6 intake is:

K   A.   serum biotin.
    B.   urinary biotin.
    C.   serum tocopherol.
    D.   urinary xanthurenic acid excretion.
    ANSWER: D   p. 541

Chapter 15   Nutrition Assessment   7

For question 28:
Mrs. Smith is a 32 year old female who is 8 months pregnant. You note that her hematocrit level is 33% and her hemoglobin level is 11.0 g/100 ml.

28. These findings reveal:

AP   A.   folate anemia.
      B.   iron deficiency.
      C.   protein-energy malnutrition.
      D.   normal hemoglobin and hematocrit levels for third trimester.
      ANSWER: D   p. 545

Objective 6 Define and distinguish between the types of nutritional anemias.

29. In relation to nutritional anemias, the finding of macrocytic RBCs from a test of mean corpuscular volume suggest:

K   A.   folate anemia.
    B.   vitamin B_{12} anemia.
    C.   iron-deficiency anemia.
    D.   folate or vitamin B_{12} anemia.
    ANSWER: D   p. 544

30. Tests that detect iron deficiency include all of the following *except*:

K   A.   serum ferritin.
    B.   serum albumin.
    C.   mean corpuscular volume.
    D.   erythrocyte protoporphyrin.
    ANSWER: B   p. 544

31. Serum folate levels reveal:

K   A.   folate stores.
    B.   vitamin B_{12} status.
    C.   liver stores of folate.
    D.   current folate intake.
    ANSWER: D   p. 547

32. A Schilling's test is used to detect:

K   A.   serum folate level.
    B.   mean corpuscular volume.
    C.   Vitamin B_{12} malabsorption.
    D.   percent transferrin saturation.
    ANSWER: C   p. 547

8   Chapter 15   Nutrition Assessment

33. Vitamin B$_{12}$ deficiency often results from:

K   A.   malabsorption.
     B.   protein energy malnutrition.
     C.   low intake of dairy products.
     D.   low intake of green leafy vegetables.
     ANSWER: A   p. 547

34. Which of the following would most likely be found in the chart of an elderly woman with a diagnosis of macrocytic anemia?

C   A.   An order for tests of vitamin B$_{12}$ and folate status
     B.   An order for iron supplements
     C.   A diet history of low in complex carbohydrate
     D.   A lab report of decreased mean corpuscular volume
     ANSWER: A   p. 547

Objective 7 Classify the types of protein energy malnutrition using the nutrition assessment process.

35. Which of the following forms of malnutrition poses *greatest* risk?

K   A.   Marasmus
     B.   Kwashiorkor
     C.   Iron deficiency anemia
     D.   Marasmic kwashiorkor
     ANSWER: D   p. 550

36. Which of the following *best* describes kwashiorkor?

K   A.   It is associated with loss of subcutaneous fat.
     B.   It is the result of extreme caloric deprivation.
     C.   It is associated with energy and protein deficiency characterized by muscular wasting and weight loss.
     D.   It is associated with protein deficiency, characterized by hypoalbuminemia and pitting edema.
     ANSWER: D   p. 551

37. The classification of PEM is made through all of the following *except*:

K   A.   biochemical analysis.
     B.   physical examination.
     C.   socioeconomic standings.
     D.   anthropometric measures.
     ANSWER: C   p. 551

38. One of the dangers of kwashiorkor is that the client:

K A. may have malnutrition that goes undetected.
   B. has no energy reserves.
   C. has skeletal muscle depletion.
   D. has a loss of subcutaneous fat.
   ANSWER: A   p. 551

Objective 8 Characterize candidates for nutritional screening.

*39. A client who may be *least* prone to a vitamin D deficiency is one who:

C A. is homebound.
   B. consistently uses sunscreen.
   C. lives where the air is polluted.
   D. takes daily outdoor walks for 10-15 minutes.
   ANSWER: D

40. Which of the following clients is at *greatest* risk of malnutrition?

C A. a body builder 5'8" and 190 lbs, taking amino acid supplements.
   B. an 85 year old woman 5'4" with a reference body weight of 122 lbs.
   C. a 30 year old woman, 5'6", 192 lbs with a recent unexplained weight loss of 25 lbs.
   D. a 15 year old boy 5'8", 132 lbs, with a good appetite going through a growth spurt.
   ANSWER: C   p. 535, 551

41. Basic nutritional screening would include all of the following *except*:

K A. weighing the client.
   B. observing the client.
   C. obtaining a food record.
   D. checking blood glucose levels.
   ANSWER: D   p. 551

42. Which of the following medications places a client at risk for a poor nutritional status?

AP A. Ibuprofen, occasional use
   B. Sulcrafate
   C. Birth control pills
   D. Cromolyn sodium
   ANSWER: C   p. 523

10   Chapter 15   Nutrition Assessment

For question 43:
Jane Albert is a 44 year old who is hospitalized for a bunionectomy. On her chart you note that she is described as well nourished. You also note that she is 5'4" and weighs 145 lbs.

43.   Is Mrs. Albert a candidate for nutritional screening?

AP/AN
    A.   Yes, because she is overweight
    B.   Yes, because she is going to have a bunionectomy
    C.   No, because her weight reveals adequate nutrition
    D.   No, because a bunionectomy is a minor surgical procedure
    ANSWER: A   p. 552

*44. What is the minimum number of servings of fruit per day recommended by the Daily Food Guide?

C   A.   1-2
    B.   2-4
    C.   3-5
    D.   6-11
    ANSWER: B

45.   Which of the observations by the nurse would indicate the need for a complete nutrition assessment?

AP   A.   Refusal to eat breakfast
    B.   Weight loss of 10% in two weeks
    C.   Weight gain of 2 lbs. in seven days
    D.   Increased consumption of dairy products
    ANSWER: B   p. 552

Objective 9 Use the nutritional assessment process to calculate protein and kcal requirements for adults.

For question 46:
Mrs. Klein is a 52 year old woman with pneumonia and fever. She weighs 125 lbs.

46.   The amount of protein she requires is:

AP/AN
    A.   45-60 grams
    B.   65-74 grams
    C.   85-113 grams
    D.   125-134 grams
    ANSWER: C   p. 556

*   Answers marked with an asterisk are found in earlier chapters of the book. These questions are comprehension or application level questions.

CHAPTER 16
NUTRITION CARE STRATEGIES

MULTIPLE CHOICE

Objective 1 Define the objectives of the nutrition care plan.

1. Which of the following is *not* a part of the nutrition care process?

K   A. Height and weight
     B. Hematocrit and hemoglobin
     C. Patient room number
     D. Diet order
ANSWER: C   p.569

2. Which of the following health care professionals is *not* a regular participant in developing and evaluating the nutrition care plan.

K   A. Nurse
     B. Dietitian
     C. Physical Therapist
     D. Physician
ANSWER: C   p.571

2   Chapter 16   Nutrition Care Strategies

3. A nutrition care plan is:

K   A. the client's diet prescription ordered by the physician.
       B. the dietitian's goals for determining and meeting the client's nutritional needs.
       C. the nurse's documentation of how well the client is eating.
       D. nutritional formularies showing minimum daily requirements.
       ANSWER: B   p.569

Objective 2 Formulate a nutrition care plan.

For question 4:
Joey Thomas is a 21 month old who eats only white and brown foods. His parents have tried to get him to eat fruits and vegetables to no avail. On his last visit to the pediatrician he was 33 inches tall and weighed 25 lbs. This put him in the 25th percentile for his age group. You are working with Joey's parents to help them improve his diet.

4. In the assessment phase of the care plan process, the first thing you should do is:

AN   A. collect a diet history.
        B. tell Joey's parents that he has to eat fruits and vegetables.
        C. have Joey's parents keep a food diary on Joey.
        D. ask Joey why he isn't eating properly.
        ANSWER: A   p.569

5. An appropriate intervention for getting Joey to eat a more nutritious diet is to:

AN   A. tell Joey's parents to not allow him to play until he eats his vegetables.
        B. give Joey's parents a list of white and brown foods that are high in vitamins.
        C. encourage the use of whole wheat bread over fortified white bread.
        D. supplement his diet with enteral feeding products.
        ANSWER: B   p.570

For questions 6 and 7:
Angelica Jorge is a 15 year old who sought assistance with weight loss. She was 5'1" tall and weighed 130 lbs. You instructed her on weight control and a 1700 kcal diet. After four weeks Angelica returns and has lost 12 lbs. On physical examination you note angular stomatitis.

6. These findings suggest the need to:

AN   A. decrease her caloric intake.
        B. evaluate her current status.
        C. redefine her nutritional problem.
        D. have her take multi-vitamins.
        ANSWER: B   p.571

Chapter 16 Nutrition Care Strategies   3

7. When you plan Angelica's diet it is important to do all of the following *except*:

AN   A.   plan a low fat, 2500 kcal diet.
        B.   have Angelica keep a food diary.
        C.   consider the influence of her culture.
        D.   consider her developmental level.
        ANSWER: A   p.571

For questions 8 and 9:
Mr. Whitaker is 5'8", 145 lbs. and has been diagnosed with esophageal cancer. His hematocrit is 28 and albumin level is 3.1 g/dl.

8. Which of the following would be noted in his nutritional care plan?

AN   A.   Need for a low-kcalorie diet
        B.   Need to reduce protein intake
        C.   Need to improve energy-protein status
        D.   Need to limit milk
        ANSWER: C   p. 569, 570

9. Which one of the following additional findings is *most* detrimental to Mr. Whitaker's nutritional status?

AN   A.   the loss of 25 lbs. in the last month
        B.   his preference for high sodium foods
        C.   his need to eat with a family member
        D.   a transferrin level of 275 mg/dl
        ANSWER: A   p.569

Objective 3 Identify strategies needed in the evaluation of nutrition care plans.

For question 10:
Mrs. Smith has had difficulty understanding the diet planned for her by the dietitian because she does not read. The dietitian provides her a pictorial guide.

10. This is an example of which phase of the nutrition care process?

C/AP   A.   assessment of nutrition status
          B.   determination of nutrient requirement
          C.   develop a plan to met nutritional needs
          D.   evaluation of the effectiveness of the plan
          ANSWER: C   p.571

4   Chapter 16 Nutrition Care Strategies

11. Evaluation of nutrition care plans is essential because:

C   A.   the Joint Commission of Associated Hospitals' Organization requires it.
    B.   it provides a legal record of the nutrition support provided.
    C.   clients have changing nutritional needs.
    D.   all of the above
    ANSWER: D   p. 571

12. Which of the following should you consider in the evaluation phase of the nutrition care plan?

K   A.   client's motivation.
    B.   results sought.
    C.   results achieved.
    D.   all of the above
    ANSWER: D   p.571

For question 13:
You met with Susan Gray eight weeks ago to plan a weight loss diet. At that time Susan was 5'4" and weighed 185 lbs. She was instructed to eat a 1000 kcal diet at your counseling session. Today Susan weighs 180 lbs.

13. At this phase of the nutrition care process you would:

C/AP A.   assess her nutrition status.
      B.   redefine the nutrition problem.
      C.   evaluate the nutrition plan previously developed.
      D.   refer Susan to an endocrinologist.
      ANSWER: C   p.571

Objective 4 Discuss the use of nursing diagnoses in the nutrition assessment process.

For question 14:
Mrs. Sealy is an 85 year old woman who states she has a poor appetite. She is 5'2" tall and weighs 80 lbs.

14. The correct nursing diagnosis is altered nutrition: less than body requirements because:

AP   A.   she states she has a poor appetite.
     B.   she is elderly.
     C.   her percent IBW is 73%.
     D.   her percent IBW is 82%.
     ANSWER: C   p.572

Chapter 16 Nutrition Care Strategies

For question 15:
Mr. Wilbur is 5'7" and weight 250 lbs. He was hospitalized following an automobile accident in which he fractured several bones. His albumin is 2.6 g/dl. His diet order for the past week has been clear liquids.

15. The most appropriate nursing diagnosis is:

AP/AN
    A.   altered nutrition: more than body requirements.
    B.   altered nutrition: less than body requirements.
    C.   altered nutrition: high risk for more than body requirements.
    D.   altered nutrition: high risk for less than body requirements.
    ANSWER: B   p.572

For question 16:
Mrs. Maples is a 42 year old woman. She is 5'2" and weight 147 lbs. She is admitted to the hospital after suffering a significant burn injury. Upon physical exam you note mild edema and angular stomatitis. Upon admission the nurse obtains the following diet history indicating her usual intake:

Breakfast	1 chocolate doughnut
	8 oz. black coffee
Lunch	1 peanut butter and jelly sandwich
	15 potato chips
	12 oz. Coke
Dinner	1 cup macaroni and cheese
	½ cup corn with butter
	½ cup applesauce
	12 oz. Coke
Snack	3 oz. M&Ms

After a week, her lab reports revealed:
Albumin 2.8 grams/dl
Prealbumin 5 mg/dl

16. What is the most appropriate nutrition nursing diagnosis:

AN   A.   altered nutrition: more than body requirements.
        B.   altered nutrition: less than body requirements.
        C.   altered nutrition: high risk for more than body requirements.
        D.   altered nutrition: high risk for less than body requirements.
        ANSWER: B   p.572

Chapter 16 Nutrition Care Strategies

Objective 5 Compare and contrast the nutrition care process to nutrition nursing diagnoses.

17. What part of the nursing process corresponds to "nutritional problems" in the nutritional care process?

AP/AN
    A.   goals
    B.   nursing diagnoses
    C.   objective data
    D.   nursing prescriptives
    ANSWER: B   p.571

For questions 18 and 19:
Jane Collins has just delivered her first infant and plans to breastfeed him. She expresses self-doubts about her abilities, and her infant is fretful. Jane is being cared for by a nurse and a dietitian.

18. Jane's care should include:

AN
    A.   nursing and nutrition plans that complement and reinforce each other.
    B.   only a nursing care plan since this is really an emotional problem.
    C.   only a nutrition care plan since breast milk reflects Jane's nutrition.
    D.   plans that are very different since nursing and nutrition differ in focus.
    ANSWER: A   p.572

19. What would be the appropriate nursing diagnosis for Infant Collins?

C
    A.   Altered nutrition: more than body requirements
    B.   Altered nutrition: less than body requirements
    C.   Altered nutrition: high risk for more than body requirements
    D.   Altered nutrition: high risk for less than body requirements
    ANSWER: D   p.572

Objective 6 Outline the goals of diet therapy.

20. Goals of diet therapy should be:

K
    A.   specific to individual clients.
    B.   independent of medical therapies.
    C.   designed for weight loss.
    D.   the sole responsibility of the dietitian.
    ANSWER: A   p.572

Chapter 16 Nutrition Care Strategies   7

21. Which of the following *best* describes diet therapy?

K   A. Providing vitamins and mineral supplements to prevent diseases
     B. Prescribing nutritional supplements to clients that you think may have possible nutrient deficiencies
     C. Providing nutrients to clients in a form they can use
     D. Providing support during weight modification programs
     ANSWER: C   p.572

22. Diet modifications usually work best if they:

K   A. are understood by the client.
     B. are independent of medical therapies.
     C. represent real change from the usual diet.
     D. are nutritious.
     ANSWER: A   p.572

Objective 7 Describe the use of diet manuals in client care activities.

23. What kind(s) of information can be found in a diet manual?

K   A. Foods not allowed on diets
     B. Sample menus
     C. Rationale for use of diets
     D. All of the above
     ANSWER: D   p.577

For question 24:
Your client is on a 1200 kcal, 2 gram sodium diet. You find each diet in the diet manual but not the combined diet.

24. Where could you *best* find information regarding this diet?

K   A. The national formulary
     B. The client's physician
     C. The client's dietitian
     D. There are no resources; you have to improvise.
     ANSWER: C   p.577 Appendix M

8   Chapter 16 Nutrition Care Strategies

For question 25:
A client has just been admitted to your unit at 11:30 pm on Saturday. He states he is hungry and wants something to eat. You note he is on a low-fat diet but have questions regarding what is allowed.

25.   Your *best* resource at this time of night is the:

C/AP   A.   diet manual
        B.   client's physician
        C.   client's dietitian
        D.   nursing supervisor
        ANSWER: A   p.576

Objective 8 Identify communication skills necessary for implementing the steps in the nutrition care process.

26.   When a client on a 2 gram sodium diet requests food from home, the nurse should:

C   A.   support him in his effort by saying, "I wouldn't eat that food either".
        B.   tell him to request that the physician change his diet order.
        C.   explore his concerns about hospital food.
        D.   tell him he may not have food from home.
        ANSWER: C   p.579

27.   Which of the following is an open-ended question?

C/AP   A.   "Do you eat cereal for breakfast?"
        B.   "Would you prefer cereal or pancakes for breakfast?"
        C.   "What kinds of foods do you usually eat and when do you eat them?"
        D.   "Did you eat all of your breakfast today?"
        ANSWER: C   p.580

28.   Good communication is characterized by all of the following *except*:

K   A.   being an active listener.
        B.   establishing a trusting relationship.
        C.   giving advice.
        D.   maintaining eye contact.
        ANSWER: C   p.580

Chapter 16 Nutrition Care Strategies 9

Objective 9 Identify factors that can affect communication.

For questions 29 and 30:
Mrs. Jones delivered twin girls seven days ago. One of the girls (Ruby) is healthy but the second one (Mary) was born with severe birth defects which will require repeated hospitalizations to correct. Mrs. Jones had planned to breast feed but circumstances have made her change her mind. Ruby is currently on infant formula. Mary is fed by nasogastric tube. You are responsible for teaching Mrs. Jones how to feed Mary prior to discharge.

29. Which of the following will effect Mrs. Jones' ability to learn?

AP
- A. Her motivation
- B. Her learning abilities
- C. Her emotions
- D. All of the above

ANSWER: D   p.584,585

30. In order to improve communication with Mrs. Jones the acute care health care professional will do all of the following *except*:

K/C
- A. express empathy.
- B. express sympathy.
- C. refer her to a home health agency for continued teaching and support.
- D. assess readiness to learn.

ANSWER: B   p.585

Objective 10 Characterize the methods by which health care professionals communicate the nutrition needs of clients.

31. The nurse should clarify which of the following diet orders?

K
- A. 1200 kcal
- B. Reduced fat
- C. 2 grams of sodium
- D. Lactose free

ANSWER: B   p.577

32. The health care professional that works directly with clients to assess their nutritional status and plan appropriate diets is the:

K
- A. nurse.
- B. physician.
- C. clinical dietitian.
- D. diet clerk.

ANSWER: C   p. 576

10 Chapter 16 Nutrition Care Strategies

For question 33:
Mrs. Wilson is 5'2" and weighs 162 lbs. The physician orders a 2000 kcal weight reduction diet.

33. The nurse should:

AN A. reinforce this diet to the client because it is realistic.
    B. question the order because the kcal level is too high.
    C. question the order because she is close to her ideal body weight.
    D. question the order because the calorie level is too low.
    ANSWER: B   p.577

34. Who benefits when health care professionals make team rounds on clients?

K   A. The client
    B. The health care professionals
    C. The client's family
    D. All of the above
    ANSWER: D   p.586

35. The main reason nurses, dietitians, and physicians document their plans of care in the clients' chart is to:

C   A. communicate these plans with other health care professionals.
    B. meet accreditation requirements.
    C. protect themselves legally.
    D. all of the above.
    ANSWER: D   p.586

CHAPTER 17
LIFE CYCLE NUTRITION: PREGNANCY, LACTATION, AND INFANCY

MULTIPLE CHOICE

1. What is the placenta?

K   A.   An organ from which the infant receives nourishment
        B.   A muscular organ within which the infant develops before birth
        C.   The developing infant from the eighth week after conception until birth
        D.   The developing infant during its second through eighth week after conception
        ANSWER: A   p. 593

2. What organ of the pregnant woman is central to the exchange of nutrients for waste products with the fetus?

K   A.   Uterus
        B.   Vagina
        C.   Placenta
        D.   Amniotic sac
        ANSWER: C   p. 593

Chapter 17 Life Cycle Nutrition: Pregnancy, Lactation, and Infancy

3. What is the name given to the human organism two to eight weeks after fertilization and the stage at which the digestive system is formed?

K   A. Fetus
     B. Embryo
     C. Mesoderm
     D. Ectoderm
ANSWER: B   p. 594

4. All of the following statements are specific to the critical periods of cell division EXCEPT

AP A. malnutrition during pregnancy can affect fetal cell division.
     B. malnutrition during critical periods can have irreversible effects.
     C. high-nutrient-density food fed after the critical period can remedy a growth deficit.
     D. whatever nutrients are needed during a critical period must be supplied at that time.
ANSWER: C   p. 594

5. What is the term given to the developing infant from the eighth week after conception until birth?

K   A. Ovum
     B. Fetus
     C. Zygote
     D. Embryo
ANSWER: B   p. 594

6. What organ functions to prepare the mother's breasts for lactation?

K   A. Uterus
     B. Ovaries
     C. Placenta
     D. Amniotic sac
ANSWER: C   p. 594

7. At what stage of pregnancy does an embryo show a beating heart and a complete central nervous system?

K   A. 8 weeks
     B. 12 weeks
     C. 20 weeks
     D. 29 weeks
ANSWER: A   p. 594

Chapter 17 Life Cycle Nutrition: Pregnancy, Lactation, and Infancy 3

8. The duration of pregnancy is generally divided into equal periods of

K
   A. 4 weeks, called quarters.
   B. 9 weeks, called quartiles.
   C. 4 months, called semesters.
   D. 3 months, called trimesters.
ANSWER: D   p. 594

9. During development of the fetus, what organ(s) are the first to reach maturity?

K
   A. Heart and lungs
   B. Liver and kidneys
   C. Gastrointestinal tract
   D. Central nervous system and brain
ANSWER: D   p. 595

10. What term is given to the time period during which irreversible damage to the fetus may occur from specific events such as malnutrition?

K
   A. First trimester
   B. Critical period
   C. Fertility period
   D. Conceptual period
ANSWER: B   p. 595

11. Risks from malnutrition before conception include all of the following EXCEPT

K
   A. it may lead to cessation of menstruation.
   B. it affects ovulation but not sperm quality.
   C. it may result in a poorly developed placenta.
   D. it results in more complications during pregnancy in overweight as well as underweight women.
ANSWER: B   p. 595-596

12. Which of the following is a characteristic of agents known to affect reproduction?

K
   A. Drugs approved by the F.D.A. are safe for use in pregnancy
   B. Major birth defects have occurred in women taking the acne medicine Accutane
   C. Hormone activity and sperm quality are not much affected by paternal drug intake
   D. Major irregularities in fertilization have been demonstrated in women ingesting caffeine
ANSWER: B   p. 596

4   Chapter 17   Life Cycle Nutrition: Pregnancy, Lactation, and Infancy

13. Edema in a pregnant woman who does not have high blood pressure or protein in the urine is

AP
   A. expected and normal.
   B. a sign of dietary deficiencies.
   C. very rare and life threatening.
   D. a warning signal of a difficult labor.
   ANSWER: A   p. 597

14. What is the recommended <u>increase</u> in energy intake for the second and third trimester of pregnancy?

K
   A. 200 kcal/day
   B. 300 kcal/day
   C. 450 kcal/day
   D. 440 kcal/day
   ANSWER: B   p. 597

15. Adaptational responses in the woman who becomes pregnant include all of the following EXCEPT

K
   A. an increase in calcium absorption.
   B. a 2-fold increase in blood volume.
   C. an increase in serum albumin concentration.
   D. a decline in blood hemoglobin concentration.
   ANSWER: C   p. 597-599

16. All of the following are normal physiological responses to pregnancy EXCEPT

K
   A. breast size increases.
   B. blood volume increases.
   C. body water level decreases.
   D. joints become more flexible.
   ANSWER: C   p. 597

17. Over the course of the <u>entire</u> pregnancy, approximately how much <u>extra</u> energy does the average pregnant woman need to consume?

AP
   A. 10,500 kcal
   B. 26,000 kcal
   C. 39,000 kcal
   D. 55,000 kcal
   ANSWER: D   p. 597

Chapter 17 Life Cycle Nutrition: Pregnancy, Lactation, and Infancy 5

18. In the U.S., what is the minimum daily amount of protein that should be consumed by a 135-pound woman during pregnancy?

AP   A. 49 g
B. 59 g
C. 108 g
D. 135 g
ANSWER: B   p. 597

19. Which of the following statements characterizes energy needs during pregnancy?

K   A. The need is proportionally greater than for most other nutrients
B The increase needs are similar at the beginning and end of pregnancy
C. The needs increase by similar amounts in teenagers and 30 year-old women
D. The increased need could be supplied by eating just 1 extra slice of bread per day
ANSWER: D   p. 597

20. For women 25 years and older who are pregnant, an increased intake of about 50% is recommended for all of the following minerals EXCEPT

K   A. calcium.
B. potassium.
C. magnesium.
D. phosphorus.
ANSWER: B   p. 598-599

21. Of the following nutrient needs, which is considered the most difficult to meet in pregnancy?

K   A. Iron
B. Protein
C. Vitamin D
D. Vitamin B_6
ANSWER: A   p. 598

22. Which of the following nutrients are required in higher amounts during pregnancy due to their roles in the synthesis of red blood cells?

AP   A. Protein and chromium
B. Calcium and vitamin K
C. Folate and vitamin B_{12}
D. Vitamin E and vitamin C
ANSWER: C   p. 599

6   Chapter 17 Life Cycle Nutrition: Pregnancy, Lactation, and Infancy

23. During pregnancy, which of the following nutrients show a dramatic increase in absorption?

K   A.   Salt and sugar
    B.   Protein and fat
    C.   Calcium and iron
    D.   Thiamin and ascorbic acid
    ANSWER: C   p. 599-600

24. Studies report that folate supplements for women may lower the incidence of neural tube defects of infants when the vitamin is taken only during the

K   A.   last trimester of pregnancy.
    B.   second trimester of pregnancy.
    C.   second and third trimesters of pregnancy.
    D.   month before conception through the first trimester of pregnancy.
    ANSWER: D   p. 599

25. Which of the following is a feature of calcium nutrition in pregnancy?

K   A.   The RDA increases by over 100%
    B.   Intestinal absorption increases by over 100%
    C.   Supplements are recommended for most women due to the increased needs
    D.   Transfer of calcium from maternal stores to the fetus increases rapidly at the beginning of the second trimester
    ANSWER: B   p. 599

26. Which of the following nutrients taken as a prenatal supplement has been found to be associated with a lower incidence of neural tube defects?

K   A.   Iron
    B.   Folate
    C.   Calcium
    D.   Cobalamin
    ANSWER: B   p. 599

27. All of the following reflect a state of iron nutrition in pregnancy EXCEPT

K   A.   absorption of the mineral increases three-fold.
    B.   the mineral is well-conserved during this period.
    C.   stores of the mineral diminish slowly during this period.
    D.   most women enter pregnancy with adequate stores of the mineral.
    ANSWER: D   p. 600

Chapter 17 Life Cycle Nutrition: Pregnancy, Lactation, and Infancy 7

28. All of the following are features of zinc nutrition in pregnancy EXCEPT

K
    A. the RDA increases by 10 mg/day.
    B. a secondary deficiency may develop when iron supplements are taken.
    C. the mineral is needed for nucleic acid synthesis and thus cell development.
    D. low blood zinc concentrations of the pregnant woman correlate with low birthweights.
ANSWER: A   p. 600

29. Examine the following menu for a pregnant woman.

BREAKFAST   LUNCH

2 scrambled eggs   2 pieces (4 oz) fried
1 crushed wheat   chicken
  English muffin   2 wheat rolls w/butter
1 cup orange juice   1/2 cup mashed potatoes and
                           gravy
                           iced tea

SUPPER

3 oz pork chop
1 ear corn on the cob
Lettuce and tomato salad with 2 tbsp dressing
2 cups low fat milk

According to the recommended food intake for pregnancy, which of the following food groups is the only one that is provided in sufficient amounts by this menu?

AP
    A. Milk
    B. Meats
    C. Vegetables
    D. Bread/cereal
ANSWER: B   p. 601

30. A craving for non-food substances is known as

K
    A. pica.
    B. bulimia.
    C. toxemia.
    D. hyperemesis.
ANSWER: A   p. 601

Chapter 17 Life Cycle Nutrition: Pregnancy, Lactation, and Infancy

31. Which of the following statements reflects current knowledge of food choices in pregnancy?

K   A. A craving for pickles is a strong indicator that the body needs salt
      B. Careful and appropriate selection of foods can meet all nutrient needs for most women
      C. A craving for milk is a strong indicator that the body needs calcium and/or phosphorus
      D. Cravings and aversions to certain foods are probably the result of altered taste and smell sensitivities induced by hormones
ANSWER: D   p. 601

32. What is the normal range of weight gain during pregnancy?

K   A. 10-18 lbs
      B. 19-24 lbs
      C. 25-30 lbs
      D. 35-40 lbs
ANSWER: C   p. 602

33. What is the average number of pounds gained during a healthy pregnancy?

K   A. 15
      B. 25
      C. 35
      D. 45
ANSWER: B   p. 602

34. The component of weight gain during pregnancy that is similar to the average weight of the infant at birth is the

AP   A. placenta.
      B. amniotic sac fluid.
      C. maternal fat stores.
      D. uterus and supporting muscles.
ANSWER: C   p. 602

35. Which of the following is a characteristic of body weight changes associated with pregnancy?

K   A. Weight gain is generally steady throughout pregnancy for normal-weight women
      B. Most women are unable to lose all of the weight that was gained during pregnancy
      C. Sudden, large, weight gain in pregnancy may signal the development of hypotension
      D. Overweight pregnant women should gain as much weight as underweight pregnant women
ANSWER: B   p. 602

Chapter 17 Life Cycle Nutrition: Pregnancy, Lactation, and Infancy   9

36. Which of the following accounts for most of the weight gain during pregnancy?

K
    A.   Lean tissue
    B.   Bone tissue
    C.   Blood volume
    D.   Adipose tissue
    ANSWER: A   p. 602

37. To maintain physical fitness during pregnancy, all of the following activities are considered acceptable EXCEPT

K
    A.   saunas.
    B.   swimming.
    C.   playing single's tennis.
    D.   45-minute balanced exercise sessions 3 times/week.
    ANSWER: A   p. 603

38. To help alleviate pregnancy-related nausea, all of the following actions are recommended EXCEPT

AP
    A.   eat dry toast or dry crackers.
    B.   avoid milk when feeling nauseated.
    C.   avoid orange juice when feeling nauseated.
    D.   eat large, infrequent meals so as to limit contact time with food.
    ANSWER: D   p. 603

39. Common problems of pregnancy include all of the following EXCEPT

K
    A.   nausea.
    B.   heartburn.
    C.   constipation.
    D.   low blood pressure.
    ANSWER: D   p. 603

40. Which of the following is the most likely explanation for the behavior of a pregnant women who awakens at 2:00 A.M. craving pickles and chocolate sauce?

AP
    A.   She needs attention and support
    B.   She drank too much coffee the previous night
    C.   She drank too much alcohol the previous night
    D.   She needs nutrients that are found in high amounts in pickles and chocolate sauce
    ANSWER: A   p. 604

Chapter 17 Life Cycle Nutrition: Pregnancy, Lactation, and Infancy

41. Which of the following is one of the recommendations to treat pregnancy-associated heartburn?

K   A.   Eat many small meals
      B.   Drink fluids only with meals
      C.   Lie down within 15 minutes after eating
      D.   Exercise within 30 minutes after eating
ANSWER: A   p. 604

42. Which of the following defines a low birthweight infant?

K   A.   3½ lbs or less
      B.   4 lbs or less
      C.   5½ lbs or less
      D.   6½ lbs or less
ANSWER: C   p. 605

43. Which of the following is the most potent single indicator of an infant's future health status?

K   A.   Infant's birthweight
      B.   Mother's weight before pregnancy
      C.   Mother's weight gain during pregnancy
      D.   Mother's nutrition status prior to pregnancy
ANSWER: A   p. 605

44. All of the following are features of eclampsia EXCEPT

K   A.   edema.
      B.   diabetes.
      C.   proteinuria.
      D.   high blood pressure.
ANSWER: B   p. 606

45. Which of the following is a characteristic of gestational diabetes?

K   A.   It predicts risk of diabetes for the infant
      B.   It occurs in over one-half of normal weight women
      C.   It leads to permanent diabetes in only about 5% of the women
      D.   It should be treated, in part, with a diet rich in carbohydrates
ANSWER: D   p. 606

46. Pregnancy-induced hypertension typically develops during the

K   A.   first half of pregnancy.
      B.   second half of pregnancy.
      C.   first month after delivery.
      D.   first trimester of pregnancy.
ANSWER: B   p. 606

47. Which of the following nutrients has been found to lower the risk of pregnancy-induced hypertension when supplied as a supplement at the appropriate time during pregnancy?

K   A.   Iron
       B.   Folate
       C.   Calcium
       D.   Vitamin B_{12}
ANSWER: C   p. 607

48. What is the name of the condition characterized by high blood pressure, edema, and protein in the urine of a pregnant woman?

K   A.   Eclampsia
       B.   Gestational diabetes
       C.   Teratogenic hypertension
       D.   Pregnancy-induced blood pressure crisis
ANSWER: A   p. 607

49. What is the percentage of babies born to teenagers in the U.S.?

K   A.   5
       B.   10
       C.   20
       D.   30
ANSWER: C   p. 607

50. Which of the following is a characteristic associated with adolescent pregnancy?

K   A.   The recommended weight gain is approximately 35 lbs
       B.   The incidence of stillbirths and preterm births is 5-10% lower compared with adult women
       C.   The incidence of pregnancy-induced hypertension is 5-10% lower as compared with older women
       D.   The time in labor is usually shorter than older women because there are fewer overweight teenagers
ANSWER: A   p. 607

51. Which of the following recommendations concerning pregnant women has been issued by the U.S. Surgeon General?

K   A.   They should drink absolutely no alcohol
       B.   They should refrain from drinking hard liquor only
       C.   They are permitted to ingest no more than 2 drinks per day
       D.   They are permitted to ingest small amounts of alcohol during the first 3 months but none thereafter
ANSWER: A   p. 608

12   Chapter 17 Life Cycle Nutrition: Pregnancy, Lactation, and Infancy

52. Which of the following describes the use of aspirin by the pregnant woman?

K A. It is highly teratogenic when taken during the first 3 months of pregnancy
   B. It is the medication of choice to treat many complications of pregnancy
   C. It can lead to excessive blood loss at delivery when taken during the last 3 months of pregnancy
   D. It promotes the absorption of dietary iron by lowering the pH of stomach contents which keeps iron in the ferrous state
   ANSWER: C   p. 608

53. Relationships between the use of tobacco products and complications of pregnancy include all of the following EXCEPT

K A. chewing tobacco during pregnancy leads to lower birthweight infants.
   B. smoking during pregnancy increases the risk of sudden infant death syndrome.
   C. taking zinc supplements prevents the development of pregnancy-induced hypertension in smokers.
   D. smoking just 2 cigarettes in succession during pregnancy adversely affects fetal breathing.
   ANSWER: C   p. 608-609

54. All of the following substances and practices should be totally eliminated during pregnancy EXCEPT

AP A. dieting.
   B. cigarette smoking.
   C. alcohol consumption.
   D. artificial sweeteners.
   ANSWER: D   p. 608-609

55. In general, what are the consequences of nutritional deprivation in the lactating mother?

K A. Cessation of lactation
   B. Reduced quality of milk
   C. Reduced quantity of milk
   D. Reduced quality and quantity of milk
   ANSWER: C   p. 611

56. Which of the following describes one of the findings from studies of lactating women who exercised compared with sedentary lactating women?

K A. They produced more milk
   B. They had similar energy intakes
   C. They produced more nutrient-dense milk
   D. They had a slightly greater amount of body fat
   ANSWER: A   p. 611

57. Which of the following statements describes an association between nutrient intake and lactation?

K   A. Milk production is related to fluid intake
      B. Ingestion of garlic may lead to an off-flavor of the milk
      C. The energy RDA for milk production calls for an additional 1,000 kcal
      D. Inadequate protein intake lowers the protein concentration of the milk
      ANSWER: B   p. 611

58. Under which of the following circumstances would it be acceptable for a mother to breastfeed?

AP   A. She has alcohol abuse
      B. She has a drug addiction
      C. She has an ordinary cold
      D. She has a communicable disease
      ANSWER: C   p. 612-613

59. Which of the following reflects one of the influences of alcohol intake on lactation?

K   A. It does not pass into the milk
      B. It mildly stimulates milk production
      C. It adversely affects milk production
      D. It passes into the milk but is degraded by enzymes in breast tissue
      ANSWER: C   p. 612

60. What would be a normal body weight after 1 year for a healthy infant with a birthweight of 8 lbs?

AP   A. 12 lbs
      B. 16 lbs
      C. 24 lbs
      D. 35 lbs
      ANSWER: C   p. 613

61. All of the following are characteristics of cow's milk use in infant nutrition EXCEPT

K   A. it is higher in total protein than breast milk.
      B. it is higher in bioavailable iron than breast milk.
      C. it causes gastrointestinal bleeding in infants less than 6 months old.
      D. it contains protein that is more difficult to digest than the protein from breast milk.
      ANSWER: B   p. 615-617

14   Chapter 17 Life Cycle Nutrition: Pregnancy, Lactation, and Infancy

62. When expressed per kilogram body weight, the nutrient needs of infants are markedly higher than for adults for all of the following nutrients EXCEPT

AP A. iron.
    B. folate.
    C. calcium.
    D. vitamin D.
    ANSWER: B   p. 615

63. Breast milk as the sole source of nutrition during the first 4 to 6 months in healthy infants is satisfactory for all nutrients with the possible EXCEPTIONS OF

K   A. iron and folate.
    B. zinc and vitamin A.
    C. calcium and vitamin C.
    D. fluoride and vitamin D.
    ANSWER: D   p. 615-616

64. What is colostrum?

K   A. Clot in the bloodstream
    B. Major protein in breast milk
    C. Hormone that promotes milk production
    D. Milk-like substance secreted right after delivery
    ANSWER: D   p. 616-617

65. Which of the following is an advantage of breastfeeding compared with formula feeding?

K   A. There is no limit to the supply
    B. It provides immunological protection
    C. The mother can be sure the baby is getting enough milk
    D. It is the only way to develop a true loving relationship with the baby
    ANSWER: B   p. 616-617

66. What is the factor in breast milk that binds iron and prevents it from supporting the growth of the infant's intestinal bacteria?

K   A. Colostrum
    B. Lactoferrin
    C. Lactalbumin
    D. Bifidus factor
    ANSWER: B   p. 616

Chapter 17 Life Cycle Nutrition: Pregnancy, Lactation, and Infancy   15

67. What is the chief protein in human breast milk?

K   A. Casein
     B. Albumin
     C. Lactose
     D. Lactalbumin
     ANSWER: D   p. 616

68. Which of the following vitamin-mineral supplements need NOT be prescribed for an infant breastfed beyond 6 months of age?

K   A. Iron
     B. Fluoride
     C. Vitamin D
     D. Vitamin E
     ANSWER: D   p. 616

69. Which of the following is associated with the bifidus factor?

K   A. Increased iron absorption
     B. Increased bacterial growth
     C. Decreased allergy protection
     D. Decreased hormone production
     ANSWER: B   p. 617

70. To gradually replace breast milk with infant formula or other foods appropriate to an infant's diet is to

K   A. feed.
     B. wean.
     C. nurse.
     D. breastfeed.
     ANSWER: B   p. 617

71. Which of the following should NOT be used to feed an infant?

K   A. Whole milk
     B. Ready-to-feed formula
     C. Liquid concentrate formula
     D. Powdered formula or evaporated milk formula
     ANSWER: A   p. 618

72. Features of infant formulas include all of the following EXCEPT

K   A. they contain antibodies.
     B. they breed bacteria in bottles left at room temperature.
     C. they typically contain over twice the amount of iron compared with breast milk.
     D. they contain fat and carbohydrate at concentrations resembling those in breast milk.
     ANSWER: A   p. 618-619

16   Chapter 17 Life Cycle Nutrition: Pregnancy, Lactation, and Infancy

73. Which of the following defines nursing bottle tooth decay?

K   A. Caries development resulting from frequent use of non-sterile bottles and nipples
      B. Bacterial attack of teeth due to severe tooth misalignment from sucking on oversized bottle nipples
      C. Marked tooth decay of an infant due to prolonged exposure to carbohydrate-rich fluids from a bottle
      D. Tooth decay resulting from constant exposure to food due to inability of the infant to swallow in normal fashion
ANSWER: C   p. 618-619

74. In comparison with cow's milk, breast milk contains

AP   A. less protein and minerals.
       B. less lactose and vitamin C.
       C. more fat and less carbohydrate.
       D. more energy and less vitamin E.
ANSWER: A   p. 619

75. Approximately how many kcal are contained in a liter of human breast milk?

K   A. 200
      B. 400
      C. 640
      D. 1200
ANSWER: C   p. 619

76. Approximately how many grams of protein are found in a quart of human breast milk?

K   A. 3
      B. 9
      C. 15
      D. 34
ANSWER: B   p. 619

77. What term defines the condition of infant tooth deterioration resulting from chronic exposure to carbohydrate-rich fluids from a bottle?

K   A. Juice bottle erosion
      B. Suckling enamelosis
      C. Formula-induced gingivitis
      D. Nursing bottle tooth decay
ANSWER: D   p. 619

Chapter 17 Life Cycle Nutrition: Pregnancy, Lactation, and Infancy   17

78.   Low-fat or nonfat milk should not be given routinely to a child until after the age of

K   A.   two weeks.
      B.   three months.
      C.   one year.
      D.   two years.
      ANSWER: D   p. 620

79.   The metabolic bone disease osteopenia is common in

K   A.   preterm infants.
      B.   overweight infants.
      C.   overweight mothers.
      D.   late-for-gestational age infants.
      ANSWER: A   p. 620

80.   Which of the following feeding practices is recommended for preterm infants?

K   A.   They should be fed exclusively on breast milk
      B.   They should be fed breast milk as well as special formula
      C.   They should be fed on breast milk enriched in a 1 to 1 ratio with cow's milk
      D.   They should be fed only on special formula because breast milk nutrient content is too
           low
      ANSWER: B   p. 620

81.   During the first year of life, cow's milk is considered an inappropriate food due to all of the
      following EXCEPT

K   A.   it is too low in iron.
      B.   it is too low in sodium.
      C.   it is too high in protein.
      D.   it is too low in vitamin C.
      ANSWER: B   p. 620

82.   During the first few months of life, which of the following nutrients is poorly digested?

K   A.   Fat
      B.   Starch
      C.   Protein
      D.   Lactose
      ANSWER: B   p. 620

83.   Which of the following represents a good age to introduce solid foods to infants?

AP   A.   Two weeks
      B.   Two months
      C.   Five months
      D.   One year
      ANSWER: C   p. 621

18   Chapter 17 Life Cycle Nutrition: Pregnancy, Lactation, and Infancy

84.   Which of the following nutrients need to be supplied first by solid foods in a baby's diet?

K   A.   Vitamin C and iron
      B.   Vitamin A and zinc
      C.   Vitamin B$_{12}$ and fluoride
      D.   Vitamin E and magnesium
      ANSWER: A   p. 621

85.   At what age does the normal infant first develop the ability to swallow solid food?

K   A.   3-5 weeks
      B.   26-32 weeks
      C.   4-6 months
      D.   9-12 months
      ANSWER: C   p. 621

86.   What adverse side effect is most likely to develop in infants who are not given solid foods before one year of age?

K   A.   Delayed growth
      B.   Impaired speech
      C.   Mental dysfunction
      D.   Impaired eye coordination
      ANSWER: A   p. 621

87.   What should be the first food introduced to the infant?

K   A.   Yogurt
      B.   Egg white
      C.   Rice cereal
      D.   Finely chopped meat
      ANSWER: C   p. 621

88.   Which of the following is an indication that the infant is first ready for solid food?

K   A.   He can roll over
      B.   Her age is 9 months
      C.   His birthweight has increased by 100%
      D.   She consumes 16 ounces of milk or formula daily and refuses any more
      ANSWER: C   p. 621

89.   Why should new foods be introduced to an infant one at a time?

K   A.   It prevents overfeeding
      B.   Any allergic reactions can be detected
      C.   Immunological protection hasn't been developed
      D.   The swallowing reflex is not under voluntary control
      ANSWER: B   p. 622

90. Of the following cereals, which is MOST likely to result in an allergic reaction upon first feeding?

AP
A. Oat
B. Rice
C. Corn
D. Wheat
ANSWER: D   p. 622

91. Which of the following is a feature of iron nutrition in the very young?

K
A. Iron deficiency is most prevalent in children aged 2 to 3 years old
B. The supply of stored iron becomes depleted after the birthweight triples
C. Infants with iron-deficiency anemia demonstrate abnormal motor development
D. Serum ferritin concentrations fall in infants who start drinking whole milk at 3 months of age but not at 6 months of age
ANSWER: C   p. 622

92. What should be the parent's response when a one-year-old child wants to clumsily spoon-feed himself?

AP
A. Punish the child
B. Let the child eat with his fingers instead
C. Gently take the spoon back and feed the child with it
D. Let the child try to feed himself so that he will learn
ANSWER: D   p. 623-624

93. Which of the following is the primary factor in the development of milk anemia?

K
A. Impaired absorption of iron
B. Excessive intake of cow's milk
C. Low iron content of breast milk
D. Insufficient intake of whole cow's milk
ANSWER: B   p. 623

94. According to many experts, what MINIMUM level of alcohol intake increases the risk of giving birth to an infant with fetal alcohol syndrome?

K
A. 1 drink/day
B. 2 drinks/day
C. 4 drinks/day
D. 7 drinks/week
ANSWER: A   p. 626-627

Chapter 17 Life Cycle Nutrition: Pregnancy, Lactation, and Infancy

95. Which of the following statements describes a relationship between alcohol intake and development?

K A. Birth defects are most severe when the woman drinks around the time of conception
   B. Infants born with fetal alcohol syndrome typically show immediate signs of brain impairment
   C. Eating well and maintaining adequate nutrient stores will prevent alcohol-induced placenta damage
   D. Toxicity to the fetus begins to occur when fetal blood alcohol levels rise above maternal blood alcohol levels
   ANSWER: A   p. 626-627

96. In what period during pregnancy would most damage occur from alcohol consumption?

K A. Before conception
   B. First trimester
   C. Second trimester
   D. Third trimester
   ANSWER: B   p. 627

Essay Questions

595-596   97. Describe the consequences of malnutrition on conception and early pregnancy.

597-600   98. What nutrients are needed in larger amounts during pregnancy and what physical changes account for the increased needs?

603   99. What are several benefits of exercise specifically for the pregnant woman? What types of exercise should be avoided and why?

Chapter 17 Life Cycle Nutrition: Pregnancy, Lactation, and Infancy

603-604   100.   What steps can be taken to minimize the development and discomfort of nausea, heartburn, and constipation during pregnancy?

606   101.   Define gestational diabetes. How is it managed?

606-607   102.   Explain the development of pregnancy-induced hypertension and the consequences if not properly managed.

607   103.   Describe the risks associated with adolescent pregnancy.

608-609   104.   What practices should be avoided during pregnancy and why?

Chapter 17 Life Cycle Nutrition: Pregnancy, Lactation, and Infancy

615-617,619   105.   Compare and contrast major differences in nutrient content of breast milk and cow's milk.

620-623   106.   Discuss guidelines for introducing first foods to an infant.

620   107.   Discuss the special nutritional needs of the preterm infant and ways to meet these needs.

626-628   108.   Explain how maternal alcohol intake affects growth and development of the fetus.

CHAPTER 18
LIFE CYCLE NUTRITION: CHILDHOOD, ADOLESCENCE, AND AGING

MULTIPLE CHOICE

1. Which of the following changes in body structure usually takes place between the ages of 1 and 2 years?

K   A. Weight doubles
    B. Weight triples
    C. Length of body doubles
    D. Length of long bones increase
    ANSWER: D   p. 630

2. Which of the following provides the most important information about a child's health?

K   A. Growth chart
    B   Blood lipid profile
    C   Long-bone size and density
    D   Onset of walking and talking
    ANSWER: A   p. 630

3. The best way to be sure children are growing normally is to

K   A. use growth equations.
    B. keep track of nutrient intakes.
    C. compare their heights and weights to their peers.
    D. compare their current heights and weights with previous measurements.
    ANSWER: D   p. 630

Chapter 18 Life Cycle Nutrition: Childhood, Adolescence, and Aging

4. Which of the following is associated with energy metabolism of the preschool child?

K   A. Food intake is remarkably similar from meal to meal
     B. Overweight individuals have appetites similar to normal weight individuals
     C. Energy needs per kg body weight increase from 1 year of age to 5 years of age
     D. A 1-year old who needs 1,000 kcal/day would require only about 1300 kcal at 3 years of age
     ANSWER: D   p. 630-631

5. Approximately how many kcal per day does an average 3-year old need to obtain?

K   A. 500
     B. 800
     C. 1300
     D. 2400
     ANSWER: C   p. 631

6. A large amount of concentrated sweets in a child's diet is most likely to lead to

AP A. apathy.
     B. dental caries.
     C. hyperactivity.
     D. growth inhibition.
     ANSWER: B   p. 631-640

7. How much more total energy does a normal 10 year old need vs. a 1-year old?

AP A. 25%
     B. 50%
     C. 100%
     D. 200%
     ANSWER: C   p. 631

8. When children are allowed to eat freely from a variety of foods, what percentage of their total energy intake is derived from sugar?

K   A. 5
     B. 10
     C. 15
     D. 25
     ANSWER: D   p. 631

9. Studies of U.S. and Canadian children show that most are meeting their recommended intakes for all nutrients EXCEPT

K A. vitamin C.
  B. zinc and iron.
  C. vitamin D and calcium.
  D. magnesium and vitamin B_1.
  ANSWER: B p. 631

10. What is the most common nutrient deficiency among Canadian and U.S. children?

K A. Iron
  B. Calcium
  C. Vitamin C
  D. Vitamin D
  ANSWER: A p. 632

11. A child who drinks a lot of milk at the expense of other foods is at high risk of showing signs of

AP A. anemia.
  B. rickets.
  C. hyperkeratosis.
  D. ariboflavinosis.
  ANSWER: A p. 632

12. The consumption of milk by children should not exceed 4 cups per day in order to lower the risk for

AP A. solute overload.
  B. iron deficiency.
  C. vitamin A toxicity.
  D. vitamin D toxicity.
  ANSWER: B p. 632

13. An adverse reaction to food that does NOT signal the body to form antibodies is termed a

K A. food allergy.
  B. food intolerance.
  C. mild food challenge.
  D. transient food episode.
  ANSWER: B p. 632-633

4   Chapter 18   Life Cycle Nutrition: Childhood, Adolescence, and Aging

14. Which of the following foods are most often the cause of allergies?

AP
    A. Eggs, peanuts, and milk
    B. Bananas, juice, and cola
    C. Apples, noodles, and rice
    D. Pears, oatmeal, and chocolate
    ANSWER: A   p. 633

15. A child who develops antibodies to a certain food is said to have a

AP
    A. food allergy.
    B. food intolerance.
    C. specific inducible episode.
    D. transient immune suppression.
    ANSWER: A   p. 633

16. Which of the following is a characteristic of a food allergy?

K
    A. It always elicits symptoms in the person
    B. It always involves the production of antibodies
    C. It usually shows up immediately after exposure to the allergic food
    D. It is usually elicited from very small, simple molecules as well as large, complex molecules
    ANSWER: B   p. 633

17. What is the term given to the child with apparent hyperactivity produced by a combination of insufficient sleep and overstimulation?

K
    A. Food hypersensitivity
    B. Fetal alcohol syndrome
    C. Caffeine hypersensitivity
    D. Tension-fatigue syndrome
    ANSWER: D   p. 634

18. Which of the following is a characteristic of iron deficiency in children?

K
    A. It affects brain function before anemia sets in
    B. It rarely develops in those with high intakes of milk
    C. It is the primary factor in tension-fatigue syndrome
    D. Mild deficiency enhances mental performance by lowering physical activity level thereby leading to increased attention span
    ANSWER: A   p. 634

Chapter 18 Life Cycle Nutrition: Childhood, Adolescence, and Aging 5

19. Which of the following is characteristic of children who regularly eat breakfast or skip breakfast?

K   A. Breakfast-skippers actually show lower scores on IQ tests than those who eat breakfast
      B. Attention spans are similar but a significant number of breakfast-skippers show hyperglycemia
      C. Breakfast-skippers initially show decreased mental performance but with time they adapt and show almost identical achievements
      D. Breakfast-skippers who change to eating breakfast show a temporary improvement in mental concentration but also a moderate degree of hypoglycemia
ANSWER: A   p. 636

20. Which of the following is the most likely reason that teachers promote the consumption of midmorning snacks for children?

AP   A. It provides an opportunity to learn about nutrition
      B. It meets federally mandated school nutrition guidelines
      C. It provides carbohydrate for maintenance of blood glucose and brain function
      D. It helps decrease the symptoms of attention deficit hyperactivity disorder in 5% of school-age children
ANSWER: C   p. 636

21. All of the following are characteristics of hyperactivity in children EXCEPT

K   A. it impairs learning ability.
      B. it is managed, in part, by prescribing stimulant drugs when necessary.
      C. it occurs in approximately 5% of those who are young and school-age.
      D. it responds favorably to dietary manipulations such as limiting sugar intake.
ANSWER: D   p. 636-637

22. Which of the following two conditions are associated with television's influence?

K   A. Obesity and poor dental health
      B. Drug abuse and teenage pregnancy
      C. Anorexia and nutrient deficiencies
      D. Hyperactivity and lower body weight
ANSWER: A   p. 637

23. Which of the following is a feature of nutrition and behavior in children?

AP   A. Watching television for 5 hours per day increases the prevalence for obesity by 10%
      B. The adverse effects from caffeine intake first appear typically after drinking 6 cans of cola per day
      C. Television commercials featuring snack foods have not been found to affect children's food preferences
      D. Most children are able to control their intake of cola beverages since they are more sensitive to the stimulating effects of caffeine
ANSWER: A   p. 637

Chapter 18 Life Cycle Nutrition: Childhood, Adolescence, and Aging

24. The influence of cholesterol in the health of children is described by all of the following EXCEPT

K
- A. cholesterol intake should be limited beginning at 2 years of age.
- B. elevated blood cholesterol levels are usually found only in obese individuals.
- C. approximately 90% of individuals with high blood cholesterol will retain this abnormality as adults.
- D. serum cholesterol is higher in individuals viewing television for 2 hours per day compared with more active individuals.

ANSWER: C   p. 637-638

25. To lower the risk of obesity in children, which of the following practices should parents institute for their children?

K
- A. Serve them smaller portions
- B. Make them clean their plates
- C. Serve them 3 meals a day without dessert
- D. Serve them more beverages and less solid food

ANSWER: A   p. 638

26. Which of the following should be done to ensure that young people eat well?

K
- A. Control the availability of food
- B. Control the consumption of food
- C. Prohibit eating except at mealtime
- D. Provide an emotional climate that discourages snacking

ANSWER: A   p. 638-640

27. Which of the following is an effective strategy for dealing with obesity in a child?

AP
- A. Institute new eating habits such as teaching the individual to clean the food plate
- B. Encourage the individual to eat quickly and then excuse him/her self from the table
- C. Take control and strongly encourage the individual to lose weight by dieting and regular exercise
- D. Teach the individual to serve him/her self small portions and to take second helpings if desired

ANSWER: D   p. 638

28. A rule of thumb for apportioning vegetables for a preschool child is

K
- A. one hundred grams total.
- B. one-half cup per vegetable.
- C. one tablespoon for each year.
- D. one-fourth cup per vegetable.

ANSWER: C   p. 639

Chapter 18 Life Cycle Nutrition: Childhood, Adolescence, and Aging   7

29. Which of the following practices is NOT among the recommendations to help children develop an interest in vegetables?

K   A.   Serve vegetables warm, not hot
    B.   Serve vegetables separately on the plate
    C.   Serve vegetables undercooked and crunchy
    D.   Serve vegetables with the promise that after they are eaten, dessert will follow
    ANSWER: D   p. 639

30. Which of the following is NOT among the recommended methods for introducing new foods to children?

K   A.   Offer foods one at a time
    B.   Offer foods in small amounts
    C.   Create a pleasant eating atmosphere
    D.   Present the new food at the end of the meal
    ANSWER: D   p. 639

31. If a child is reluctant to try a new food, it is best to

K   A.   send the child to his/her room.
    B.   quietly remove it and try again at another time.
    C.   withhold dessert until all food on the plate is eaten.
    D.   encourage other family members to coax the child to eat it.
    ANSWER: B   p. 639-640

32. Even in preschoolers whose habits are being established, existing dietary attitudes are relatively resistant to change. How should wise parents react?

K   A.   Be patient and persistent
    B.   Impose their own eating habits on the children
    C.   Exert continuous pressure to initiate good food habits
    D.   Wait until the children start school to initiate changes
    ANSWER: A   p. 639-640

33. The single most effective way to teach nutrition to children is by

AP A.   example.
    B.   punishment.
    C.   singling out only hazardous nutrition practices for attention.
    D.   explaining the importance of eating new foods as a prerequisite for dessert.
    ANSWER: A   p. 641

8   Chapter 18 Life Cycle Nutrition: Childhood, Adolescence, and Aging

34. Which of the following foods are LEAST likely to promote dental caries in children?

AP
A. Potato chips, pie, and cookies
B. Popcorn, pretzels, and corn chips
C. Chocolate milk and fruited yogurt
D. Fruit packaged in syrup and fruit juices
ANSWER: B   p. 641

35. What minimum fraction of the RDA for children 10-12 years of age should be provided by public school lunches?

K
A. 1/8
B. 1/4
C. 1/3
D. 1/2
ANSWER: C   p. 643

36. The adolescent growth spurt

K
A. affects the brain primarily.
B. decreases total nutrient needs.
C. affects every organ except the brain.
D. begins and ends earlier in girls than in boys.
ANSWER: D   p. 643

37. Which of the following is a characteristic of the adolescent period?

K
A. Obesity occurs more often in black females
B. Appetite for red meat increases in females to meet iron needs
C. Males need more nutrient-dense foods because of their faster development
D. Males are at greatest risk for calcium insufficiency due to high intake of soft drinks
ANSWER: A   p. 644

38. Approximately what fraction of an average teenager's daily energy intake is derived from snacks?

AP
A. 1/4
B. 1/3
C. 1/2
D. 2/3
ANSWER: A   p. 645

39. Users of hard drugs or narcotics face all of the following problems EXCEPT

AP
A. they tend to overeat during "high" periods.
B. they spend money for drugs rather than food.
C. they often have hepatitis, which causes taste changes.
D. they often develop infectious diseases which increase needs for nutrients.
ANSWER: A   p. 646

Chapter 18 Life Cycle Nutrition: Childhood, Adolescence, and Aging 9

40. What percentage of high school seniors report exposure to an illicit drug?

K   A. 10
     B. 30
     C. 60
     D. 95
ANSWER: C   p. 646

41. Which of the following is a characteristic of marijuana use?

K   A. Appetite for sweet foods is increased
     B. Regular use leads to excessive weight gain
     C. Smoking it dulls the sense of taste and smell
     D. The active ingredient is cleared from the body within 24 hours
ANSWER: A   p. 646

42. Associations between cigarette smoking and nutrition include all of the following EXCEPT

K   A. hunger sensations are blunted by smoking.
     B. smokers have lower body weights than nonsmokers.
     C. smokers degrade vitamin C faster than nonsmokers.
     D. there seem to be no foods that are protective against lung cancer.
ANSWER: D   p. 647

43. What is the life expectancy of males and females in the U.S.?

K   A. 65-70 years
     B. 71-78 years
     C. 79-84 years
     D. 85-89 years
ANSWER: B   p. 647

44. Which of the following is a proposed mechanism for energy restriction and improvement of longevity in animals?

K   A. Reduction of body fat level
     B. Increase in the metabolic rate
     C. Enhancement of lipid oxidation
     D. Acceleration of growth and development
ANSWER: A   p. 648

45. All of the following environmental factors are known to promote aging EXCEPT

AP A. exercise.
     B. diseases.
     C. lack of nutrients.
     D. extremes of heat and cold.
ANSWER: A   p. 649-650

10   Chapter 18   Life Cycle Nutrition: Childhood, Adolescence, and Aging

46. Studies of adults show that longevity is related, in part, to all of the following EXCEPT

K
    A. weight control.
    B. regularity of meals.
    C. short periods of sleep.
    D. no or moderate alcohol intake.
ANSWER: C   p. 649

47. What would be the physiological age of a 75-year old woman whose physical health is equivalent to that of her 50 year-old daughter?

AP
    A. 25 years
    B. 50 years
    C. 70 years
    D. 125 years
ANSWER: B   p. 649

48. What type of effect would best describe a theoretical 8-fold increase in the risk for cardiovascular disease for an obese person who smokes, despite the risk being just 2-fold each for smoking and obesity?

AP
    A. Genetic
    B. Synergistic
    C. Antagonistic
    D. Dual stressor
ANSWER: B   p. 649

49. Which of the following identifies a relationship between illness and genetics, fitness and stress?

K
    A. Cancer risk is influenced primarily by genetics
    B. Vascular diseases are influenced primarily by nutrition
    C. Exercise has a greater influence on death rate than does heredity, smoking, hypertension, or obesity
    D. Tolerance to physical stress increases with age, thereby enhancing the body's ability to resist certain fatal diseases
ANSWER: C   p. 649-650

50. What are the thickenings that occur to the lenses of the eye, thereby affecting vision, especially in the elderly?

K
    A. Keratoids
    B. Retinitis
    C. Cataracts
    D. Rhodopolids
ANSWER: C   p. 650-651

Chapter 18 Life Cycle Nutrition: Childhood, Adolescence, and Aging 11

51. What nutrients appear to be protective of cataract formation?

K   A. Iron and calcium
B. Chromium and zinc
C. Vitamin B_{12} and folate
D. Vitamin C and vitamin E
ANSWER: D   p. 651

52. Which of the following foods seems to aggravate arthritis in some people?

K   A. Milk
B. Iodized salt
C. Canned fruit
D. Refined cereals
ANSWER: A   p. 651

53. Which of the following types of diets has been shown to prevent or reduce arthritis inflammation?

K   A. High in simple sugars, low in canned fruit
B. High in animal protein, low in canned fruit
C. Low in polyunsaturated fat, high in oleic acid
D. Low in saturated fat, high in eicospentaenoic acid
ANSWER: D   p. 651

54. Which of the following describes the nutrient needs of older people?

K   A. They vary according to individual histories
B. They remain the same as in young adult life
C. They increase, therefore supplementation is required
D. They decrease for vitamins and minerals due to changes in body composition
ANSWER: A   p. 652

55. At what period in life does the body first become physically capable of reproduction?

AP   A. Puberty
B. Adolescence
C. Body fat level of 15-22%
D. Age 12 years in females and 14 years in males
ANSWER: A   p. 652-653

56. Factors to be considered in determining the RDA of elderly include all of the following EXCEPT

K   A. RDA should be aimed at maintenance of optimal functioning.
B. RDA should be aimed at levels that may prevent age-related diseases.
C. RDA should take into account the decreased intake of food in older people.
D. RDA should take into account medications that older people are likely to take.
ANSWER: D   p. 652-653

12   Chapter 18   Life Cycle Nutrition: Childhood, Adolescence, and Aging

57.   Which of the following is a feature of elderly people and water metabolism?

K   A.   They do not feel thirsty or recognize dryness of the mouth
      B.   They have a higher total body water content compared with younger adults
      C.   They show increased frequency of urination which results in higher requirements
      D.   They frequently show symptoms of overhydration such as mental lapses and disorientation
      ANSWER: A   p. 652

58.   Which of the following has been associated with regular physical activity in older adults?

K   A.   Retention of sodium
      B.   Increase in blood LDL
      C.   Improved muscle tone but not mobility
      D.   Decrease in frequency of nighttime urination
      ANSWER: D   p. 653

59.   Which of the following describes food preferences of the elderly?

K   A.   About 95% enjoy fruit
      B.   About 20% eat no vegetables
      C.   About 90% dislike all vegetables
      D.   About 60% refrain from eating fruit
      ANSWER: B   p. 653

60.   A condition that increases the likelihood of iron deficiency in older people is

AP   A.   lack of intrinsic factor.
      B.   loss of iron due to more frequent running activity.
      C.   blood loss from yearly physical testing procedures.
      D.   poor iron absorption due to reduced stomach acid secretion and/or use of antacids.
      ANSWER: D   p. 654

61.   Which of the following statements describes one aspect of mineral nutrition of older adults?

K   A.   Zinc intake is adequate for about 95% of this group
      B.   Calcium intakes of females are near the RDA for this group
      C.   Iron-deficiency anemia in this population group is less common than in younger adults
      D.   Calcium allowances for this group have recently been increased by the Committee on Dietary Allowances
      ANSWER: C   p. 654

Chapter 18 Life Cycle Nutrition: Childhood, Adolescence, and Aging   13

62. Older people should probably take vitamin and mineral supplements when their daily energy intake first drops below

K   A.   1000 kcal.
    B.   1200 kcal.
    C.   1500 kcal.
    D.   2000 kcal.
    ANSWER: C   p. 655

63. Characteristics associated with the use of nicotine gum as a antismoking aid include all of the following EXCEPT

K   A.   it is successful only 25% of the time.
    B.   side effects include nausea and hiccups.
    C.   the nicotine is absorbed primarily from the mouth.
    D.   alkaline foods interfere with absorption of the nicotine.
    ANSWER: D   p. 655

64. Aspirin is best known to alter the requirements or utilization of

K   A.   iron and folate.
    B.   zinc and chromium.
    C.   biotin and cobalamin.
    D.   calcium and phosphorus.
    ANSWER: A   p. 656

65. Goals of the federal Nutrition Program for the elderly include the provision of all of the following EXCEPT

K   A.   transportation services.
    B.   high-cost nutritious meals.
    C.   opportunity for social interaction.
    D.   counseling and referral to other social services.
    ANSWER: B   p. 657

66. Studies of the eating habits of older adults demonstrate all of the following EXCEPT

K   A.   more men than women had poor-quality diets.
    B.   adults living alone consumed insufficient amounts of food.
    C.   malnutrition was associated with a lower level of education.
    D.   men living with spouses ate higher quality diets than men living alone.
    ANSWER: A   p. 657

14   Chapter 18   Life Cycle Nutrition: Childhood, Adolescence, and Aging

67. Which of the following is a characteristic of caffeine in nutrition?

K   A. It increases the risk of ulcer development
B. It diminishes the utilization of vitamin B_{12}
C. It is a suspected cause of anxiety in some people
D. It enhances the action of adenosine resulting in a worsening of chest pain in people with heart disease
ANSWER: C   p. 661-663

68. Which of the following is NOT a common source of caffeine for people?

K   A. Diuretics
B. Pain relievers such as Dristan
C. Sodas such as 7-Up and orange
D. Weight-loss aids such as Dexatrim
ANSWER: C   p. 661-662

69. All of the following are dietary sources of caffeine EXCEPT

K   A. cola.
B. coffee.
C. legumes.
D. chocolate.
ANSWER: C   p. 662

70. What is the standard chemical used to remove caffeine from coffee beans?

K   A. Nitric acid
B. Sodium propionate
C. Methylene chloride
D. Polybrominated biphenyl
ANSWER: C   p. 663

71. All of the following are used to decaffeinate coffee beans EXCEPT

K   A. water.
B. nitric oxide.
C. ethyl acetate.
D. methylene chloride.
ANSWER: B   p. 663

Essay Questions

632-633   72. Discuss the effects of food allergies and food intolerance on nutritional status.

Chapter 18 Life Cycle Nutrition: Childhood, Adolescence, and Aging   15

634-635   73.   Give examples of how nutrient deficiencies affect behavior in children.

639-640   74.   Explain the appropriate procedure for introducing new foods to children.

645   75.   Describe the typical eating patterns of teenagers and suggest appropriate changes to foster better eating habits.

646-647   76.   List 6 nutrition problems associated with drug abuse.

649-650   77.   Discuss the roles of genetics, fitness, and stress on longevity.

651   78.   Explain the relationship between diet and arthritis treatment. List at least 8 foods or nutrients that are known to have no beneficial effects on arthritis.

16   Chapter 18 Life Cycle Nutrition: Childhood, Adolescence, and Aging

652-655   79.   Give several reasons for the decline in nutritional status consequent to aging.

653-654   80.   List nutrients of special consideration for older adults and present reasons for their concern.

654   81.   List the factors that increase iron deficiency in older adults.

661-663   82.   a.   Describe the association between caffeine intake and disease.

              b.   List major sources of caffeine intake.

CHAPTER 19
NUTRITION AND ILLNESS

MULTIPLE CHOICE

Objective 1 Describe the relationship between illness and nutritional status.

1. Stress is defined by Whitney, Catalado, and Rolfes as:

K   A.   emotional strain.
       B.   an alteration in homeostasis.
       C.   any threat to a person's well-being.
       D.   a defense response to illness.
       ANSWER: C   p. 667

2. Sources of stress can be:

K   A.   infections.
       B.   a check-up.
       C.   a pleasant experience.
       D.   all of the above
       ANSWER: D   p. 667

Chapter 19 Nutrition and Illness

*3. Short term "stress" affects one's nutrition status by:

C   A.   increasing blood glucose levels.
      B.   increasing stores of glucagon.
      C.   burning fat.
      D.   using protein stores.
      ANSWER: A

Objective 2 Assess the primary and secondary effects of illness on nutritional status.

4. Illness can effect nutrition status by altering:

K   A.   appetite.
      B.   digestion.
      C.   metabolism.
      D.   all of the above
      ANSWER: D   p. 668

5. Illness can effect nutritional status by all of the following _except_:

K   A.   diminishing appetite to meet decreased metabolic needs.
      B.   causing nausea and vomiting.
      C.   causing food aversions.
      D.   altering renal excretion.
      ANSWER: A   p. 668

6. Individuals who are at risk for decubitus ulcers are those who are:

K   A.   overweight.
      B.   elderly.
      C.   hypoalbuminemic.
      D.   all of the above.
      ANSWER: D   p. 669

OBJECTIVE 3 Describe how appropriate nutrition status and nutrition support can affect the outcome of an illness.

7. An individual with protein energy malnutrition, receiving a clear liquid diet, is at risk for all of the following _except_:

K   A.   delayed wound healing.
      B.   infectious diseases.
      C.   decubitus ulcers.
      D.   increase in muscle mass.
      ANSWER: D   p. 670

Chapter 19 Nutrition and Illness

OBJECTIVE 4 Discuss the synergistic cycle that can occur with illness, poor nutrition, and an impaired immune status.

8. Delivery of nutrients directly into the gastrointestinal tract:

K
- A. prevents malnutrition.
- B. provides antibodies.
- C. prevents diarrhea.
- D. preserves the intestinal barrier.

ANSWER: D   p. 676

9. Factors that can impair the immune system are all of the following *except*:

K
- A. stress.
- B. malnutrition.
- C. disease.
- D. E coli in the lower GI tract.

ANSWER: D   p. 667

10. Enteral feeding is preferable to parenteral feeding for all of the following *except*:

K
- A. it is associated with fewer serious complications.
- B. it encourages translocation of microbes.
- C. it is less expensive.
- D. it is less invasive.

ANSWER: C   p. 676

11. T-cells are vital in the immune process because they:

K
- A. produce antibodies.
- B. destroy specific antigens.
- C. are part of the cells' secretions.
- D. provide the first line of defense.

ANSWER: B   p. 674

OBJECTIVE 5 Describe common drug-nutrient interactions.

12. Which of the following individuals is *least* likely to experience a drug-nutrient interaction?
AP/AN
- A. A 56 year old using nystatin, an anti-fungal agent
- B. a 40 year old on a multi-drug regimen for hypertension
- C. A 26 year old taking isoniazid (INH) for tuberculosis
- D. A 37 year old taking astenizole (Hismanal) for allergies

ANSWER: A   p. 677, 678

4   Chapter 19 Nutrition and Illness

13. Clients taking methotrexate and pyrimethamine can develop a deficiency of:

AP   A.   protein
        B.   tyramine
        C.   folate
        D.   vitamin K
        ANSWER: C   p. 680

14. Mrs. George has hypoalbuminemia. Since she is on several drugs you are concerned for all of the following reasons *except*:

C   A.   more free drug will be stored in the spleen.
       B.   excess free drug may result in an exaggerated effect.
       C.   decreased free drug may result in a reduced effect.
       D.   with normal therapeutic doses she may have symptoms of toxicity.
       ANSWER: D   p. 676

15. Tetracycline should not be taken with milk products or antacids because:

K   A.   protein inhibits absorption of the drug.
       B.   milk and antacids increase gastric motility, thereby increasing absorption.
       C.   milk and antacids decrease gastric motility causing buildup of the drug.
       D.   minerals in these products bind with the drug molecules and decrease absorption.
       ANSWER: D   p. 678

For question 16:
Mr. Coats is taking warfarin (Coumadin). When you take a dietary history you note that he eats large amounts of bananas, oranges, liver, and oatmeal.

16. Which of these foods could contribute to a food and drug interaction?
AP/AN
       A.   Bananas
       B.   Oranges
       C.   Liver
       D.   Oatmeal
       ANSWER: C   p. 359, 679

17. Which of the following foods would be appropriate for a client on a MAO inhibitor?

AP   A.   Green peppers
       B.   Cheddar cheese
       C.   Sausage
       D.   Chocolate
       ANSWER: A   p. 679

Chapter 19 Nutrition and Illness

*18. Clients taking lithium should:

    C   A. have a high sodium intake.
           B. have a low sodium intake.
           C. have a constant sodium intake.
           D. not regulate sodium intake.
           ANSWER: C   Appendix E

19. Clients taking warfarin should not increase their intake of:

    C   A. calcium.
           B. carbohydrate.
           C. vitamin K.
           D. protein.
           ANSWER: C   p.679

20. Aspirin can affect the body's use of which of the following vitamins?

    K   A. A
           B. C
           C. Folate
           D. Pyridoxine
           ANSWER: C   p.680

21. Calcium can do which of the following?

    K   A. decrease absorption of a drug by altering gastric pH.
           B. decrease absorption of a drug by binding with drug molecules.
           C. delay absorption of a drug.
           D. displace a drug from plasma protein carriers.
           ANSWER: B   p. 677

22. Antacids can interfere with absorption of:

    K   A. iron.
           B. aluminum.
           C. folate.
           D. monoamines.
           ANSWER: A   p. 678

23. A client taking griseofulvin should be asked if he takes it with food because food:

           A. enhances the absorption of griseofulvin.
           B. delays the absorption of griseofulvin.
           C. increases the metabolism of griseofulvin.
           D. increases the risk of diarrhea.
           ANSWER: A   p. 677

6   Chapter 19   Nutrition and Illness

24. An effect of amphetamines is to:

K
   A. diminish appetite.
   B. increase saliva.
   C. enhance food intake.
   D. diminish food allergies.
   ANSWER: A   p. 677

OBJECTIVE 6 Discuss the impact nonprescription drugs have on nutritional status.

25. Which of the following non-prescription drugs is *least* likely to affect a person's nutritional status?

K
   A. Bulk forming laxatives
   B. Aspirin
   C. Antihistamines
   D. Acetaminophen
   ANSWER: D   p. 678

OBJECTIVE 7 Discuss the role health care professionals have in identifying and preventing drug nutrient interactions.

26. When assessing a client for possible nutrient-drug interactions, the health care professional should consider the client's:

K
   A. age.
   B. diet and drug history.
   C. use of OTC drugs.
   D. all of the above
   ANSWER: D   p. 681

27. Which of the following statements would alert you that a client needs teaching regarding food/drug interactions?

AP
   A. "A glass of wine before dinner stimulates my appetite."
   B. "I always take my tetracycline with a glass of chocolate milk."
   C. "Since I'm taking birth control pills I take a multivitamin."
   D. "Since I take warfarin (Comadin), I watch my intake of vitamin K."
   ANSWER: B   p. 677

OBJECTIVE 8 Plan interventions to alleviate eating problems associated with hospitalized adults and children.

28. Strategies to help sick children eat include all of the following except:

K   A. letting the child eat with other children.
      B. serving small portions.
      C. arranging for procedures to be done right after mealtime.
      D. encouraging the child to eat foods high in nutrients first.
      ANSWER: C   p. 688

For question 29:
Mrs. Garza is two days post-operative. She has been eating approximately 50% of her bland diet for the past two days.

29. Which of the following interventions should you try first to encourage increased food intake?

AN   A. have Mrs. Garza's family bring food from home.
       B. encourage Mrs. Garza to select foods she like from the diet menu.
       C. have Mrs. Garza eat alone so she can eat in a peaceful atmosphere.
       D. give Mrs. Garza IM pain medication 30 min prior to meals.
       ANSWER: B   p. 683

30. Hospitalized clients may complain about their food for all of the following reasons *except*:

      A. to vent fear and frustration.
      B. to exercise some control.
      C. the food is different from what they are used to.
      D. hospital food is prepared several days before it is served.
      ANSWER: D   p. 683

CHAPTER 20
NUTRITION AND SEVERE STRESS

MULTIPLE CHOICE

Objective 1 Compare and contrast the metabolic effects of starvation vs stress.

1. The role of glucagon in physiological stress is to:

K   A.   promote storage of amino acids.
      B.   stimulate triglyceride synthesis.
      C.   increase fluid retention.
      D.   stimulate gluconeogenesis
      ANSWER: D   p.694

2. During stress, which of the following physiological responses would be expected?

K   A.   Hypoglycemia
      B.   Decrease in calorie requirements
      C.   Negative nitrogen balance
      D.   Sodium depletion
      ANSWER: C   p.695

2   Chapter 20 Nutrition and Severe Stress

3. Which of the following physiological stressors lowers kcal requirements?

K   A.   Elective surgery
     B.   Infection
     C.   Fasting
     D.   Soft tissue trauma
     ANSWER: C   p.695

4. Mr. Smith is a 50 year old man who sustained multiple broken bones in a car accident. Upon assessment he is hyperglycemic and edematous. The health care professional should:

    A.   call the physician.
    B.   suspect undiagnosed diabetes.
    C.   institute a low kcal, low sodium diet.
    D.   recognize these signs are associated with stress.
    ANSWER: D   p.695

5. The predominant source of endogenous glucose during severe stress is:

K   A.   amino acids.
     B.   glycerol.
     C.   free fatty acids.
     D.   ketones.
     ANSWER: A   p.693

Objective 2 Discuss the effects of severe stress on an individual with protein-energy malnutrition (PEM).

6. Which of the following systems is among the first to suffer the effects of PEM?

K   A.   Skin
     B.   GI tract
     C.   Kidney
     D.   Cardiac
     ANSWER: B   p.697

For question 7:
Mr. Watson is a 50 year old man who is 5'10" and weighs 145 lbs. He has lost 25 lbs. over the past month and reports "not wanting to eat after his wife died." His serum albumin is 4.0 g/dl and his total lymphocyte count is normal.

7. Which subtype of PEM is suggested by these assessment data?

AP   A.   Chronic malnutrition/marasmus
       B.   Acute malnutrition/kwashiorkor
       C.   Mixed malnutrition
       D.   No malnutrition identified
ANSWER: A   p. 699

8. Which of the following is an expected finding in acute malnutrition/kwashiorkor?

K   A.   Significant weight loss
     B.   Depleted body fat evidenced by decrease in tricep skinfold
     C.   Depleted somatic protein evidenced by a decrease in midarm muscle mass
     D.   Decrease in serum albumin
ANSWER: D   p. 699

9. Of the following, the person suffering a severe stress at greatest risk for dying while hospitalized is someone with the diagnosis of?

K   A.   kwashiorkor.
     B.   marasmus.
     C.   kwashiorkor/marasmus.
     D.   none of the above.
ANSWER: C   p. 698

Objective 3 Outline the nutritional needs during stress.

10. The initial task for the health care team for a client under major stress is to:

     A.   institute total parenteral nutrition to prevent negative nitrogen balance.
     B.   place a nasogastric tube to begin enteral nutrition support.
     C.   restore fluid and electrolyte balance.
     D.   calculate calorie needs via indirect calorimetry.
ANSWER: C   p. 700

4   Chapter 20   Nutrition and Severe Stress

11. An estimate of the non-protein kcal needs of a 70 kg man who has undergone bypass surgery would be:

AP A. 1525-1700
    B. 1750-2100
    C. 2450-2800
    D. 2950-3175
    ANSWER: B   p. 700

12. How many grams of protein would a 120 lb. woman require after major physiological stress?

AP A. 55-80
    B. 82-109
    C. 156-173
    D. 180-240
    ANSWER: B   p. 701

13. High levels of which fatty acid suppress the immune system?

C   A. Linoleic
    B. Stearic
    C. Linolenic
    D. Oleic
    ANSWER: A   p. 701

14. To improve the intake of clients with stress induced anorexia, health care professionals should do all of the following *except*:

    A. serve a variety of foods.
    B. increase activity.
    C. administer IV dextrose.
    D. provide easy to eat high kcal foods.
    ANSWER: C   p. 702

Objective 4 Analyze the barrier associated with nutrient delivery during stress.

15. In many cases, feeding directly into the small intestine immediately post-stress is:

AP A. contraindicated, as stress decreases GI motility.
    B. dangerous, as the risk of aspiration is high.
    C. avoided, as it is very expensive.
    D. advantageous, as it prevents gut atrophy.
    ANSWER: D   p. 703

16. Of the following groups of foods, which is *most* appropriate on a clear liquid diet?

C
- A. Chicken broth, custard, jello
- B. Apple juice, lemonade, ice cream
- C. Strained oatmeal, custard, hard candy
- D. Coffee, broth, popsicle

ANSWER: D   p. 704

For question 17:
Mrs. Cousins is a 56 year old who had an uncomplicated hip replacement yesterday and complains of severe pain. Her lab work is WNL. She is 5'6" and weighs 145 lbs. She is receiving 5% glucose in NS. Her oral nutrition intake for the last two days has been minimal. Because of sedation, oral intake is anticipated to remain low.

17. The most appropriate nutritional intervention for her now would be:

AP
- A. supplemental formula.
- B. high protein shakes.
- C. tube feedings or parenteral nutrition.
- D. low-fiber diet.

ANSWER: A   p. 702

18. Barriers to adequate nutrition during severe stress can include all of the following *except*:

K
- A. decreased energy.
- B. pain.
- C. increased GI motility.
- D. anorexia.

ANSWER: C   p. 702

Objective 5 Outline a nutrition strategy to help prevent refeeding syndrome associated with PEM.

19. Which of the following diets would prevent refeeding syndrome in a client who has PEM?

K
- A. High-kcalorie, moderate-carbohydrate, low-sodium, lactose-free
- B. High-kcalorie, high-protein, moderate-carbohydrate
- C. Low-kcalorie, moderate-carbohydrate, low-sodium, lactose-free
- D. Low-kcalorie, high potassium, high-carbohydrate

ANSWER: C   p. 706

Chapter 20 Nutrition and Severe Stress

For question 20:
Jane Smith is a 55 year old black woman. She has had an appendectomy and her diet order is "as tolerated". As she is advanced to a full liquid diet, she complains of gas, cramping, bloating and diarrhea.

20. Based on her symptoms, the health care professional should:
AP/AN
    A.   recommend total parenteral nutrition.
    B.   recommend enteral nutrition.
    C.   provide a lactose-free full liquid diet.
    D.   explain that her stomach will adjust.
    ANSWER: C   p. 705

For question 21:
Jill Merwin is a 21 year old woman with a history of anorexia nervosa admitted to the intensive care unit with an abdominal gunshot wound. She is 5'2" and weighs 81 lbs. Following resuscitation, her diet order is for a 3500 kcal, high-carbohydrate, high-protein, formula to be delivered by vein.

21. Jill's most likely response to this diet will be:

AP   A.   rapid recovery.
        B.   boredom with the type of food.
        C.   the refeeding syndrome.
        D.   constipation.
        ANSWER: C   p. 706

Objective 6 Design a plan to meet the nutrient needs of clients experiencing the following stressors:
        Infection/Fever
        Trauma
        Organ Transplant
        Burn

For question 22:
Bill Martin is a 33 year old accountant recently hospitalized for meningitis. Prior to admission, Bill ate a well-balanced diet, exercised regularly and donated blood through his corporate program. Upon admission his hematocrit is 33 and his hemoglobin is 9. He also had a decreased mean corpuscular volume, confirming iron (microcytic) anemia.

22. The health care professional should expect that:

AP   A.   an iron supplement will be ordered to raise his hemoglobin.
        B.   folate and B_{12} supplements will be ordered for macrocytic anemia.
        C.   iron supplements could worsen the meningitis.
        D.   a Schilling test will be ordered to rule out pernicious anemia.
        ANSWER: C   p. 707

Chapter 20 Nutrition and Severe Stress   7

23. Mr. Caldwell has had a kidney transplant. Which of the following statements indicates the need for further education?

AP
  A. "I plan to go out Saturday night for raw oysters."
  B. "I will wash my hands before I eat."
  C. "I will cook my meat to well done."
  D. "I will avoid homemade eggnog and Caesar salad."
  ANSWER: A   p. 711

24. A client with a 15% BSA burn should receive:

K
  A. total parenteral nutrition.
  B. tube feeding.
  C. a regular diet.
  D. a full liquid diet.
  ANSWER: C   p. 712

25. In general, clients with burns need supplements above the RDA of:

K
  A. thiamin and riboflavin.
  B. folic acid and pyridoxine.
  C. ascorbic acid and retinol.
  D. iron and magnesium.
  ANSWER: C   p. 713

26. A client with a temperature of 101.6° F has a increase in his/her BMR by:

K
  A. 26%.
  B. 21%.
  C. 13%.
  D. 7%.
  ANSWER: B   p. 700

27. An appropriate total parenteral nutrition solution for a stressed client provides:

K
  A. dextrose only.
  B. animo acids only.
  C. lipid and amino acids.
  D. dextrose, amino acids and lipids.
  ANSWER: D   p. 701

28. During the immediate post-burn period the treatment of an extensive burn focuses on:

K
  A. calculating the protein loss.
  B. providing IV dextrose for caloric support.
  C. replacing lost fluids and electrolytes.
  D. providing supplemental lipids.
  ANSWER: C   p. 711

CHAPTER 21
ENTERAL NUTRITION

MULTIPLE CHOICE

Objective 1 Compare and contrast the following nutritional formulas and their indications for use: blenderized, complete, hydrolyzed, intact, modular

1. Which one of the following formulas is *not* nutritionally complete?

K   A.   Hydrolyzed
       B.   Modular
       C.   Protein isolate
       D.   Polymeric
       ANSWER: B   p. 730

2. Which of the following formulas is usually *highest* in residue?

K   A.   Blenderized
       B.   Hydrolyzed
       C.   Monomeric
       D.   Polymeric
       ANSWER: A   p. 730

Chapter 21   Enteral Nutrition

3. The best method of nutrition support for a client with severe secretory diarrhea is often:

AP
   A.   blenderized food.
   B.   lactose free tube feeding.
   C.   intact or polymeric formula.
   D.   parenteral nutrition.
   ANSWER: D   p. 726

4. The best way to serve flavored liquid supplements is:

K
   A.   cold with a straw.
   B.   room temperature.
   C.   in the original container.
   D.   by a feeding tube.
   ANSWER: A   p. 725

5. Which of the following formulas has the greatest amount of free water?

C
   A.   1 kcal/ml
   B.   1.5 kcal/ml
   C.   1.5 kcal/ml, high protein
   D.   2.0 kcal/ml
   ANSWER: A   p. 736

Objective 2 Identify the indications and contraindications for enteral tube feeding.

For question 6:
Mr. Heiman has multiple sclerosis with dysphagia. He is 5'8" and weighs 127 lbs.

6. The most appropriate method of nutrition support for him would be:

AP
   A.   total parenteral nutrition.
   B.   peripheral parenteral nutrition.
   C.   liquid supplements.
   D.   gastrostomy feedings.
   ANSWER: D   p. 726

7. Tube feeding is preferable to intravenous feeding because it:

K
   A.   costs less.
   B.   maintains gut function.
   C.   may help prevent bacterial translocation.
   D.   does all of the above
   ANSWER: D   p. 727

Objective 3 Describe the selection criteria for a feeding tube.

For question 8:
Mr. Smith is 63 years old with Alzheimer's disease.

8. He has an order for a feeding tube because he refuses to eat and is becoming malnourished. Which of the following feeding tubes would be a good choice?

AP/AN
    A. Nasogastric
    B. Nasoduodenal
    C. Gastrostomy
    D. Jejunostomy
    ANSWER: C   p. 727,729

9. Which of the following is the most appropriate feeding tube site for a 30 year old man with multiple sclerosis and severe dysphagia?

AP/AN
    A. Nasogastric
    B. Esophagostomy
    C. Gastrostomy
    D. Jejunostomy
    ANSWER: D   p. 729

Objective 4 Explain and interpret the assessment data that would be collected for a client on a tube feeding.

10. Daily assessment data to be collected on a client on a tube feeding should include all of the following *except*:

K   A. intake and output.
    B. weights.
    C. fat fold measurements.
    D. assessing breath sounds.
    ANSWER: C   p. 739

For question 11:
Mr. Thomas is receiving an enteral feeding product at 60 cc/hr by continuous drip. At 2:00 pm it is time to hang additional feeding product since there are only 40 cc left in the feeding bag.

11. When you check the residual you note that there is 50 cc of gastric contents, and so you should:

AN   A. stop the feeding and contact the physician.
    B. stop the feeding, irrigate the tube and then contact the physician.
    C. continue the feeding but decrease the rate to 50 cc/hr.
    D. continue the feeding as ordered.
    ANSWER: D   p. 744

4   Chapter 21   Enteral Nutrition

For question 12:
Mr. Seymour is a 56 year old man with cancer who is 5'8" tall and weighs 130 lbs. His appetite has been poor and he is started on bolus feeding of a 1 kcal/ml formula. Within 24 hours he has increased his weight by 2.5 lbs.

12. The appropriate intervention is to:

AN   A.   realize he needs more calories.
     B.   recognize this represents a likely fluid gain.
     C.   change to intermittent feedings.
     D.   increase the protein content of his feeding.
     ANSWER: B   p. 736

Objective 5 Describe ways to identify and alleviate the complications of tube feedings and feeding tubes.

13. Prior to starting a tube feeding you should elevate the client's head at least 30° in order to:

K   A.   prevent aspiration.
     B.   prevent gastric distention.
     C.   promote client comfort.
     D.   facilitate feeding process by increasing gravity flow.
     ANSWER: A   p. 744

14. Possible complications of a nutritionally complete tube feeding include all of the following *except*:

K   A.   aspiration.
     B.   hypoproteinemia.
     C.   dehydration.
     D.   fluid overload.
     ANSWER: B   p. 743

For question 15:
Mr. Jones has a closed head injury and is comatose. He has been on a tube feeding for the last two weeks. At report the day nurse stated that he had clear vesicular breath sounds. At 5:00 pm you auscultate pulmonary crackles.

15. Possible causes for this finding are all of the following *except*:

AP   A.   aspiration pneumonia.
     B.   misplaced feeding tube.
     C.   prolonged bedrest.
     D.   hypernatremia.
     ANSWER: D   p. 743

Chapter 21 Enteral Nutrition

For question 16:
Claire Wilson is an 80 year woman on a tube feeding. Upon assessment, her blood pressure is 90/72, serum sodium 146 mEq/l and a potassium level of 5.6 mEq/l.

16. These findings indicate:

AP/AN
    A. hypertension.
    B. overhydration.
    C. hyponatremia.
    D. dehydration.
    ANSWER: D   p. 736

17. Possible causes of diarrhea in a tube fed client are all of the following *except*:

C   A. lactose.
    B. bacterial contamination.
    C. opiates.
    D. hypertonic solutions.
    ANSWER: C   p. 742

Objective 6 Describe how age and development influence the enteral feeding process.

For questions 18 and 19:
Joey Small is a one month old premature infant who is to receive tube feeding.

18. An appropriate choice of insertion for a feeding tube would be:

C/AP   A. nasogastric.
    B. orogastric.
    C. gastrostomy.
    D. jejunostomy.
    ANSWER: B   p. 738

19. Potential complications resulting from Joey's tube feeding could include all the following *except*:

C/AP   A. aspiration.
    B. delay in sucking development.
    C. decreased oxygenation.
    D. pump damage.
    ANSWER: D   pp. 737, 738

6   Chapter 21   Enteral Nutrition

For question 20:
Tom Teenager is a 15 year old who is eating some but must also receive enteral feeding for malnutrition associated with Crohn's disease.

20.   To help Tom carry on normal activities, the health care team might try:

AP   A.   Bolus feedings.
       B.   feeding at night only.
       C.   neon colored feeding tube.
       D.   all of the above
       ANSWER: B   p. 738

Objective 7 Describe the steps associated with formula preparation and administration.

For question 21:
Mr. Thomas is receiving an enteral feeding product at 60 cc/hr by continuous drip. At 2:00 pm it is time to hang an additional feeding product since there is only 40 cc left in the feeding bag.

21.   If you decide to continue the feeding you should:

AP   A.   pour new feeding into the bag with the remaining 40 cc.
       B.   let the remaining feeding infuse prior to adding new product.
       C.   add 20 cc of feeding because your shift ends at 3:00 pm.
       D.   check your institutions policy regarding hang time.
       ANSWER: B   pp. 734,735

For question 22:
Mrs. Arthur is receiving an enteral feeding product that contains 1 kcal/cc at 60 cc/hr. She is not on fluid restrictions.

22.   How much additional water will she need each 24 hour period?

AP   A.   250 cc
       B.   775 cc
       C.   1276 cc
       D.   no additional water is need
       ANSWER: B   p. 736

For question 23:
Mr. Simpson is receiving 50 ml/hr of a 1 kcal/ml lactose free enteral product given by continuous infusion.

23.   How many milliliters water is Mr. Simpson receiving from the formula?

AP   A.   720
       B.   930
       C.   1020
       D.   1200
       ANSWER: C   p. 736

For question 24:
Mrs. Smith, a client with congestive heart failure, requires 2000 kcal/day. She is receiving a formula with 2 kcal/ml by continuous drip.

24. How many milliliters of formula will be given each hour?

AP   A.   33
        B.   42
        C.   66
        D.   83
ANSWER: B   p. 736

25. The delivery of up to 400 ml of formula within 10 minutes is termed:

K   A.   minimal residual.
      B.   intermittent feeding.
      C.   bolus feeding.
      D.   continuous drip.
ANSWER: C   p. 736

Objective 8   Describe the administration of medications via a feeding tube.

26. A client who would be the *least* likely to develop diarrhea on a tube feeding is one:

C   A.   with a serum albumin level of 4.0 g/dl
      B.   receiving potassium chloride
      C.   receiving an elixir diluted with sorbitol
      D.   taking magnesium containing antacids
ANSWER: A   pp. 742, 746

27. Which of the following nursing interventions is appropriate for the delivery of medications through a feeding tube?

    A.   Flush feeding tube with water before and after medication
    B.   Give only time release medications through the feeding tube
    C.   Discontinue the tube feeding every hour to enhance drug absorption
    D.   Rinse feeding tube with a solution of meat tenderizer and sterile water before and after medication is administrated
ANSWER: C   p. 745

CHAPTER 22
PARENTERAL NUTRITION

Objective 1 Identify the components of a parenteral nutrition solution

1. The protein in a TPN solution is primarily in the form of:

K   A. amino acids.
    B. protein hydrolysate.
    C. short chain fatty acids.
    D. intact protein.
    ANSWER: A   p. 753

2. If available, the advantage of using a lipid emulsion containing fish oils would be:

K   A. prevention of fat emboli.
    B. elevation of triglycerides.
    C. enhancement of immune system.
    D. increase in serum albumin.
    ANSWER: C   p. 754

3. Which of the following vitamins is *not* found in IV adult multivitamin solutions?

K   A. C
    B. D
    C. E
    D. K
    ANSWER: D   p. 754

1

Chapter 22 Parenteral Nutrition

Objective 2 Describe the selection criteria for using simple IV solutions versus total parenteral nutrition

4. The purpose of an IV of D_5W is to:

K   A.   provide adequate calories.
      B.   decrease the incidence of diarrhea.
      C.   provide fluid.
      D.   prevent aspiration.
      ANSWER: C   p. 755

5. A client receiving 3000 kcal per day via parenteral nutrition should:

K   A.   have it administered via peripheral vein.
      B.   receive dextrose and amino acids only.
      C.   have it administered in bolus form.
      D.   be given nutrition by the central venous route.
      ANSWER: D   p. 757

6. The purpose of short term infusion of simple IV solutions is all of the following *except*:

K   A.   maintain acid-base balance.
      B.   maintain fluid and electrolyte balance.
      C.   provide complete nutritional support.
      D.   provide fluid and kcal support.
      ANSWER: C   p. 755

For question 7:
Judy Smith is a 36 year old who just had a bowel resection. She is expected to be NPO for approximately seven days.

7. Which of the following would be appropriate nutrition support?

AP   A.   Peripheral total parenteral nutrition
       B.   Central total parenteral nutrition
       C.   Simple IV solutions with amino acids
       D.   Enteral feeding via nasogastric tube
       ANSWER: B   p. 756

Objective 3 Compare and contrast the indications for use of peripheral vs. central total parenteral nutrition

For question 8:
Susan Taylor is a 59 year old accountant who sustained multiple abdominal injuries in a motor vehicle accident. She is allergic to sulpha drugs, eggs and seafood.

8. Her nutritional needs will most likely be met by:

AP   A.   peripheral total parenteral nutrition.
      B.   central total parenteral nutrition.
      C.   peripheral total parenteral nutrition with fat emulsions.
      D.   central total parenteral nutrition with fat emulsions.
      ANSWER: B   p. 758

For question 9:
Joan Sussman is in her second trimester of pregnancy and has experienced hyperemesis gravidarum for 14 days.

9. At this point she is a candidate for:

AP   A.   peripheral total parenteral nutrition.
      B.   central total parenteral nutrition.
      C.   peripheral total parenteral nutrition with fat emulsion.
      D.   central total parenteral nutrition with fat emulsion.
      ANSWER: D   p. 758

Objective 4 Calculate the kcal and protein content of IV solutions

10. How many grams of amino acids would be provided to a client receiving 2,000 ml of a 5% amino acid solution?

AP   A.   50 gm
      B.   100 gm
      C.   200 gm
      D.   400 gm
      ANSWER: B   p. 756

11. The amount of kcal in 3 liters of D_5W is:

AP   A.   150.
      B.   510.
      C.   600.
      D.   660.
      ANSWER: B   p. 755

Chapter 22 Parenteral Nutrition

For question 12:
Mr. Adams is on a TPN solution containing 2000 kcal from dextrose and amino acids.

12. The addition of a lipid solution should provide *no* more than:

AP A. 80 kcal.
    B. 200 kcal.
    C. 400 kcal.
    D. 1000 kcal.
    ANSWER: D   p. 754

Objective 5 Explain the possible TPN complications and related interventions

13. Which of the following nursing interventions is *not* indicated for a client receiving TPN?

C   A. Monitor weights
    B. Maintain I & O records
    C. Speed up the flow rate if the solution gets behind to meet the day's volume
    D. Check blood glucose
    ANSWER: C   p. 759

For question 14:
Mr. Rodriguez has been stable on a standard TPN solution for three weeks. During this time his blood glucose has been 150 mg/dl. You check his blood glucose at 10:00 am and it is 240 mg/dl.

14. The most likely explanation is:
AP/AN
    A. the dextrose in the TPN solution.
    B. hypocalcemia.
    C. refeeding syndrome.
    D. infection
    ANSWER: D   p. 760

15. Which of the following measurements should be done daily for a client receiving TPN?

K   A. Weights
    B. Serum calcium
    C. Serum ammonia
    D. CBC
    ANSWER: A   p. 761

Chapter 22 Parenteral Nutrition   5

For question 16:
Sue Watson is receiving 3 liters of a standard TPN solution with 500 ml of a 10% IV lipid emulsion to be hung piggyback three times per week. As the lipid emulsion is being infused for the first time, Ms. Watson becomes chilled and begins wheezing.

16. The *most* appropriate intervention is to:

AP   A.   continue the TPN and the emulsion as this is a normal and temporary reaction.
       B.   continue the TPN and emulsion but call the doctor *stat*.
       C.   remove the TPN and the emulsion and notify the doctor when he arrives in 30 minutes.
       D.   continue the TPN, remove the emulsion and call the doctor *stat*.
       ANSWER: D   p. 754

For question 17:
Mary Jones, a 69 year old diabetic, has been receiving TPN with fat emulsions. She complains of a backache, chills, nausea and chest pain.

17. The *most* likely cause of these symptoms is:

       A.   an infection.
       B.   hypoglycemia.
       C.   hyperglycemia.
       D.   a reaction to the fat emulsions.
       ANSWER: D   p. 754

18. The benefits of cyclic infusion of TPN include:

K   A.   maintenance of high insulin levels.
      B.   increase in fat stores.
      C.   use of body fat for energy.
      D.   achievement of a negative nitrogen balance.
      ANSWER: C   p. 760

Objective 6 Review the special concerns associated with the administration of parenteral nutrition in infants and children

For question 19:
Courtney Troxclair, age three months, has necrotizing enterocolitis. Prior to initiation of TPN blood tests show:

     total protein 7.5 g/dl
     blood urea nitrogen 10 mg/dl
     blood glucose 80 mg/dl
     hematocrit of 44%
     bilirubin 5 mg/dl

6   Chapter 22   Parenteral Nutrition

19. Based on these findings the TPN solution should contain low levels of:

AN A. dextrose.
    B. amino acids.
    C. lipids.
    D. iron.
    ANSWER: C   p. 754

20. Risks for premature infants receiving TPN are due to their:

K   A. inability to concentrate serum ammonia.
    B. immature organ systems.
    C. low body water volume.
    D. increased membrane permeability.
    ANSWER: B   p. 761

21. Which of the following would be the *best* method of delivery of long-term TPN to a 14 year old?

C   A. Cyclic infusion
    B. Peripheral total parenteral infusion
    C. Central total parenteral infusion
    D. Central total parenteral infusion with lipids five times a week
    ANSWER: A   pp. 760-761

Objective 7 Explain the transition process associated with the discontinuation of TPN

For question 22:
Greg Thomas is a twelve year old who is being weaned off of TPN. In addition to TPN Greg is on a soft diet. Greg is 5'2" weighs 110 lbs. His caloric count reveals he is consuming 1700 kcal/dl.

22. Which intervention is appropriate at this time?

AP A. The TPN should be discontinued.
    B. Oral feeding should be doubled.
    C. Enteral feeding should be considered.
    D. TPN should be increased to provide an additional 1100 kcal.
    ANSWER: A   p. 762

23. When long term TPN is discontinued, oral feedings are gradually reintroduced because of all of the following reasons *except*:

K   A. intestinal villi may have shrunk.
    B. malabsorption may occur.
    C. bloating may occur.
    D. albumin levels may have dropped.
    ANSWER: D   pp. 747,762

Objective 8 Discuss the unique challenge of delivering and monitoring parenteral nutrition in the community setting

24. An advantage to cyclic parenteral infusion often used in home parenteral programs is:

K   A. a decrease in the cost of solution.
     B. the elimination of the need for a pump.
     C. a decrease in the incidence of fatty infiltration of the liver.
     D. the ease with which clients can prepare IV solutions.
     ANSWER: C   p. 759

25. Which of the following clients would *not* be a candidate for in-home cyclic TPN?

K   A. An 86 year old with congestive heart failure
     B. A 36 year old with Crohn's disease
     C. A 52 year old with cancer
     D. An 18 year old with radiation enteritis
     ANSWER: A   p. 758, 764

CHAPTER 23
NUTRITION AND DISORDERS OF THE UPPER GI TRACT

Objective 1 Describe the rationale and dietary therapy required for clients with chewing difficulties.

1. A client with difficulties with chewing are usually started on a:

K   A.   mechanical soft diet.
       B.   enteral feedings.
       C.   pureed diet.
       D.   full liquid diet.
ANSWER: A   p. 775

2. A technique to help ease the task of chewing is:

K   A.   providing fluids with the meal.
       B.   limiting fluids during the meal.
       C.   serving cold foods.
       D.   limiting sugars in the diet.
ANSWER: A   p. 776

3. Which of the following foods would be best for a client with problems chewing?

C   A.   Roast beef, green salad, and an apple
       B.   Casserole, mashed potatoes, and canned peaches
       C.   Swiss steak, new potatoes, and fresh fruit cup
       D.   Baked chicken, garden salad, carrot sticks, and apple pie
ANSWER: B   p. 776

Chapter 23 Nutrition & Disorders of the Upper GI Tract

4. Of the following menus, which is the most appropriate for a client with mouth ulcers?

AP/AN
- A. Orange juice, toast, scrambled eggs
- B. Tomato juice, chef's salad with Italian dressing
- C. Cottage cheese, sliced peaches, banana bread
- D. Chicken broth, jello, grapefruit juice

ANSWER: C   p. 776

Objective 2 Discuss the conditions commonly associated with dysphagia and the appropriate dietary therapy.

5. Of the following, the best choice for enteral feeding of a client with dysphagia is:

AN
- A. nasogastric.
- B. gastrostomy.
- C. jejunostomy.
- D. orogastric.

ANSWER: C   p. 778

6. All of the following conditions may lead to dysphagia *except*:

AP
- A. head injury.
- B. brain tumor.
- C. AIDS.
- D. T7 fracture.

ANSWER: D   p. 777

7. Signs and symptoms of dysphagia include:

K
- A. drooling.
- B. weight loss.
- C. refusing to swallow food.
- D. all of the above

ANSWER: D   p. 777

8. Which of the following beverages is most appropriate for a client with dysphagia?

AP
- A. Water
- B. Chicken broth
- C. Iced tea
- D. Pear nectar

ANSWER: D   p. 776

Chapter 23 Nutrition & Disorders of the Upper GI Tract 3

For question 9:
The home health care nurse is visiting Paul Cantu, a 82 year old man, recovering from a stroke. Upon assessment, the nurse observes that Mr. Cantu has lost weight, frequently clears his throat and exhibits drooling.

9. The nurse should suspect:

AP   A.   reduced saliva flow.
          B.   dysphagia.
          C.   reflux esophagitis.
          D.   peptic ulcer disease.
          ANSWER: B   p. 777

10. Which of the following clients is likely to experience dysphagia?

AP   A.   A 38 year old pregnant woman
          B.   A 52 year old executive with heart burn
          C.   An 82 year old man with Alzheimer's disease
          D.   A 28 year old man with a hiatal hernia
          ANSWER: C   p. 777

Objective 3 Describe the role diet plays in the prevention and treatment of reflux esophagitis.

11. Interventions that can help eliminate distress from reflux esophagitis include:

K   A.   lying down for 30 minutes after meals.
        B.   fluid intake with meals.
        C.   small frequent feedings.
        D.   pureed diet.
        ANSWER: C   p. 779

12. Which of the following foods does *not* affect cardiac sphincter pressure?

C   A.   Chocolate
        B.   Sausage
        C.   Peppermint candy
        D.   Whole wheat bread
        ANSWER: D   p. 779

13. Management of reflux esophagitis includes all of the following *except*:

K   A.   neutralizing gastric acid.
        B.   giving a bland diet.
        C.   performing surgery.
        D.   dilating the esophageal sphincter.
        ANSWER: D   p. 779

Chapter 23 Nutrition & Disorders of the Upper GI Tract

For question 14:
Mrs. Nichol is 5'2", weighs 103 lbs., and suffers from a hiatal hernia. She smokes and occasionally drinks wine. Today she is being prepared for discharge.

14. Which of the following statements by Mrs. Nichol indicates the need for further discharge instructions?

C   A. "I should lose weight to reduce my symptoms."
     B. "I will avoid wine."
     C. "I will go to the lung association classes."
     D. "I will eat small, frequent meals."
     ANSWER: A   p. 779

Objective 4 Outline dietary and pharmacological interventions needed for management of:
     indigestion
     nausea and vomiting
     gastritis
     peptic ulcer disease

Indigestion
15. Which of the following foods is included on a low-fiber diet?

K   A. Pinto beans
     B. Granola
     C. Grapefruit sections
     D. Prune juice
     ANSWER: C   p. 782

16. Indigestion is also called:

K   A. dysphagia.
     B. dyspnea.
     C. dysgeusia.
     D. dyspepsia.
     ANSWER: D   p. 781

17. Which of the following menus best represent a low-fiber diet?

AP   A. Peanut butter & jelly sandwich, apple, and a doughnut
      B. Yogurt, carrots & celery sticks, and fresh raspberries
      C. Roast beef sandwich, banana, and apple juice
      D. Bean burrito, lettuce & tomato, and grape juice
      ANSWER: C   p. 782

Chapter 23 Nutrition & Disorders of the Upper GI Tract 5

Nausea & Vomiting

18. Dietary interventions for nausea include all of the following *except*:

K   A.   ice cream.
       B.   cold fluids.
       C.   dry toast.
       D.   small meals.
       ANSWER: A   p. 783

19. A client suffering from chronic nausea should eat:

C   A.   a hot breakfast in the morning.
       B.   tuna salad sandwich at lunch.
       C.   dry toast or crackers.
       D.   bagels with cream cheese.
       ANSWER   C   p. 783

Gastritis
For question 20:
Sam Evans has gastritis and has been experiencing nausea and vomiting for the last three days.

20. Appropriate management would include:

C   A.   liberal bland diet.
       B.   antacids.
       C.   simple IV therapy.
       D.   diet high in vitamin B_{12}.
       ANSWER: C   p. 784

Peptic ulcer

21. The dietary management of acute gastritis includes:

K   A.   avoiding antacids.
       B.   switching to decaffeinated coffee.
       C.   increasing aspirin for pain.
       D.   avoiding alcohol.
       ANSWER: D   p. 784

22. All of the following are used in the management of peptic ulcer disease *except*:

K   A.   histamine blockers.
       B.   antibiotics.
       C.   low-fiber diets.
       D.   antacids.
       ANSWER: C   p. 785

Chapter 23 Nutrition & Disorders of the Upper GI Tract

Objective 5 Outline common nutritional problems and related therapies associated with gastric surgery.

For question 23:
Mr. McInnis recently had a partial gastrectomy for peptic ulcer disease.

23. Which of the following statements suggests that he understands the dietary guidelines to prevent dumping syndrome?

C A. "I will eat ice cream for a snack."
  B. "I will drink fluids between meals."
  C. "I will avoid peanut butter."
  D. "I will have raisin bran for breakfast."
  ANSWER: B p. 788

24. The postgastrectomy diet includes:

K A. fluid with meals.
  B. refined carbohydrates.
  C. high in water insoluble fiber.
  D. an emphasis on fats and proteins.
  ANSWER: D pp. 787-788

25. Anemia after a gastrectomy is usually associated with all of the following <u>except</u>:

K A. blood loss.
  B. malnutrition.
  C. iron deficiencies.
  D. deficiency of vitamin B_6.
  ANSWER: D pp. 787-788

For question 26:
Mrs. Chang had gastric surgery six months ago. Since that time her diet has been advanced although she continues to experience dumping syndrome and frequent nausea and vomiting. Mrs. Chang's lab work reveals a hemoglobin of 14 g/dl and a hematocrit of 38%.

26. The most valid inference from these data is that Mrs. Chang has:

AN A. bleeding from the colon.
  B. steatorrhea.
  C. anemia.
  D. folate deficiency.
  ANSWER: C p. 791

Chapter 23 Nutrition & Disorders of the Upper GI Tract

27. A sign of dumping syndrome is:

K   A.   tachycardia.
      B.   hyperglycemia.
      C.   hypervolemia.
      D.   edema.
ANSWER: A   pp. 785-786

28. All of the following meet the guidelines for a post-gastrectomy diet *except*:

K   A.   liquids with meals.
      B.   decrease simple sugar.
      C.   small frequent meals.
      D.   pectin added to meals.
ANSWER: A   p. 787

29. Microcytic anemia may develop after a gastrectomy because:

K   A.   surgery alters B_{12} absorption.
      B.   folate rich foods are avoided.
      C.   iron is absorbed poorly.
      D.   lactose is absorbed poorly.
ANSWER: C   p. 787

30. Clients experiencing "blind loop syndrome" after gastric resection are most likely to exhibit:

K   A.   microcytic anemia.
      B.   steatorrhea.
      C.   scurvy.
      D.   hypoalbuminemia.
ANSWER: B   p. 789

CHAPTER 24
NUTRITION AND DISORDERS OF THE LOWER GI TRACT

Objective 1 Delineate the nutritional management of motility disorders such as diarrhea and irritable bowel syndrome.

For question 1:
Mrs. Johnson is a 36 year old female who enters the emergency room complaining of severe diarrhea of a four hour duration. Physical assessment findings reveal warm dry skin; decreased turgor; dry mucous membranes; and vital signs of T-99.6, P-104, R-24.

1. The nurse caring for Mrs. Johnson should:

AP   A.   recommend over the counter (OTC) antidiarrheal agents.
       B.   instruct Mrs. Johnson to remain NPO until the diarrhea subsides.
       C.   encourage a diet high in pectin.
       D.   evaluate for possible fluid and electrolyte replacement.
ANSWER: D   p. 799

2. Clients with irritable bowel syndrome should avoid foods such as nuts and apples because they:

AP   A.   contain raffinose and stachyose.
       B.   aggravate lactose intolerance.
       C.   have a high fat content.
       D.   promote rapid gastric emptying.
ANSWER: A   p. 798-799

2 Chapter 24 Nutrition & Disorders of the Lower GI Tract

3. Oral rehydration solutions used in the treatment of diarrhea contain:

K A. vitamins.
  B. minerals.
  C. protein.
  D. electrolytes.
  ANSWER: D p. 798

Objective 2 Describe the nutritional management of fat malabsorption.

4. How many servings of fat are allowed on a 35 gm fat-restricted diet?

K A. 0
  B. 1
  C. 2
  D. 3
  ANSWER: D p. 801

5. MCT oil is commonly used in malabsorption syndromes because:

K A. it is high in essential fatty acids.
  B. the absorption occurs in the large intestine.
  C. it does not require bile or pancreatic lipase for digestion and absorption.
  D. it can be delivered parenterally.
  ANSWER: C p. 802

6. Which of the following menus *best* meets the objectives of a low fat diet for a client with steatorrhea?

AP A. Tuna fish salad, crackers, ice cream, tea
  B. Baked chicken, macaroni and cheese, biscuits, milk
  C. Pork tenderloin, baked potato, applesauce, tea
  D. Sirloin steak, potato salad, broccoli augratin, milk
  ANSWER: C p. 801

7. Which is the *best* dessert for a client on a low fat diet?

C A. Pudding
  B. Ice milk
  C. Cherry pie
  D. Sherbert
  ANSWER: D p. 801

Chapter 24 Nutrition & Disorders of the Lower GI Tract

Objective 3 Analyze, with rationale, the appropriate management of conditions associated with malabsorption syndrome.

8. An ileostomy is characterized by:

K   A.   formed stool.
    B.   bloody drainage.
    C.   absence of the small intestine.
    D.   loss of fluid and electrolytes.
    ANSWER: D   p.811

9. An appropriate food for a client with celiac disease is:

C   A.   peanut butter and jelly sandwich.
    B.   oatmeal cookies.
    C.   applesauce.
    D.   cheese and crackers.
    ANSWER: C   p. 813

10. Short gut syndrome commonly results in:

C   A.   hyperglycemia.
    B.   hypocalcemia.
    C.   hypokalemia.
    D.   hyperphosphatemia.
    ANSWER: B   p. 810

11. The purpose of a nasogastric tube for a client with acute pancreatitis is:

K   A.   to provide clear liquids.
    B.   for suction.
    C.   for medication delivery.
    D.   to begin enteral support.
    ANSWER: B   p. 803

12. Serum amylase levels are monitored in clients with pancreatitis to:

AP A.   establish the presence of lactose intolerance.
    B.   assess pancreatic function.
    C.   improve protein status.
    D.   evaluate need for drug therapy.
    ANSWER: B   p. 803

Chapter 24 Nutrition & Disorders of the Lower GI Tract

13. The characteristics of diet therapy for pancreatitis include all the following *except*:

K   A. elimination of fat.
     B. monitoring of vitamin B_{12} status.
     C. serving of small frequent meals.
     D. avoidance of alcohol.
     ANSWER: A   p. 804

14. Patients diagnosed with chronic pancreatitis should be cautioned to avoid:

C   A. large meals, fatty foods, and alcohol.
     B. red meats, sweets, and complex carbohydrates.
     C. carbohydrates, low-fat dairy products, and coffee.
     D. high protein foods, food with a high sucrose content, and caffeine.
     ANSWER: A   p. 805

15. An indication for enteral tube feeding a client with cystic fibrosis is:

K   A. inadequate sodium chloride intake.
     B. the need for water miscible forms of fat soluble vitamins.
     C. weight loss than 85% of IBW.
     D. steatorrhea.
     ANSWER: C   p. 805

16. The most appropriate diet therapy for clients with cystic fibrosis is to:

K   A. reduce fat to less than 35 grams per day.
     B. supply missing enzymes.
     C. limit kcalories to 1200 per day.
     D. restrict sodium.
     ANSWER: B   p. 806

17. Which of the following enteral formulas is *most* appropriate for a client with Crohn's disease?

K   A. Polymeric
     B. Intact
     C. Hydrolyzed
     D. Modular
     ANSWER: C   p. 808

Chapter 24 Nutrition & Disorders of the Lower GI Tract

For question 18:
Hakeem is a 22 year old man with Crohn's disease. He is 5'8" and weighs 128 lbs. upon assessment, he has steatorrhea and reports "having gas and diarrhea" when he consumes milk.

18. Based on these data, his diet order should be high kcalorie, high protein and:

   A. iron restricted.
   B. fat and lactose restricted.
   C. folate and selenium enriched.
   D. no other restriction or enrichment.
   ANSWER: B   p. 809

19. Which of the following conditions results in fat malabsorption but with no need for a severe dietary fat restriction?

C A. Celiac disease
   B. Pancreatitis
   C. Cystic fibrosis
   D. Crohn's disease
   ANSWER: C   p. 805

20. Nutritional assessment of a client with Crohn's disease would include all of the following *except*:

C/AP A. serum albumin levels.
   B. hematocrit and hemoglobin levels.
   C. serum amylase
   D. serum iron levels.
   ANSWER: C   p. 808

21. Ulcerative colitis involves which section(s) of the gastrointestinal tract?

K A. Large intestine
   B. Small intestine
   C. Jejunum and rectum
   D. Biliary tract
   ANSWER: A   p. 809

22. Diet recommendations for a client with ulcerative colitis may include all of the following *except*:

K A. high fiber diet.
   B. high protein diet.
   C. high kcalorie diet.
   D. low fat diet.
   ANSWER: A   p. 809

Chapter 24 Nutrition & Disorders of the Lower GI Tract

For question 23:
Mrs. Jones has ulcerative colitis and is scheduled for surgery in two days. Her nutrition status has been deteriorating.

23. Which of the following therapies is recommended for nutritional support?

C   A. High-kcalorie, high-protein diet
      B. Enteral feedings
      C. Total parenteral nutrition
      D. Clear liquid diet
      ANSWER: C   p. 810

24. Which of the following substances is thought to stimulate adaptation of intestine after a small bowel resection?

K   A. Glutamine
      B. Raffinose
      C. Stachyose
      D. Oxalate
      ANSWER: A   p. 810

25. Immediately after intestinal surgery the primary nutritional effort should be to:

K   A. increase protein levels.
      B. replace fluids and electrolytes.
      C. provide kcalories.
      D. decrease gas formation.
      ANSWER: B   p. 811

For question 26:
Mrs. Ellis has celiac disease. She is 5'4" and weight 120 lbs. A nutritional assessment reveals recent poor compliance with a gluten-free diet and an albumin level of 2.8 gm/dl.

26. Mrs. Ellis' weight signals a future problem because she is:

AN   A. underweight for height.
      B. probably dehydrated.
      C. likely to go into tetany.
      D. probably edematous.
      ANSWER: D   p. 813

Objective 4 Describe the nutritional management of diverticular disease.

27. Which of the following foods would be the *least* appropriate for a person with diverticulosis?

K   A.   Whole-wheat bread
      B.   Low-fat milk
      C.   Raw carrots
      D.   Strawberries
      ANSWER: D   p. 815

28. Dietary recommendations for a person with diverticulosis include a:

K   A.   high-fiber diet.
      B.   gluten-restricted diet.
      C.   low-fat diet.
      D.   diet without restrictions.
      ANSWER: A   p. 815

29. Clients with diverticular disease should:

      A.   avoid foods with seeds.
      B.   avoid high fiber foods.
      C.   restrict fluids.
      D.   increase fiber content quickly.
      ANSWER: A   p. 815

CHAPTER 25
NUTRITION AND DISORDERS OF THE LIVER

Objective 1 Describe the metabolic alterations associated with hepatitis and the appropriate nutritional therapy.

1. A client with hepatitis who has persistent anorexia and nausea should be started on:

K   A.   parenteral nutrition.
      B.   enteral nutrition.
      C.   IV glucose solution.
      D.   a low protein diet.
ANSWER: B   p. 824

2. A client with a fatty liver is at risk for:

K   A.   heart disease.
      B.   diabetes.
      C.   intolerance to sun.
      D.   cirrhosis.
ANSWER: D   p. 824

Chapter 25 Nutrition and Disorders of the Liver

Objective 2 Discuss the physiological and metabolic consequences of cirrhosis and the necessary dietary alterations.

3. Which of the following findings would be unexpected in a client with cirrhosis?

K   A.   Portal hypertension
       B.   Esophageal varices
       C.   Hypoammonemia
       D.   Ascites
       ANSWER: C   p. 825

4. For a client with ascites, the nurse should expect a reduction of dietary:

K   A.   sodium.
       B.   potassium.
       C.   calcium.
       D.   magnesium.
       ANSWER: A   p. 826

5. The purpose for limiting animal protein in the diet of clients with cirrhosis is to decrease their blood levels of:

K   A.   ammonia.
       B.   nitrogen.
       C.   glucose.
       D.   cholesterol.
       ANSWER: A   p. 827

6. When signs and symptoms of hepatic encephalopathy appear the nurse should anticipate:

K   A.   an increase in dietary protein.
       B.   a restriction of protein intake.
       C.   the use of agents to slow peristalsis.
       D.   a reduction of dietary branch chain amino acids.
       ANSWER: B   p. 827

7. The purpose of lactulose in the medical treatment of hepatic encephalopathy is to:

K   A.   aid in milk digestion.
       B.   provide a source of fat soluble vitamins.
       C.   reduce serum ammonia levels.
       D.   elevate serum albumin levels.
       ANSWER: C   p. 827

Chapter 25 Nutrition and Disorders of the Liver   3

8. Which of these statements by an adult male with alcoholic cirrhosis of the liver indicates the greatest need for further education?

C   A.   "I will not eat a 8 oz. steak every night."
    B.   "I will eat hard candy and drink soft drinks for extra calories."
    C.   "I will limit my drinking to a glass of wine a few times per week."
    D.   "I will limit my sodium intake if I develop ascites."
    ANSWER: C   p. 829

9. Which food is highest in aromatic amino acids?

K   A.   Yogurt
    B.   Whole wheat bread
    C.   Green beans
    D.   Hamburger
    ANSWER: D   p. 829

10. Aromatic amino acids may be limited in the diets of clients with hepatic encephalopathy because they:

C   A.   reduce the synthesis of albumin.
    B.   elevate bilirubin levels.
    C.   may contribute to neurological decline.
    D.   cause a false positive on hemacult test for blood in the stool.
    ANSWER: C   p. 829

11. Clients in hepatic coma should receive:

C   A.   nothing by mouth.
    B.   100 grams of protein to regenerate albumin levels.
    C.   a polymeric, high nitrogen enteral products.
    D.   protein as dictated by neurological status.
    ANSWER: D   p. 830

12. Which of the following groupings approximates 40 grams of protein?

AP/ A.   8 oz. milk, 2 slices bread, 1 oz. meat
AN B.   5 oz. meat, 2 slices bread
    C.   1 egg, 1 oz. meat, 8 oz. milk, 1 slice bread
    D.   8 oz. milk, 8 oz. yogurt, 2 slices bread
    ANSWER: B   p. 830

13. Supplements of which vitamin decrease prothrombin time?

C   A.   A
    B.   D
    C.   K
    D.   E
    ANSWER: C   p. 830

Chapter 25 Nutrition and Disorders of the Liver

14. An alcoholic patient has an increased need for which of the following?

K
- A. Fats and potassium
- B. Vitamin C and sodium
- C. Protein and simple sugars
- D. B vitamins and magnesium

ANSWER: D   p. 830

15. Which of the following is the most appropriate snack for a patient with ascites?

C/AP
- A. Canned tomato soup
- B. Hard candy
- C. Potato chips
- D. Ham sandwich

ANSWER: B   p. 831-832

16. Which of the following diet orders would be appropriate for a client with esophageal varices?

C
- A. NPO
- B. High protein
- C. Soft
- D. Clear liquids

ANSWER: C   p. 833

17. Clients with poor nutrition status and bleeding esophageal varices should be provided with:

C
- A. duodenal tube feedings.
- B. a soft diet.
- C. parenteral nutrition.
- D. gastrostomy feedings.

ANSWER: C   p. 833

18. Which nutritional intervention should be encouraged for a client with cirrhosis and steatorrhea?

AP
- A. Increasing the intake of polyunsaturated fat
- B. Reducing calorie intake by 20%
- C. Limiting vitamin B intake per day
- D. Limiting fat intake

ANSWER   D   p. 830

Chapter 25 Nutrition and Disorders of the Liver 5

Objective 3 Calculate the kcal and protein requirements of clients with liver disease.

For question 19:
Jane Watson is a 40 year old woman suffering from cirrhosis. She is 5'4" and weighs 130 lbs.

19. What are her approximate daily calorie and protein requirements for optimal nutrition?

AP   A.   1200 calories
     B.   1800 calories
     C.   2000 calories
     D.   2200 calories
ANSWER: D   p. 830

20. What is Jane's protein requirement for optimal nutrition?

AP   A.   40-46 g
     B.   47-52 g
     C.   53-58 g
     D.   60-65 g
ANSWER: D   p. 830

Objective 4 Plan diets/meals for clients needing sodium restriction in liver disease.

21. Which of the following foods would be an appropriate choice on a 1000 mg sodium diet?

AP   A.   Instant oatmeal
     B.   Sauerkraut
     C.   Carrots
     D.   Tomatoes
ANSWER: D   p. 832

22. Which of the following would be the best choice for a client with ascites on a 2000 mg sodium diet?

AN   A.   Eggs, bacon, and toast with butter
     B.   Chicken salad sandwich, celery, and an orange
     C.   Barbecue chicken, canned mixed vegetables, and pumpkin pie
     D.   Shredded wheat cereal, 1% milk, and toast with butter
ANSWER: D   p. 832

23. Sodium levels for clients with ascites are restricted to:

K   A.   250-500 mg
    B.   501-750 mg
    C.   751-1000 mg
    D.   1000-2000 mg
ANSWER: D   p. 831

Chapter 25 Nutrition and Disorders of the Liver

24. Which of the following meals is *most* appropriate for clients with cirrhosis requiring a sodium restriction?

AN A. Roast beef, rice, zucchini, ice tea
    B. Ham sandwich, apple, milk
    C. Cheese omelette, toast with jelly, orange juice
    D. Turkey, beets, spinach salad with oil and vinegar, tea
    ANSWER: A   p. 832

25. On a 2 gram sodium diet the daily intake of regular milk is generally limited to:

C   A. 4 oz.
    B. 8 oz.
    C. 16 oz.
    D. 32 oz.
    ANSWER: C   p. 832

Objective 5 Describe the alterations in the nutritional assessment process seen in clients with disorders of the liver.

26. The **best** indicator that liver function is improving in a client with cirrhosis is:

K   A. weight gain.
    B. weight loss.
    C. increased abdominal girth.
    D. arm anthropometrics.
    ANSWER: B   p. 835

27. During hospitalization alcoholics need:

K   A. extra kcalories.
    B. low sodium diet.
    C. intravenous alcohol.
    D. extra fat.
    ANSWER: A   p. 835

CHAPTER 26
NUTRITION, DIABETES, AND HYPOGLYCEMIA

Objective 1 Differentiate between the pathophysiology of insulin-dependent and noninsulin-dependent diabetes mellitus.

1. People with IDDM need insulin because they:

K   A.   have become insulin resistant.
       B.   have developed hyperinsulinemia.
       C.   no longer synthesize insulin.
       D.   digest insulin with GI enzymes.
ANSWER: C   p. 844

2. All of the following conditions are present in diabetic clients with NIDDM except:

K   A.   being over age 40 at onset.
       B.   currently taking insulin.
       C.   being 20% over IBW.
       D.   no longer producing insulin.
ANSWER: D   p. 844, 845

Chapter 26 Nutrition, Diabetes, and Hypoglycemia

3. Which of the following *best* describes clients with NIDDM?

K   A. Usually lean
     B. Rapid onset of symptoms
     C. Weight loss needed
     D. Ketosis prone
     ANSWER: C   p. 845

4. The hallmark for NIDDM is:

K   A. insulin deficiency.
     B. insulin resistance.
     C. absence of receptor sites for insulin.
     D. beta cell exhaustion.
     ANSWER: B   p. 845

Objective 2 List the physiological tests that measure glucose control.

5. Glycosylated hemoglobin (A1C) can best described as a:

K   A. by-product of fat metabolism.
     B. a reflection of mean blood glucose concentration over two months.
     C. end-product of protein metabolism formed in the liver.
     D. summary of hemoglobin rates for Type I diabetes.
     ANSWER: B   p. 851

Objective 3 Plan a diet for a client with IDDM.

6. Which of the following foods is considered a meat exchange on a diabetic diet?

K   A. Bacon
     B. Peanuts
     C. Ham
     D. Yogurt
     ANSWER: C   p. 36-43

7. Which of the following foods is *not* found in the vegetable exchange group?

K   A. Potatoes
     B. Green beans
     C. Broccoli
     D. Tomato juice
     ANSWER: A   p. 36-43

Chapter 26 Nutrition, Diabetes, and Hypoglycemia

8. Alcoholic beverages such as rum, gin and vodka are best substituted for which exchange on a diabetic diet?.

K
   A. fruit
   B. fat
   C. bread
   D. milk
ANSWER: B   p. 856

9. For a diabetic diet, a croissant containing 17 grams of carbohydrate and 30 grams of fat should be counted as:

AP
   A. 1 bread and 4 fats
   B. 1 fruit and 6 fats
   C. 1 bread and 6 fats
   D. 1 fruit and 4 fats
ANSWER: C   p. 36-43

Objective 4 Describe the desired balance between activity, insulin, and food intake in IDDM.

For question 10:
Mrs. Barclay's physician has prescribed 6U Reg and 15U NPH for control of her diabetes. Mrs. Barclay is 5'3", weighs 112 lbs., and is an active woman who plays handball three times per week.

10. While preparing her for discharge the nurse should tell Mrs. Barclay that:

AP
   A. she does not need to eat extra food for exercise as her diet is designed to cover strenuous activity.
   B. she should eat three meals only to cover the action of her insulin.
   C. she should not rotate her injection sites.
   D. if she drinks alcoholic beverages, she is at risk of hypoglycemia.
ANSWER: D   p. 856

Objective 5 Develop a plan for detecting and treating hyperglycemia and hypoglycemia in a diabetic client.

11. When NPH insulin is administered once daily, before breakfast, hypoglycemic reactions are *most likely* to occur:

C/AP
   A. 2 hours after the drug is injected.
   B. at midday (before lunch).
   C. before the third meal of the day (supper).
   D. at bedtime.
ANSWER: C   p. 852

4   Chapter 26 Nutrition, Diabetes, and Hypoglycemia

12.   Symptoms of hypoglycemia include:

AP   A.   confusion and irritability.
     B.   increased thirst and polyuria.
     C.   Kussmaul breathing.
     D.   warm-flushed skin.
     ANSWER: A   p. 864

13.   Which of the following represents an appropriate snack at the beginning of an episode of hypoglycemia?

C   A.   6-8 lifesavers
     B.   8 oz. orange juice with 1 teaspoon sugar
     C.   10 saltine crackers
     D.   1 piece of chewing gum
     ANSWER: A   p. 864

For question 14:
While you are making rounds at the beginning of the evening shift (4PM), Mrs. Davis complains of feeling dizzy. When taking her pulse, you note that her hand trembles slightly and feels cool and moist.

14.   It is most likely that Mrs. Davis is experiencing:

C   A.   a relapse into ketoacidosis.
     B.   hypoglycemia.
     C.   respiratory alkalosis from hyperventilation.
     D.   hyperglycemia.
     ANSWER: B   p. 852, 864

For question 15:
A 50 year old woman with uncontrolled NIDDM is admitted to the hospital for the initiation of insulin therapy. She received 25U of NPH insulin at 8:00 am. At 4:00 pm she is complaining of diaphoresis, rapid heart rate and shakiness.

15.   The first thing the nurse should do is:

C   A.   give her ½ c. orange juice.
     B.   call the physician.
     C.   give her skim milk and two crackers.
     D.   check her blood sugar.
     ANSWER: D   p.

Chapter 26 Nutrition, Diabetes, and Hypoglycemia

16. Evaluate the following two statements:

K   1. The Somogyi response is *best* described as rebound hypoglycemia.
      2. Gradually increasing the amount of insulin will prevent it.

      A.   1 is true; 2 is false
      B.   1 is false; 2 is true
      C.   1 and 2 are both true
      D.   1 and 2 are both false
      ANSWER: D   p. 862

For question 17:
Mrs. Decker is 5'2" tall and weighs 147 lbs. She has NIDDM and is controlled with diet alone. Her doctor has prescribed an 1100 kcal diet for her which she states she is following. Her current complaint is "feeling shaky" at about 10:00 am.

17. An appropriate nursing intervention is to:

C   A.   request the doctor change her kcal level to 1400.
      B.   advise her to eat hard candy when she feels shaky.
      C.   review the signs and symptoms of hyperglycemia.
      D.   explain to her she is experiencing hunger.
      ANSWER: D   p. 845

For question 18:
Mildred Jones is a 28 year old woman with insulin-dependent diabetes. She is admitted to the hospital for the treatment of the Somogyi effect.

18. The health care provider should expect the blood glucose levels for Mildred to:

AP   A.   progressively rise from bedtime to the morning hours.
       B.   decrease during sleeping hours with hypoglycemia around 3:00 am and rise until dawn.
       C.   be normal throughout the sleeping hours and rise suddenly at dawn.
       D.   rise at bedtime, be elevated throughout the night and decrease at dawn.
       ANSWER: B   p. 862

19. All of the following are associated with diabetic ketoacidosis *except*:

K   A.   dehydration.
      B.   blood glucose level less than 65 mg/dl.
      C.   electrolyte depletion.
      D.   Kussmaul respirations.
      ANSWER: B   p. 847,848

Chapter 26 Nutrition, Diabetes, and Hypoglycemia

20. On the cellular level, diabetic ketoacidosis is a form of:

K A. hypertrophy.
   B. starvation.
   C. hypoglycemia.
   D. hyperplasia.
   ANSWER: B   p. 847

21. During an acute illness, clients with IDDM should:

C A. decrease their medications if their appetite is poor.
   B. decrease the fluid intake to prevent nausea.
   C. drink fluids with sugar if the blood glucose is greater than 240 mg/dl.
   D. monitor urine for ketones.
   ANSWER: D   p. 847, 863

For question 22:
Mrs. Carter, age 30, is admitted to the hospital with pneumonia. Her glucose levels range from 240 gm/dl to 350 gm/dl. She is unable to tolerate her regular diabetic diet. She has taken NPH 35U daily for a year.

22. The best approach is to provide:

AN A. a regular house diet.
   B. sugar free liquids.
   C. sugar containing liquids.
   D. a lower dose of insulin.
   ANSWER: C   p. 864

Objective 6 Describe the special needs of children and the elderly with IDDM.

For question 23:
Claude Wilkins, age 80, has IDDM. At last clinical visit, his glycosolated hemoglobin was 16%.

23. Which of the following drugs is most likely to contribute to this level of glycosolated hemoglobin?

AP A. propranolol
   B. hydrochlorothiazide
   C. ibuprofen
   D. digoxin
   ANSWER: B   Appendix E

Chapter 26 Nutrition, Diabetes, and Hypoglycemia

24. An appropriate kcal level for a 6 year old child with IDDM is:

K   A. 1000.
      B. 1200.
      C. 1400.
      D. 1600.
      ANSWER: D   p. 865

For question 25:
Jane Watson is a 16 year old with IDDM. At clinic she reports all fasting blood sugars to be within the 100-150 mg/dl range and no postprandial blood glucoses greater than 180 mg/dl. Her glycosolated hemoglobin level is 18%.

25. The most likely explanation is:

AN   A. chronic hypoglycemia.
       B. Somogyi effect.
       C. noncompliance.
       D. adolescent growth spurt.
       ANSWER: C   p. 865

Objective 7 Plan a diet for a client with NIDDM.

For question 26:
Mr. Sanchez is a 52 year old male is being discharged from the hospital. He participates freely in the discussion during discharge instructions about NIDDM.

26. Which statement indicates some understanding of his nutrition plan?

C   A. "I should avoid dried beans and peas because they have too much starch."
     B. "Green peas and green beans are both in the vegetable exchange group."
     C. "Sausage won't make my blood sugar go up but it will clog my arteries."
     D. "If I don't want to drink 8 oz. of skim milk, I can drink 4 oz. of whole milk instead."
     ANSWER: C   p. 36-43

For question 27:
Mrs. Lucas is 5'2" tall and weighs 142 lbs. She has been recently diagnosed as having NIDDM.

27. The appropriate kcal level for Mrs. Lucas for weight reduction is:

C   A. 1100.
     B. 1400.
     C. 1600.
     D. 1800.
     ANSWER: A   p. 857

Chapter 26 Nutrition, Diabetes, and Hypoglycemia

For question 28:
Hector Martinez is a 70 year old Hispanic man recently diagnosed with NIDDM. He is having difficulty understanding the exchange system and has limited financial resources.

28. Which of the following strategies is *most* likely to help him control his diabetes?
AP/AN
    A.   Emphasis how important it is to follow only the exchange system
    B.   Try an alternate diet approach
    C.   Give him a printed exchange list of traditional Hispanic foods
    D.   Encourage him to join a spa and exercise
    ANSWER: B   p. 868

For question 29:
Mrs. Billings was recently diagnosed with NIDDM. She is 5'8" and weighs 200 lbs. and lives a sedentary life style. During the interview, she tells you her lowest weight in her adult life is 160 lbs.

29. What is the *most* appropriate kcal level for the management of her diabetes?

C   A.   1400
       B.   1600
       C.   1800
       D.   2000
       ANSWER: A   p. 857

Objective 8 Describe the desired balance between activity, drug therapy, and food intake in NIDDM.

For question 30:
Mr. Merwin is a 45 year old man with NIDDM. He is 5'9" tall and weighs 210 lbs. His diabetes is currently controlled with diet alone.

31. Which of the following will help to improve insulin resistance?

C   A.   Weight reduction
       B.   Hard candy for hypoglycemic attack
       C.   Antioxidants
       D.   Three meals plus a morning, afternoon, and bedtime snack
       ANSWER: A   p. 867

Chapter 26 Nutrition, Diabetes, and Hypoglycemia

32. Evaluate the following two statements.

1. Physiological stress, such as surgery, causes an increase in blood glucose.
2. Clients with noninsulin-dependent diabetes may temporarily require insulin during times of physiological stress.

K A. 1 is true, 2 is false
   B. 1 is false, 2 is true
   C. both 1 and 2 are true
   D. both 1 and 2 are false
   ANSWER: C   p. 863

For question 33:
Mrs. Barclay has NIDDM and you are preparing her for discharge. She tells you that she loves red beans and rice and knows that she must eliminate them from her diet because they will elevate her blood glucose level.

33. You should explain to her that:
AN/AP
   A. she can enjoy ⅓ c. beans mixed with ⅓ c. rice in exchange for 2 slices of bread.
   B. red beans are eliminated because they are high in complex carbohydrates.
   C. red beans are high in water soluble fiber and should be avoided.
   D. peas are a better choice than red beans.
   ANSWER: A   p. 36-43

For question 34:
Mrs. Filbert, age 56, has been diagnosed with IDDM. During discharge instruction she makes a number of statements.

34. Which one indicates some understanding of her diabetes management?

C A. "If my blood glucose is between 100-180 mg/dl I should not exercise."
   B. "If I eat high fat foods my blood sugars will be elevated."
   C. "Adding cheese or peanut butter to my bedtime snack may prevent hypoglycemia during the night."
   D. "Red beans can be exchanged for broccoli on my diet."
   ANSWER: C   p. 36-43, 854, 862

For question 35:
Mr. Lilly, a 42 year old male, tells you that he used to take "pills" for his diabetes but is now taking insulin.

35. What is the most likely reason that he no longer takes oral hypoglycemics?

K A. They are only effective in juvenile-onset diabetes
   B. His body now stimulates enough insulin to meet his needs
   C. They suppress insulin release
   D. They were not controlling his blood glucose
   ANSWER: D   p. 845

Chapter 26 Nutrition, Diabetes, and Hypoglycemia

Objective 9 Describe the prenatal care for women with existing diabetes and gestational diabetes.

36. The prenatal care for women who develop gestational diabetes can include:

K   A.   insulin until delivery.
      B.   high protein intake.
      C.   reduced carbohydrate intake.
      D.   a weight reduction diet.
      ANSWER: A   p. 871

37. IDDM women who are attempting to become pregnant should be aware that diabetes contributes to all of the following **except**:

K   A.   diabetes in the infant.
      B.   a high rate of infertility.
      C.   fluctuations in insulin needs during pregnancy.
      D.   congenital malformations
      ANSWER: A   p. 869, 870

Objective 10 Describe the nutritional assessment for a diabetic client.

38. The essential nutrition assessment parameters for the person newly diagnosed with diabetes include all of the following except:

K   A.   body weight.
      B.   diet history.
      C.   midarm muscle circumference.
      D.   blood glucose levels.
      ANSWER: C   p. 874

For question 39:
Jane Smith is a 36 year old client with IDDM who has experienced frequent episodes of hypoglycemia.

39. The most helpful tool for evaluating her management of her disease is:

K   A.   glycosylated hemoglobin level.
      B.   blood glucose monitoring records.
      C.   triglyceride levels.
      D.   fasting blood sugar level.
      ANSWER: B   p. 874

CHAPTER 27
NUTRITION AND DISORDERS OF THE HEART AND BLOOD VESSELS

Objective 1 Identify modifiable and non-modifiable risk factors for coronary heart disease.

1. Which of the following conditions is modifiable as a risk factor for coronary heart disease?

K A. Hypertension
  B. Gender
  C. Diabetes mellitus
  D. High LDL cholesterol
  ANSWER: D   p. 882

2. Based on the limited data provided, which of the following individuals has the lowest risk for developing coronary heart disease?

AP A. A 40 year old man with controlled hypertension
  B. A 50 year old post-menopausal woman
  C. A 45 year old woman who is 5'2" and weighs 125 lbs.
  D. A 35 year old woman with a LDL to HDL ratio of 5.0
  ANSWER: C   p. 883-885

Chapter 27 Nutrition and Disorders of the Heart and Blood Vessels

3. Which of the following is a NCEP risk factor for coronary artery disease?

K   A. Being female
     B. Body weight 20% less than ideal
     C. HDL greater than 35 mg/dl
     D. LDL cholesterol greater than 160 mg/dl
     ANSWER: D   p. 883-885

4. Clients with diabetes are likely to have low levels of:

K   A. LDL.
     B. triglycerides.
     C. total cholesterol.
     D. HDL.
     ANSWER: D   p. 885

Objective 2 Describe recommendations for detecting and improving blood lipids using the following strategies:
    screening
    diet
    physical activity

For question 5:
Mrs. Thomas gave blood two weeks ago. Today she has received a postcard from the blood bank listing her blood type and indicating that her cholesterol level was 230 mg/dl. Mrs. Thomas asks you if she is at risk for developing heart disease.

5. The best information to give her is that she should:

C   A. ask her physician to retest her lipid level.
     B. begin a low-fat diet.
     C. consult her physician about drug therapy to lower her cholesterol level.
     D. begin an exercise program.
     ANSWER: A   p. 887

6. A Step II diet to control cholesterol allows a total fat intake of less than _____% of total kcalories with saturated fat intake being no more than _____%.

	Total Fat	Saturated Fat
K A.	30	15
B.	30	7
C.	25	10
D.	20,	3

ANSWER: B   p. 889

7. A total cholesterol of 221 mg/dl would be classified as:

K   A. desirable.
     B. normal.
     C. borderline high.
     D. high.
     ANSWER: C   p. 883

8. Recent research suggests that supplementing which vitamin decreases the risk of heart disease?

K   A. Pyridoxine
     B. Thiamin
     C. Tocopherol
     D. Riboflavin
     ANSWER: C   p. 885

9. Recommendations to lower cholesterol via physical exercise are that:

K   A. weight lifting is the most effective exercise.
     B. women should exercise to lower their HDL.
     C. men should use diet and exercise to increase HDL.
     D. exercise does not lower LDL.
     ANSWER: C   p. 889

10. The effect of diets rich in omega-3 fatty acids is a(n):

K   A. decrease in serum cholesterol.
     B. decrease in platelet aggregation.
     C. increase in serum triglycerides.
     D. tendency to form thrombi.
     ANSWER: B   p. 882

Objective 3 Discuss the nutritional problems and their appropriate interventions for a client with a cardiovascular or pulmonary disease.

11. A recommendation for clients with hypertension is a low sodium diet that contains:

K   A. high potassium and high calcium.
     B. low potassium and high calcium.
     C. low potassium and low calcium.
     D. high potassium and low calcium.
     ANSWER: A   p. 894,895

4   Chapter 27 Nutrition and Disorders of the Heart and Blood Vessels

12. The purpose of an intravenous infusion immediately after a myocardial infarction is to:

C   A.   provide an energy source.
    B.   prevent dehydration.
    C.   provide fuel to the heart muscle.
    D.   prevent a fluid shift.
    ANSWER: B   p. 898

13. Early dietary interventions after a myocardial infarction include:

K   A.   low fat diet.
    B.   low fiber diet.
    C.   high calorie diet.
    D.   high fiber diet
    ANSWER: B   p. 899

14. Dietary guidelines for the management of hypertension emphasize:

K   A.   avoidance of calcium rich food.
    B.   a diet rich in fresh fruits and vegetables.
    C.   6 oz. wine per day.
    D.   avoidance of starchy foods.
    ANSWER: B   p. 893,894

15. Prior to feeding someone post-stroke, the health care professional should assess the client for:

C   A.   food intolerance.
    B.   salt sensitivity.
    C.   dysphagia.
    D.   hydration status.
    ANSWER: C   p. 900

16. Dietary interventions for a client with congestive heart failure are aimed at all of the following *except*:

C   A.   reducing the workload of the heart.
    B.   preventing fluid overload.
    C.   increasing the metabolic rate.
    D.   restricting sodium intake.
    ANSWER: C   p. 901,902

17. Clients on long-term steroid therapy for COPD are at risk for developing which of the following nutrient electrolyte imbalances?

AN
- A. low sodium, low protein, and high potassium.
- B. low calcium, low protein, and low potassium.
- C. high calcium, high protein, and low sodium.
- D. high sodium, high potassium, and high calcium.

ANSWER: B   Appendix E, Table E-1

18. Dietary interventions for a client in respiratory failure include controlling carbohydrate intake, because carbohydrates:

C
- A. fuel infections.
- B. impaire the immune function.
- C. decrease oxygenation.
- D. generate carbon dioxide.

ANSWER: D   p. 905

19. Overfeeding should be avoided in clients with respiratory failure primarily because:

AP
- A. albumin levels will decrease.
- B. serum cholesterol will increase.
- C. CO_2 production will increase.
- D. protein energy malnutrition will result.

ANSWER: C   p. 905

20. Clients who are on ventilators should receive:

K
- A. continuous parenteral support.
- B. an individualized diet based on indirect calorimetry.
- C. a protein restricted diet.
- D. a high potassium diet.

ANSWER: B   p. 905

For questions 21:
Mr. Goldman is a 55 year old man who has suffered a myocardial infarction. His total cholesterol level is 242 mg/dl, LDL 172 mg/dl, HDL 35 mg/dl, and triglycerides 400 mg/dl (high).

21. Which statement by Mr. Goldman suggests some accurate recall of dietary instructions?

C
- A. "I should drink a glass of wine every day to raise my HDL cholesterol."
- B. "I'm supposed to eat 300 mg of cholesterol per deciliter."
- C. "I must eliminate red meat from my diet."
- D. "Avoidance of saturated fat is a primary concern."

ANSWER: D   p. 888

Chapter 27 Nutrition and Disorders of the Heart and Blood Vessels

22. Clients with edema associated with congestive heart failure usually have orders for:

C   A.   cholesterol restriction and bile acid sequesterants.
       B.   saturated fat restriction and corticosteroids.
       C.   sodium restriction and diuretics.
       D.   carbohydrate restriction and insulin.
       ANSWER: C   p. 901

23. The term for protein energy malnutrition associated with congestive heart failure is:

K   A.   cardiac cachexia.
       B.   anorexia nervosa.
       C.   dyspnea.
       D.   tachycardia.
       ANSWER: A   p. 901

24. The goal of dietary intervention in congestive heart failure is to provide:

C   A.   extra calories for rapid weight gain.
       B.   adequate nutrients with limited work for the heart.
       C.   a decrease in calories and protein.
       D.   large meals to maximize rest periods for the client.
       ANSWER: B   p. 902

Objective 4 Plan a diet for a client with a cardiovascular or pulmonary disease.

For question 25:
Mr. Kline is a 36 year old black male with hypertension. He is currently taking a potassium sparing diuretic to help lower his blood pressure.

25. Which of the following meals would be most appropriate for Mr. Kline?

AP   A.   Vegetable soup (canned), ½ c. chocolate pudding, and carrot sticks
        B.   Ham sandwich, potato salad, and frozen yogurt with strawberries
        C.   Cheese sandwich, garden salad, and dried apricots
        D.   Chicken, Caesar salad, French bread, and an apple
        ANSWER: D   p. 895-898

For question 26:
Interventions for post-myocardial infarction usually include a low-fat, low-kcalorie salt-restricted diet.

26. If a client continues to have pain post-MI you should:

AP   A.   encourage a liquid diet.
        B.   suggest small, frequent feedings.
        C.   restrict sodium even further.
        D.   ask for an order for enteral feedings.
        ANSWER: B   p. 899

Chapter 27 Nutrition and Disorders of the Heart and the Blood Vessels   7

27. Which of the following groups of foods are *most* appropriate for a hypertensive client on a low-fat 2 gm sodium, high-potassium diet?

AP
    A. Macaroni and cheese; carrot and raisin salad; and chocolate layer cake
    B. Fried shrimp; French fries; spinach salad with Italian dressing; and fresh strawberries
    C. Cheese omelette; buttermilk biscuits; and apple pie
    D. Hamburger patty; lettuce and tomato with vinegar and oil; and baked potato with margarine
    ANSWER: D   p. 154-164,888

28. Which of the following groups of foods are *most* appropriate for a low-cholesterol, low-saturated fat diet?

AP/AN
    A. Turkey breast, mashed potatoes with gravy, green beans and coconut pie
    B. Scrambled eggs, toast with jelly, orange juice, and whole milk
    C. Beef tenderloin, wild rice, peas, and angel food cake
    D. Cheeseburger with lettuce and tomato, apple, and chocolate milkshake
    ANSWER: C   p. 888

29. The food highest in saturated fat is:

AP
    A. chicken.
    B. egg yolk.
    C. lard.
    D. canola oil.
    ANSWER: C   Appendix H

30. Which of the following is an appropriate dietary restriction for a "cardiac rest" diet?

C
    A. 7 gram sodium
    B. Liberal bland
    C. Reduced kcal
    D. Low purine
    ANSWER: C   p. 899

8   Chapter 27   Nutrition and Disorders of the Heart and Blood Vessels

For question 31:
Mr. Peabody had a stroke seven days ago. Initially he was fed via tube feeding because he had dysphagia. Today the tube has been removed and his diet is advanced.

31.   Which of the following foods would be the *most* appropriate for Mr. Peabody?

AP   A.   Pureed carrots
     B.   Cubed meat
     C.   Sliced apple
     D.   Rice
     ANSWER: A   p. 777

For question 32:
Mrs. Green has congestive heart failure. She is currently taking the drugs digoxin and furosemide (diuretic) to help control the symptoms. You visit her at home and note she is eating fried chicken, green beans, and a baked potato with sour cream. She is drinking a carbonated cola.

32.   Mrs. Green's meal contains:
AP/AN
     A.   too much fat, sodium, and potassium.
     B.   too much fat, sodium, and calcium.
     C.   too much fat and sodium.
     D.   amounts of fat and minerals that require further assessment.
     ANSWER: D   p. 901-902

33.   Which of the following foods is highest in cholesterol?

AP   A.   Peanut butter
     B.   Olive oil
     C.   Canola oil
     D.   Chicken
     ANSWER: D   Appendix H

For question 34:
Mr. Bidwell, age 68, has suffered a myocardial infarction six weeks ago. On his clinic visit he tells you he has been following a Step I diet. You ask him to describe a typical dinner.

34.   Mr. Bidwell probably understands his dietary instructions if he describes a dinner of:

AP   A.   Baked chicken, macaroni and cheese, and jello
     B.   Shrimp creole, rice, salad with blue cheese dressing, and sherbet
     C.   Turkey, cranberry sauce, and angel food cake
     D.   Spare ribs, boiled potato, and coleslaw
     ANSWER: C   Appendix H

Chapter 27 Nutrition and Disorders of the Heart and the Blood Vessels

For question 35:
Mrs. Gonzales has been placed on a two gram sodium diet for her hypertension.

35. Which of the following statements suggests some understanding of this dietary restriction?

AP   A.   "I will only eat ham twice per week."
      B.   "I will use monosodium glutamate (MSG)."
      C.   "I will cook with small amounts of salt or add no salt at the table."
      D.   "I cannot eat foods seasoned with garlic powder."
      ANSWER: C   p. 896

36. How many milligrams of sodium are in a teaspoon of salt?

K   A.   500
    B.   1000
    C.   1500
    D.   2000
    ANSWER: D   p. 380, 895

37. Which of the following meals is lowest in sodium?
AP/AN
    A.   Pancakes, sausage, and orange juice
    B.   Chicken breast, baked potato, and spinach
    C.   Spaghetti with tomato sauce, carrots, and dinner roll
    D.   Cheeseburger on a bun with lettuce, tomato and ketchup, and milkshake
    ANSWER: B   p. 380

38. Which of the following is the leanest cut of beef?

K   A.   Top sirloin steak
    B.   Ribeye steak
    C.   Brisket
    D.   Hamburger meat
    ANSWER: A   p. 36-43

For question 39:
Mr. Parks owns a sandwich shop. He has hired you to help him to revise his "lunch specials" to label them "heart healthy". One popular "special" offers a 3 oz. cut of grilled sirloin on sour dough bun; a salad of ½ tomato, lettuce leaf, and ½ avocado.

39. Which of the following would be the most effective revision to recommend to Mr. Parks?
AP/AN
    A.   Substitute 3 oz. skinless chicken for sirloin
    B.   Double the amount of lettuce
    C.   Provide a choice of wheat or sour dough bun
    D.   Substitute bell pepper for avocado
    ANSWER: D   p. 36-43 Appendix H

CHAPTER 28
NUTRITION AND DISORDERS OF THE KIDNEYS

Objective 1 Differentiate between the symptoms and treatment of acute and chronic renal failure.

1. A blood urea nitrogen (BUN) of 80 mg/dl indicates:

K   A.   renal stability.
       B.   malnutritional.
       C.   azotemia.
       D.   approaching death.
ANSWER: C   p. 919

2. A client in acute renal failure who is uremic is likely to be:

K   A.   hyperactive.
       B.   hypoglycemic.
       C.   alert.
       D.   anorexic.
ANSWER: D   p. 920

Chapter 28 Nutrition and Disorders of the Kidneys

3. As glomerular filtration decreases in renal failure, so does the tolerance for:

K   A. carbohydrate.
     B. protein.
     C. fat.
     D. vitamins.
     ANSWER: B   p. 922

Objective 2 Explain the therapeutic options in acute renal failure and their impact on nutritional support.

4. A client in acute renal failure with a potassium level is 6.2 mEq/L will probably require:

C   A. IV dextrose and insulin therapy.
     B. IV normal saline with potassium.
     C. extra amounts of oral fluids.
     D. parenteral glucagon therapy.
     ANSWER: A   p. 923

5. The primary reason for giving TPN with $D_{70}W$ to clients in acute renal failure is to:

C   A. provide low kcal.
     B. provide high protein.
     C. prevent fluid overload.
     D. avoid using lipid emulsions.
     ANSWER: C   p. 924

For questions 6 and 7:
Mrs. Jones is in acute renal failure and has a potassium of 5.2 mEq/L. Her physician has ordered resin enemas.

6. Additional therapy at this time for Mrs. Jones should be a diet that is:

C   A. high in phosphorus.
     B. low in potassium.
     C. low in carbohydrates.
     D. low in phosphate binders.
     ANSWER: B   p. 923

7. When Mrs. Jones becomes oliguric and receives diuretics, her diet should be:

AP A. higher in potassium.
     B. lower in potassium.
     C. lower in sodium.
     D. higher in protein.
     ANSWER: C   p. 923

Chapter 28 Nutrition and Disorders of the Kidneys 3

Objective 3 Describe the long-term nutritional problems associated with chronic renal failure and appropriate interventions.

For question 8:
Sam Martin is a 9 year old boy in end stage renal disease. He weighs 35 kg.

8. How many kcal does Sam need to promote reasonable growth?
AP
    A. 1400
    B. 2200
    C. 2800
    D. 4000
    ANSWER: C   p. 927

9. Which of the following is an application of a dietary principle for treatment of chronic renal failure?
AP/AN
    A. Avoidance of hard candy to prevent dental caries
    B. Drinking three glasses of milk per day for extra calcium.
    C. Adding extra margarine to toast to increase calories.
    D. Eating spinach to promote elimination of potassium salts.
    ANSWER: C   p. 927

10. The fluid allowance for a client with a urine output of 800 ml is:
AP
    A. 800 ml.
    B. 1300 ml.
    C. 1800 ml.
    D. 2300 ml.
    ANSWER: B   p. 930

11. Phosphorus levels of 7 mg/dl in chronic renal failure indicate:
AP
    A. probable compliance with the diet.
    B. erythropoietin deficiency.
    C. the need to assess fluid status.
    D. the need to assess diet and drug compliance.
    ANSWER: D   p. 928

12. Clients with zinc deficiency often exhibit:
K
    A. dysphagia.
    B. dysgeusia.
    C. dyspnea.
    D. dyslipidemia.
    ANSWER: B   p. 931

Chapter 28 Nutrition and Disorders of the Kidneys

13. Which of the following medications is used to treat an elevated serum phosphate level during end stage renal disease?

K   A. Calcium carbonate
      B. Glucagon
      C. $D_{50}W$ and insulin
      D. Kayexalate
      ANSWER: A   p. 929

For question 14:
Mr. Jones has insulin dependent diabetes and end stage renal disease. He becomes hypoglycemic while on dialysis.

14. The immediate treatment for Mr. Jones should be 4 oz. of:
AP/AN
      A. unsweetened orange juice.
      B. prune juice.
      C. lemon-lime soft drink.
      D. tomato juice.
      ANSWER: C   p. 932, 933

Objective 4 Plan a diet for a client in chronic renal failure.

15. Which of the following beverages is the best choice for a client with chronic renal failure?

K   A. Sports drink
      B. Cranberry juice
      C. Orange juice
      D. Tomato juice
      ANSWER: B   p. 933

16. Which of the following is an example of a food containing protein of high biological value?

C   A. Gelatin
      B. Dried beans
      C. Peanut butter
      D. Fish
      ANSWER: D   p. 928

17. Of the following fruits, which is highest in potassium?

C/AP   A. Grapefruit
         B. Cantaloupe
         C. Apple
         D. Grapes
         ANSWER: B   p. 932

For question 18:
Mr. Bustoz is on a 60 gm protein, 2 gm Na diet.

18. Which of the following combinations meets his protein allowance?

AN   A.   3 oz. meat, 1 fruit, 1 vegetable, and 3 breads
         B.   6 oz. meat, 3 fruits, 2 vegetables, 4 breads, and 1 milk
         C.   8 oz. meat, 4 fruits, 4 vegetables, 4 breads, and 1 milk
         D.   9 oz. meat, 3 fruits, 3 vegetables, 3 breads, and 1 milk
         ANSWER: B   p. 934

Objective 5 Explain dietary guidelines following a kidney transplant.

For questions 19 through 22:
John Miller is on dialysis and his current protein allowance is 60 gm.

19. After he receives a kidney transplant, the health care professional should expect Mr. Miller's protein intake to be:

AP/AN
         A.   unchanged.
         B.   decreased to .5 gm/kg.
         C.   increased to 1.5 gm/kg.
         D.   unrestricted.
         ANSWER: C   p. 936

20. When Mr. Miller inquires if he should continue to restrict his sodium after transplant, you reply:

AP/AN
         A.   "Since your renal function has been restored you do not need to restrict your sodium intake."
         B.   "Since you are on immunosuppressants, you need to restrict your sodium level to 2-4 gm/day."
         C.   "Since you are going to be on diuretics, there is no need to restrict sodium."
         D.   "Once you are off the immunosuppressants, you will no longer need to restrict sodium intake."
         ANSWER: B   p. 936

21. Regulation of carbohydrate intake after Mr. Miller's transplant helps to control which immunosuppresant effect?

AP   A.   a catabolic effect.
         B.   glucose intolerance.
         C.   weight gain.
         D.   hyperkalemia.
         ANSWER: B   p. 936

Chapter 28 Nutrition and Disorders of the Kidneys

22. When you notice on a home visit that Mr. Miller does not wash his fruits and vegetables thoroughly, you:

AN
    A. remind him to wash produce very carefully.
    B. decide that this does not matter since he is going to cook the produce anyway.
    C. call Mr. Miller's physician for an antibiotic prescription.
    D. demonstrate to Mr. Miller the correct way to clean produce.
    ANSWER: D   p. 935,936

23. Which of the following snacks *best* meets the needs of the kidney transplant recipient?

AP
    A. Roast beef sandwich
    B. Ham and cheese sandwich
    C. Chocolate candy bar
    D. Potato chips
    ANSWER: A   p. 936

24. When a client is rejecting a new kidney, his diet therapy will most likely be:

K
    A. unchanged.
    B. changed to a high potassium diet.
    C. changed to a renal diet.
    D. changed to a high protein diet.
    ANSWER: C   p. 937

Objective 6 Explain the dietary guidelines for nephrotic syndrome.

For question 25:
Billy Lewis is a 20 year old man admitted to the hospital with nephrotic syndrome. He is 5'11", 192 lbs. and has edema. His blood values include albumin 1.7 g/dl, K+ 3.3 mEq/L, cholesterol 492 mg/dl, and triglycerides of 680 mg/dl. He is complaining of hunger and wants a snack.

25. The most appropriate food choice would be a:

AN/S
    A. sausage biscuit.
    B. grilled chicken sandwich with lettuce and tomato.
    C. peanut butter and crackers.
    D. piece of coconut cream pie.
    ANSWER: B   p. 938,939

26. Dietary guidelines for a client with nephrotic syndrome restrict all of the following *except*:

C
    A. protein.
    B. fat.
    C. sodium.
    D. calcium.
    ANSWER: D   p. 939

Chapter 28 Nutrition and Disorders of the Kidneys 7

27. A high-protein diet for a nephrotic client is contraindicated because:

AN   A. protein foods are usually high in fat.
       B. energy requirements are decreased with nephrotic syndrome.
       C. protein may accelerate nephrotic syndrome.
       D. protein levels in nephrotic syndrome are not altered.
       ANSWER: C   p. 939

28. Diets high in vitamin D and calcium are recommended for children with nephrotic syndrome to prevent:

K   A. beri beri.
      B. marasmus.
      C. nephrosclerosis.
      D. rickets.
      ANSWER: D   p. 938

Objective 7 Describe the assessment of a client with a disorder of the kidney.

For question 29:
Johanna Klien, a 12 year old, has chronic renal failure and receives dialysis three times per week. According to her dry weights over the last month, Johanna has lost six lbs.

29. What is the most likely explanation for this weight loss?

AN   A. Johanna is responding to the dialysis and is having less edema
       B. Johanna is at risk for growth failure
       C. Johanna is at risk for developing osteodystrophy
       D. Johanna's diet is too low in sodium
       ANSWER: B   p. 940, 941

30. When Glen Davis, a 46 year old dialysis client, calls you to report a blood pressure of 160/100 mm Hg, you should:

AN   A. refer him to his internist for an antihypertensive agent.
       B. ask him when the blood pressure was taken in regards to his dialysis schedule.
       C. tell him to further restrict his sodium intake.
       D. refer him to his nephrologist for an increase of his diuretic.
       ANSWER: B   p. 940

CHAPTER 29
NUTRITION AND WASTING DISORDERS: CANCER AND AIDS

Objective 1 Describe dietary factors associated with cancer.

For question 1:
Mr. Nelson asks you what he can do to prevent cancer.

1. You should recommend that he do all of the following *except*:

C   A.   avoid all food additives.
       B.   avoid excess kcalories and fat.
       C.   avoid foods that are preserved with salt.
       D.   eat a variety of foods, especially fruits and vegetables.
ANSWER: A   p. 953

2. Which of the following cancers is *not* influenced by dietary habits?

K   A.   Colorectal
       B.   Stomach
       C.   Endometrial
       D.   Prostate
ANSWER: C   p. 951

Chapter 29 Nutrition and Wasting Disorders: Cancer and AIDS

3. Research suggests that reducing the consumption of which food may reduce the risk of cancer of the colon and breast.

K   A.   fresh fruits
      B.   dietary fat
      C.   fiber
      D.   simple sugar
      ANSWER: B   p. 951

Objective 2 Describe the use of foods as cancer antipromoters.

4. Antipromoters of cancer include all of the following *except*:

K   A.   alcohol.
      B.   antioxidants.
      C.   cruciferous vegetables.
      D.   dietary fiber.
      ANSWER: A   p. 952

5. The main reason cruciferous vegetables are considered cancer antipromoters because they:

K   A.   are high in fiber.
      B.   are low in fat.
      C.   contain indoles and dithiolthiones.
      D.   support the immune system.
      ANSWER: C   p. 952

6. Dietary fiber is considered a cancer antipromoter because it:

K   A.   activates enzymes capable of destroying carcinogens.
      B.   increases the rate of peristalsis.
      C.   contains tryptophan.
      D.   decreases the risk of obesity.
      ANSWER: B   p. 952

Objective 3 Explain the nutritional consequences of cancer and cancer treatments.

For question 7:
John Taylor, age 36, recently received a bone marrow transplant. Three weeks post-transplant he experienced nausea, vomiting, taste alterations, and anorexia.

7. Mr. Taylor's symptoms suggest that:

C   A.   his immune system is trying to reject the bone marrow.
      B.   he is immunocompromised.
      C.   he is responding to pre-radiation treatments.
      D.   he has developed food aversion.
      ANSWER: A   p. 957,958

8. Altered carbohydrate metabolism in individuals with cancer contributes to all of the following *except*:

C   A. cachexia.
    B. hyperglycemia.
    C. anorexia.
    D. hypoglycemia.
    ANSWER: D   p. 961

For question 9:
Bill Freeman, age 36, was recently diagnosed with cancer.

9. Which of his statements suggest some understanding of the role of nutrition in cancer?

C   A. "Eating a diet rich in fruits and vegetables can cure cancer."
    B. "Omitting alcohol from my diet will prevent spreading."
    C. "A well-balanced diet will help me to keep my strength up."
    D. "A low-fat diet is the best diet to maintain my health."
    ANSWER: C   p. 962

10. Cancer induced causes of anorexia include all of the following *except*:

C   A. lowered metabolic rate.
    B. pain.
    C. early satiety.
    D. psychological stress.
    ANSWER: A   p. 955

Objective 4 Describe the goal of nutrition support for a client with cancer.

11. One of the goals of nutrition support for a person with cancer is to:

C   A. reverse cachexia.
    B. limit the loss of lean body mass.
    C. increase metabolism.
    D. regenerate lean body mass.
    ANSWER: B   p. 962

For question 12:
Sally Merwin has esophageal cancer. Her basal energy expenditure is estimated to be 1200 kcal.

12. Her current total energy needs should be _____ kcal:

AP A. 1200
    B. 1500
    C. 2200
    D. 2700
    ANSWER: C   p. 964

Chapter 29 Nutrition and Wasting Disorders: Cancer and AIDS

Objective 5 Describe interventions to improve nutrient intake and prevent nutrient loss in a cancer client.

13. Which of the following may help a cancer patient to alleviate a metallic taste?

C   A. Avoiding spicy foods
     B. Avoiding red meats
     C. Saving liquids for after meals
     D. Serving food hot
     ANSWER: B   p. 965

For question 14:
Mrs. Caruthers has been complaining of nausea for the past two days. You note that she has an antiemetic order as needed.

14. When would be the best time to offer her the antiemetic?

AP A. Just before meal time
     B. When she is through eating
     C. After she has vomited
     D. 30 minutes to 1 hour before meals
     ANSWER: D   p.

15. Clients with cancer can sometimes control nausea and vomiting if they:

C   A. prepare their own meals.
     B. try coffee to stimulate appetite.
     C. drink orange juice with meals.
     D. avoid spicy and high-fat foods.
     ANSWER: D   p. 965

16. The best dietary intervention for a cancer patient experiencing a metallic taste is to:

AP A. serve meat very warm.
     B. use poultry, fish, or eggs for protein.
     C. avoid all foods containing protein.
     D. provide mouth care after meals.
     ANSWER: B   p. 965

Objective 6 Explain the dietary considerations for a bone marrow recipient.

17. The rationale for providing a high-protein, high-calcium diet to a bone marrow recipient is that this diet:

K   A. prevents potassium loss.
     B. prevents steatorrhea.
     C. counteracts protein and calcium loss.
     D. helps support the immune system.
     ANSWER: C   p. 967

18. The most appropriate form of nutrition support for immunosuppressed, anorexic bone marrow transplant patients is:

AP   A.   oral supplements.
        B.   enteral feedings.
        C.   peripheral IVs of fluids and electrolytes.
        D.   total parenteral nutrition.
        ANSWER: D   p. 958

19. Bone marrow recipients may have glutamine added to their TPN. The rationale for adding glutamine to the TPN of bone marrow recipients is that glutamine:

AP   A.   helps prevent bacterial translocation.
        B.   reduces the need for insulin.
        C.   prevents steatorrhea.
        D.   improves nutrient absorption.
        ANSWER: A   p. 965

Objective 7 Explain the nutritional consequences of HIV/AIDS.

20. A high gastric pH in clients with AIDS causes poor absorption of:

K   A.   iron and calcium.
        B.   retinol and tocopherol.
        C.   pyridoxine and zinc.
        D.   selenium and manganese.
        ANSWER: A   p. 970,971

For question 21:
Jane Williams, age 60, has AIDS. During her monthly clinic visit she reports that she continues to have six loose stools most days even though she takes Lomotil and follows her diet plan. She is medium frame, 66 inches tall and weight 105 lbs. She has lost five lbs. since her last visit. Mrs. Williams tells you that she has heard from other AIDS patients that "taking the stuff that makes jelly gel is good for diarrhea." She also asks if the fingers in her intestine will ever grow back.

21. The most useful area of further assessment at this moment is:

AN   A.   her understanding of malabsorption.
        B.   possible evidence of dementia in her statements.
        C.   her choice of particular foods on her diet.
        D.   her vulnerablity for nutrition cures.
        ANSWER: A   p. 975

6   Chapter 29 Nutrition and Wasting Disorders: Cancer and AIDS

22. Thrush interferes with dietary intake for all of the following reasons *except*:

K   A.   altered taste sensations.
     B.   pain.
     C.   reduced saliva.
     D.   impaired fat absorption.
     ANSWER: D   p. 970

23. The major nutritional problems seen in clients with AIDS are:

C   A.   dysgeusia and dyspepsia.
     B.   diarrhea and malabsorption.
     C.   weight gain and iron deficiency anemia.
     D.   dyspnea and gastroesophageal reflux.
     ANSWER: B   p.

Objective 8 Describe the goals of nutrition support for a client with HIV/AIDS.

For question 24:
Terry Pike is a 28 year old with AIDS. Recently he has been experiencing severe diarrhea. Terry's physician has identified that he has an infection in the large intestines.

24. All of the following dietary modifications would be appropriate for Terry *except*:
AP/AN
     A.   a diet high in water insoluble fiber.
     B.   low-residue diet.
     C.   caffeine restrictions.
     D.   low-fat diet.
     ANSWER: A   p. 973

25. In order to decrease the occurrence of food-borne infections in people with AIDS, you should encourage them to:

AP   A.   buy only organic produce.
      B.   wash produce thoroughly.
      C.   eat only canned produce.
      D.   microwave all produce prior to eating it.
      ANSWER: B   p. 973

26. Clients with AIDS who develop severe gastrointestinal infections with intractable diarrhea are *best* fed:

C   A.   orally.
     B.   peripherally.
     C.   enterally.
     D.   parenterally.
     ANSWER: D   p. 974

Chapter 29 Nutrition and Wasting Disorders: Cancer and AIDS   7

Objective 9 Relate the nutritional assessment factors that are the key to detecting nutrient deficiencies in clients with cancer or HIV/AIDS.

27. A careful drug history, including OTC products, is taken when a client has HIV or cancer for all of the following reasons *except*:

    A. alternative therapies are common.
    B. use of alternative therapies may impair nutrition status.
    C. use of alternative therapies may contribute to drug-nutrient interactions.
    D. use of some alternative therapies is illegal.
    ANSWER: D   p. 975

28. Information about all of the following in a client with AIDS is useful for assessment of nutrition status *except*:

K   A. diarrhea.
    B. fluid intake.
    C. depression.
    D. total lymphocyte counts.
    ANSWER: D   p. 975

29. Which of the following tools is *least* helpful for assessing the nutritional status of a client with AIDS?

C   A. Change in weight
    B. 24 hour food record
    C. Serum albumin
    D. Triceps skinfold thickness
    ANSWER: D   p. 975